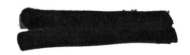

Nursing
Know-How

Charting
Patient Care

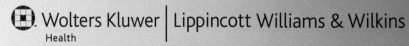

Wolters Kluwer | Lippincott Williams & Wilkins
Health

Philadelphia · Baltimore · New York · London
Buenos Aires · Hong Kong · Sydney · Tokyo

STAFF

Executive Publisher
Judith A. Schilling McCann, RN, MSN

Editorial Director
H. Nancy Holmes

Clinical Director
Joan M. Robinson, RN, MSN

Art Director
Mary Ludwicki

Editorial Project Manager
Ann E. Houska

Clinical Project Manager
Kate Stout, RN, MSN, CCRN

Editor
Patricia Nale

Copy Editors
Kimberly Bilotta (supervisor),
Jeannine Fielding, Pamela Wingrod

Designer
Donna S. Morris (project manager), Joseph
John Clark (cover design)

Digital Composition Services
Diane Paluba (manager), Joyce Rossi Biletz

Associate Manufacturing Manager
Beth J. Welsh

Editorial Assistants
Karen J. Kirk, Jeri O'Shea, Linda K. Ruhf

Indexer
Dianne L. Schneider

The clinical treatments described and recommended in this publication are based on research and consultation with nursing, medical, and legal authorities. To the best of our knowledge, these procedures reflect currently accepted practice. Nevertheless, they can't be considered absolute and universal recommendations. For individual applications, all recommendations must be considered in light of the patient's clinical condition and, before administration of new or infrequently used drugs, in light of the latest package-insert information. The authors and publisher disclaim any responsibility for any adverse effects resulting from the suggested procedures, from any undetected errors, or from the reader's misunderstanding of the text.

NKHCPC010508

Library of Congress
Cataloging-in-Publication Data

Nursing know-how. Charting patient care.
   p. ; cm.
  Includes bibliographical references and index.
  1. Nursing records—Handbooks, manuals, etc.
  [DNLM: 1. Nursing Records—Handbooks. 2. Documentation—methods—Handbooks. 3. Nursing Assessment—methods—Handbooks. 4. Patient Care Planning—Handbooks. WY 49 N9749 2009]

  RT50.N875 2009
  651.5′04261—dc22
  ISBN-13: 978-0-7817-9194-6 (alk. paper)
  ISBN-10: 0-7817-9194-4 (alk. paper)   2008004152

Contents

Contributors and consultants

Jeanette M. Anderson, RN, MSN
Nurse Consultant
Fort Worth, Tex.

Helen Christina Ballestas, RN, MS, CRRN
Faculty Nursing
New York Institute of Technology
Old Westbury

Rita Bates, RN, BS, MSN
Assistant Professor
University of Arkansas—Fort Smith

Julie Calvery, RN, MS
Instructor
University of Arkansas—Fort Smith

Cindy Cook, RN
Quality Outcomes Coordinator
Blue Ridge HealthCare, Inc.
Morganton, N.C.

MaryAnn Edelman, RN, MS, CNS
Assistant Professor—Nursing
Kingsborough Community College
Brooklyn, N.Y.

Christine Greenidge, APRN,BC, DHA
Director of Nursing Professional Practice
Montefiore Medical Center
Bronx, N.Y.

Timothy L. Hudson, BSN, MED, MS, CCRN, FACHE
Evening/Night Nursing Supervisor
U.S. Army, Martin Army Community Hospital
Fort Benning, Ga.

Merita Konstantacos, RN, MSN
Clinical Consultant
Clinton, Ohio

Kimberly Such-Smith, RN, BSN, LNC
Legal Nurse Consultant/Long-term Care Consultant
Nursing Analysis & Review
Byron, Minn.

Chris Thompson, RN, BSN
Quality Coordinator
Texoma Medical Center
Denison, Tex.

Rita Wick, RN, BSN
Education Specialist
Berkshire Health Systems
Pittsfield, Mass.

Part one

Documentation and legal issues

1 Documenting from admission to discharge

Documentation must reflect the nursing process, which is based on theories of nursing and other disciplines and follows the scientific method. This problem-solving process:

- systematically organizes nursing activities to ensure the highest quality of care
- allows you to determine problems you can help alleviate and potential problems you can help prevent
- helps you identify what kind and how much assistance a patient requires
- helps you identify the person who can best provide assistance to the patient and the desired and actual treatment outcomes.

Six-step nursing process

This flowchart shows the six steps of the nursing process and lists the forms you should use to document them.

Step 1
Assessment
Gather data from the patient's health history, physical examination, medical record, and diagnostic test results.

Documentation tools
Initial assessment form, flow sheets

Step 2
Nursing diagnosis
Make judgments based on assessment data.

Documentation tools
Nursing care plan, patient care guidelines, clinical pathway, progress notes, problem list

Step 3
Outcome identification
Set realistic, measurable goals with outcome criteria and target dates.

Documentation tools
Nursing care plan, clinical pathway, progress notes

To get a complete picture of the patient's situation, you'll need to systematically follow and document the six steps of the nursing process—assessment, nursing diagnosis, outcome identification, planning, implementation, and evaluation. (See *Six-step nursing process.*)

Fundamentals of nursing documentation

To ensure clear communication and complete, accurate documentation of nursing care, you must keep in mind the fundamentals of documentation.

Write neatly and legibly

Documentation allows you to communicate with other members of the health care team. Clean, legible documentation eases the communication process. Sloppy or illegible handwriting:
- confuses other members of the health care team and wastes time
- causes a patient potential injury if other caregivers can't understand crucial information.
    If you don't have room to document something legibly:
- leave that section blank, put a bracket around it, and write, "see progress notes"
- document the information fully and legibly in the progress notes
- indicate the date and time when cross-referencing a progress note.

Step 4
Planning
Establish care priorities, select interventions to accomplish expected outcomes, and describe interventions.
Documentation tools
Nursing care plan, patient care guidelines, clinical pathway

Step 5
Implementation
Carry out planned interventions.
Documentation tools
Progress notes, flow sheets

Step 6
Evaluation
Use objective data to assess outcome.
Documentation tools
Progress notes

Write in ink

Complete documentation in ink, not in pencil, which is susceptible to erasure and tampering. Also follow these guidelines:
- Use black or blue ink because other colors may not photocopy well.
- Don't use felt-tipped or gel ink pens on charts containing carbon paper; the pens may not produce sufficient pressure for copies.

Use correct spelling and grammar

Documentation filled with misspelled words and incorrect grammar creates the same negative impression as illegible handwriting. To avoid spelling and grammatical errors:
- keep a general and medical dictionary in documentation areas
- post a list of commonly misspelled words, especially terms and medications regularly used on the unit.

Use standard abbreviations

The Joint Commission standards and many state regulations require health care facilities to use an approved abbreviation list to prevent confusion. To make sure that your documentation meets applicable standards:
- Know and use your facility's approved abbreviations.
- Place a list of approved abbreviations in documentation areas.
- Avoid using unapproved abbreviations because they may result in ambiguity, which may endanger the patient's health. (See *Abbreviations to avoid.*)

Write clear, concise sentences

- Avoid using a long word when a short word will do.
- Clearly identify the subject of the sentence.
- Use "I," as in "I contacted the patient's family at 1300 hours, and I explained the change in his condition." Doing so differentiates your actions from those of the patient, physician, or another staff member.

Say what you mean

- Be precise. Don't use inexact qualifiers such as "appears" or "apparently" because other caregivers reading the patient's chart may conclude that you weren't sure what you were describing or doing.
- State clearly and succinctly what you see, hear, and do.
- Don't sound tentative.

Abbreviations to avoid

The Joint Commission requires every health care facility to develop a list of approved abbreviations for staff use. Certain abbreviations should be avoided because they're easily misunderstood, especially when handwritten. The Joint Commission has identified a minimum list of dangerous abbreviations, acronyms, and symbols. This do-not-use list includes the following items.

Abbreviation	Intended meaning	Misinterpretation	Correction
U or *u*	unit	Frequently misinterpreted as a "0" or a "4," causing a tenfold or greater overdose	Write "unit."
IU	international unit	Frequently misinterpreted as I.V. or 10	Write "international unit."
q.d., q.o.d.	every day, every other day	Mistaken for each other. The period after the "q" has sometimes been misinterpreted as "i," the "o" can be mistaken for "i" and the drug has been given q.i.d. rather than daily.	Write "daily" or "every other day."
Trailing zero (X.O mg) Lack of leading zero (.X mg)	10 mg, 0.1 mg	Frequently misinterpreted dosage	Never write a zero by itself after a decimal point (10.0 mg should be 10 mg) and always use a zero before a decimal point if no other number is present, such as 0.1 mg.
MS, MSO₄, MgSO₄	morphine sulfate magnesium sulfate	Confused with each other	Write "morphine sulfate" or "magnesium sulfate."

In addition to the minimum required list, the following items should also be considered when expanding the do-not-use list.

Abbreviation	Intended meaning	Misinterpretation	Correction
℥	fluid ounce	Misinterpreted as "mcg"	Use the metric equivalents.
ʒ	fluid dram	Misinterpreted as "zinc"	Use the metric equivalents.
♏	minim	Misinterpreted as "molar"	Use the metric equivalents.
Ͽ	scruple	Misinterpreted as "day"	Use the metric equivalents.
MTX	methotrexate	Misinterpreted as mustargen (mechlorethamine hydrochloride)	Write "methotrexate."

(continued)

Abbreviations to avoid *(continued)*

Abbreviation	Intended meaning	Misinterpretation	Correction
CPZ	Compazine (prochlorper-azine)	Misinterpreted as chlorpro-mazine	Write "compazine."
HCl	hydrochloric acid	Misinterpreted as potassium chloride ("H" is misinterpret-ed as "K")	Wirte "hydrochloric acid."
DIG	digoxin	Misinterpreted as digitoxin	Write "digoxin."
MVI	multivitamins without fat-soluble vitamins	Misinterpreted as multi-vitamins with fat-soluble vitamins	Write "multivitamins."
HCTZ	hydrochlorothiazide	Misinterpreted as hydrocorti-sone (HCT)	Write "hydrochlorothiazide."
ara-A	vidarabine	Misinterpreted as cytarabine (ara-C)	Write "vidarabine."
au	*auris uterque* (each ear)	Frequently misinterpreted as "OU" (*oculus uterque—* each eye)	Write "each ear."
µg	microgram	Frequently misinterpreted as "mg"	Use "mcg."
cc	cubic centimeter	Frequently misinterpreted as U (units)	Write "ml" for milliliters.
A.S., A.D., and AU	Latin abbreviations for left ear, right ear, and both ears, respectively	Frequently misinterpreted as O.S., O.D., and OU	Write "left ear," "right ear," or "both ears."
OD	once daily	Frequently misinterpreted as "O.D." (*oculus dexter—* right eye)	Write "once daily."
OJ	orange juice	Frequently misinterpreted as "O.D." (*oculus dexter—* right eye) or "O.S." (*oculus sinister—*left eye). Medica-tions that were meant to be diluted in orange juice and given orally have been given in a patient's right or left eye.	Write "orange juice."
Per os	orally	The "os" is frequently mis-interpreted as "O.S." (*oculus sinister—*left eye).	Use "PO," "by mouth," or "orally."
qn.	nightly or at bedtime	Frequently misinterpreted as "q.h." (every hour)	Write out "nightly" or "at bed-time."

Abbreviations to avoid *(continued)*

Abbreviation	Intended meaning	Misinterpretation	Correction
S.C. SQ	subcutaneous	Mistaken as SL for sublingual or "5 every"	Use "Sub-Q," "subQ," or write out "subcutaneous."
D/C	discharge or discontinue	Frequently misinterpreted as each other	Write "discharge" or "discontinue."
h.s.	half-strength or at bedtime	Frequently misinterpreted as each other	Write out "half-strength" or "at bedtime."
T.I.W.	three times per week	Frequently misinterpreted as three times per day or twice weekly	Write "three times per week."

Document promptly

■ Document observations and nursing actions as soon as possible to be more accurate.
■ Use bedside computers to document promptly.
■ Use bedside flow sheets to facilitate documentation throughout the shift. Keep these flow sheets in a secure place to maintain confidentiality.
■ Document pertinent information on a worksheet or pad that you keep in your pocket when time is an issue. Jot down key phrases and times; then transcribe the information into the patient record as soon as possible.

Document the time

■ Be specific about times in the chart. Particularly document the exact time of:
– sudden changes in the patient's condition
– significant events
– nursing actions.
■ Avoid block documentation such as "0700 to 1500." This sounds vague and implies inattention to the patient.

Document in chronological order

■ Document observations, assessments, and interventions as you make them, to keep them in chronological order and to establish the pattern of care or events.

KNOW-HOW

Watch your documentation language

At times, some of us may speak and write in a vague or judgmental manner without being aware of it. However, when you're documenting, you should conscientiously avoid including ambiguous statements and subjective judgments.

Ambiguous time periods
"Mrs. Brown asks for pain medication *every so often.*" How would you interpret "every so often"—once an hour, once per shift, or once per day? Although you can't time each and every interaction or occurrence precisely, you should document time relationships when appropriate. In this case, for example, you might document, "Mrs. Brown asked for pain medication at 0800 and again at 1300."

Ambiguous quantities
"A *large amount* of bloody drainage drained from the nasogastric tube." "A large amount" could mean 75 ml of fluid to you and 150 ml to another nurse. Document a specific measurement.

Subjective judgments
"Mr. Russo has a *good attitude.*" How do you know? Support your judgment with an objective rationale—for example, "Mr. Russo states that he intends to learn insulin injection techniques before discharge."
   Don't be afraid to give your impressions of the patient; just make sure that you support your observations—for example, "Leslie was frustrated, voicing dismay at being unable to walk around the room without help." Avoid using words such as "seems" or "appears"—they make you sound unsure of your observations.

Document accurately and completely

- Document facts, not opinions or assumptions.
- Document all relevant information relating to patient care and to the nursing process.

Document objectively

- Document exactly what you see, hear, and do. (See *Watch your documentation language.*)
- When you document a patient's statement, use his exact words and quotation marks.
- Avoid making subjective statements such as "Patient's level of cooperation has deteriorated since yesterday." Instead, include the facts that

KNOW-HOW

Signing nurses' notes

To discourage others from adding information to the nurses' notes, draw a line through any blank spaces and sign your name at the far right of the column.

1/5/08	1200	Will continue plan and request enterostomal
		therapist to assess patient's knowledge and
		acceptance of colostomy on the 2nd postop
		day. ———————————— *Nora Martin, RN*

If you don't have enough room to sign your name after the last word of your entry, draw a line from the last word to the end of the line. Then go to the next line and draw a line from the left margin toward the right margin, leaving room to sign your name on the far right side.

1/5/08	0900	Pt.'s respiratory status markedly improved after
		diuretic and O₂ therapy. Continue to monitor
		ABGs, urine output, weight, and breath sounds.
		Continue diuretic therapy as prescribed. ———
		———————————— *Nora Martin, RN*

If you need to document a lot of information but run out of room on the page, write "Continued on next page," and add your signature at the bottom of the page. Start the next page with "Continued from previous page." Then finish your notes and sign the second page as usual.

| 1/5/08 | 1500 | Morphine sulfate effective. Patient drowsy. |
| | | (continued on next page) — *Nora Martin, RN* |

1/5/08	1500	(continued from previous page)
		States that pain is now 2 on a scale of 0 to
		10. ———————————— *Nora Martin, RN*

led you to this conclusion. If you must document a conclusion, make sure to document the objective assessment data that support it.

■ Document data you have witnessed or data witnessed by a reliable source—such as the patient or another nurse. When you include information reported by someone else, cite your source.

Sign each entry

■ Sign each entry you make in your progress notes with your first name or initial, full last name, and professional licensure, such as RN or LPN. (See *Signing nurses' notes,* page 9.)

■ If you find the last entry unsigned, contact the nurse who made the entry. If you can't locate her, notify the charge nurse or manager, who will follow up on the unsigned entry.

Assessment

Assessment of a patient begins with the first encounter and continues throughout the patient's hospitalization. The initial step of the nursing process, assessment includes collecting relevant information from various sources and evaluating it to form a complete picture of your patient. Accurate assessments:

■ help guide you through the rest of the nursing process

■ help you formulate nursing diagnoses, create patient problem lists, and write nursing care plans

■ serve as a vital communication tool for other health care team members

■ form a baseline from which to evaluate a patient's progress

■ help you meet the requirements of The Joint Commission and other regulatory agencies

■ provide a means of indicating that quality care has been given (Peer review organizations and other quality assurance reviewers consider nursing assessment data as proof of quality care.)

■ serve as evidence in court.

Initial assessment

Perform an initial assessment when first meeting a patient. Before getting started, consider two questions:

■ Which information will be most relevant for this patient at this time?

■ How much time do I have to gather the information?

Collecting relevant information

In your initial patient assessment, be sure to document:

■ chief complaint as stated by the patient

■ signs and symptoms

Complying with the time frame

Your time limit for completing the initial assessment depends on the policy of your health care facility. The Joint Commission requires facilities to establish an assessment time frame for each type of patient they serve. Thus, depending on the unit where you work, the time frame for initiating the first assessment may range from 15 minutes to 12 hours.

Because many facilities offer a wide variety of care, they must establish individual assessment time frames for units or groups of units that share similar patient populations. Thus, a nurse on an intensive care or a trauma emergency unit would have a much shorter time frame for completing an initial assessment than a nurse on an elective surgical unit.

■ type of care received in another unit, such as the intensive care unit or the emergency department, if appropriate
■ date and time the assessment was performed. (See *Complying with the time frame.*)

Also consider these questions:
■ When did the problem begin?
■ Are the patient's immediate problems life-threatening?
■ Does a potential for injury exist?
■ What other influences—such as advanced age, fear, cultural differences, or lack of understanding—might affect treatment outcomes?
■ What medications does the patient take?
■ When did he take the last dose of medication?
■ Is the patient allergic to latex, medications, or foods? (See *Handling latex allergy,* page 12.)

Categorizing assessment data

Subjective information represents the patient's perception of his problem. A patient's complaint of chest pain, for example, is subjective information. Objective information is something you can observe and verify without interpretation—such as a patient's blood pressure reading. (See *Documenting subjective and objective information,* page 13.)

Sources of data

Information gathered directly from the patient (primary source data) is the most valuable because it reflects his situation most accurately.

KNOW-HOW

Handling latex allergy

Allergy to latex, a material derived from natural rubber, is a large and growing problem in the United States. Reactions range from mild dermatitis to anaphylactic shock. As part of the initial patient evaluation, you should ask each patient if he has an allergy to latex or natural rubber.

When caring for a patient with a known or suspected latex allergy, clearly document the allergy on all appropriate records (paper or electronic), and document in the body of the chart precautions you've taken to create a latex-safe environment for the patient. Also, place a "Latex precautions" label on the patient's chart, and apply an allergy identification bracelet to the patient's wrist.

Latex allergy policies may vary from one facility to another, so follow your facility's protocol. If your facility has a latex-free supply cart, be sure to document that it was placed in or outside the patient's room, according to your facility's protocol.

However, additional data about a patient can be obtained from secondary sources, including:
■ family members
■ friends
■ other members of the health care team
■ written records, such as past clinical records, transfer summaries, and personal documents such as a living will.

Gather as much information from secondary sources as possible. You'll find that it's helpful because:
■ it gives you alternative viewpoints from the patient's
■ the information may help establish a complete profile because of a patient's condition or age
■ family members and friends give important indications of family dynamics, educational needs, and available support systems
■ including people close to the patient helps alleviate their feelings of helplessness during the hospitalization.

Performing the initial assessment

An initial assessment consists of your general observations, the patient's health history, and the physical examination. It is best to document the assessment as you perform it. Assessments are performed by the registered professional nurse.

Documenting subjective and objective information

Subjective information

Subjective information includes the patient's chief complaint or concern, current health status, health history, family history, psychosocial history, medication history, activities of daily living, and a review of body systems. The patient's history, embodying his perception of his problems, is your most important source of assessment information. However, it must be interpreted carefully. When possible, document using the patient's own words. Suppose a patient complains of frequent stomach pain:

■ Find out what he considers "frequent": once per week, once per day, twice per day, or all day.
■ Find out what he means by "stomach" by asking him to point to the specific area affected. This also tells you if the pain is localized or generalized.
■ Find out how he defines "pain" by having him describe the sensation as stabbing or dull, twisting or nagging.
■ How does he rate its severity on a scale of 0 to 10?
   When documenting subjective data, be sure to:
■ Write the patient's own words in quotation marks.
■ Introduce patient statements with a phrase such as "Patient states."
■ Ask the patient to define unfamiliar words or phrases such as slang words. For clarity, record the phrase and the patient's definition.

Objective information

When documenting objective information, follow these guidelines:
■ Be specific and avoid using subjective descriptions, such as "large," "small," and "moderate."
■ Use measurements to record data clearly.
■ Specify color, size, and location when appropriate.
■ Avoid interpreting the data and reflecting your opinion.

General observations

Observations can begin as soon as you meet the patient. By looking critically at him, you can collect valuable information about his:
■ level of consciousness
■ mental state
■ emotional state
■ immediate comfort level

- mobility status
- general physical condition. (See *Making general observations.*)
  When making observations, follow these guidelines:
- Document general observations made during the interview and physical examination as well as throughout the patient's hospitalization.
- Keep your observations objective, and don't draw conclusions.
- Document the facts.

Health history

The health history organizes pertinent physiologic, psychological, cultural, and psychosocial information. (See *Conducting the interview,* pages 17 and 18.) When documenting your patient's health history, include:

- subjective data about the patient's current health status that point to actual or potential health problems
- the patient's ability and willingness to comply with health care interventions and his expectations for treatment outcomes
- details about the patient's lifestyle, family relationships, and cultural influences—all of which may affect his health care needs
- patient problems that your nursing interventions can help resolve.

Physical examination

Perform the physical examination by using the assessment techniques of inspection, palpation, percussion, and auscultation. When you document the physical examination, include:

- the scope of the physical examination
- objective data that may confirm or rule out suspicions raised during the health history interview
- findings that will enable you to plan care and start teaching the patient about his condition
- abnormal findings that require a more in-depth assessment.

A routine review for an adult patient includes a general survey of his height, weight, vital signs, and pulse oximetry as well as a review of the following body systems.

Neurologic system
After examining the neurologic system, document:

- level of consciousness, including orientation to time, place, and person and ability to follow commands
- pupillary reactions and cranial nerve function
- strength and movement of extremities.

Making general observations

Your general observations of the patient's appearance, mobility, communication ability, and cognitive function form an important part of your initial assessment. To save time, here are some specific characteristics to look for and document.

Appearance

Age
- Appears to be stated age
- Appears older or younger than stated age

Physical condition
- Physically fit, strong, and appropriate weight for height
- Deconditioned, weak, and either underweight or overweight
- Apparent limitations, such as an amputation or paralysis
- Obvious scars or rash

Dress
- Dressed appropriately or inappropriately for season
- Clean and well-kept clothes
- Soiled or torn clothes; smell of alcohol, urine, or feces

Personal hygiene
- Clean and well-groomed
- Unkempt; unshaved; dirty skin, hair, and nails
- Body odor or unusual breath odor

Skin color
- Appropriate for race
- Pale, ruddy, cyanotic, jaundiced, or tanned

Mobility

Ambulation
- Walks independently; steady gait
- Uses a cane, crutches, or walker
- Unsteady, slow, hesitant, or shuffling gait; leans to one side; can't support own weight
- Transfers from chair to bed independently
- Needs assistance (from one, two, or three people) to transfer from chair to bed

Movement
- Moves all extremities
- Has right- or left-sided weakness; paralysis
- Can't turn in bed independently
- Has jerky or spastic movements of body parts (specify)

(continued)

Making general observations *(continued)*

Communication

Speech
- Speaks clearly in English or other language
- Speaks only with one-word responses; doesn't respond to verbal stimuli
- Speech is slurred, hoarse, loud, soft, incoherent, hesitant, slow, fast, or nonsensical
- Has difficulty completing sentences because of shortness of breath or pain

Hearing
- Hears well enough to respond to questions
- Hard of hearing; wears hearing aid; must speak loudly into left or right ear
- Deaf; reads lips or uses sign language

Vision
- Sees well enough to read instructions in English or other language
- Wears corrective lenses to see or read
- Can't read
- Blind

Cognitive functions

Awareness
- Oriented to person, place, and time; aware of surroundings
- Disoriented; unaware of time, place, and person

Mood
- Responds appropriately; talkative
- Answers in one-word responses; offers information only in response to direct questions
- Hesitates in answering questions; looks to family member before answering
- Angry; states "Leave me alone" (or similar response); speaks loudly and abruptly to family members
- Maintains or avoids eye contact

Thought processes
- Maintains a conversation; makes relevant statements; follows commands appropriately
- Mind wanders; makes irrelevant statements; follows commands inappropriately

Respiratory system

After examining the respiratory system, document:
- rate and rhythm of respirations and types of breath sounds auscultated in specific lung fields

KNOW-HOW

Conducting the interview

When conducting a patient interview, show empathy, compassion, self-aware-ness, and objectivity to promote a trusting relationship with your patient.

Techniques to use

■ *Use general leads.* Broad opening questions allow the patient to relate infor-mation that he deems essential. Asking such questions as "What brought you to the hospital?" or "What concerns do you have?" encourages the patient to dis-cuss what's most important to him.

■ *Restate information.* To help clarify the patient's meaning, restate or summarize the essence of his comments. For instance, suppose a patient says, "I have pain after I eat," and you respond, "So, you have pain about three times per day." This might prompt the patient to reply, "Oh no, I eat only breakfast, and then the pain is so severe that I don't eat for the rest of the day."

■ *Use reflection.* Asking a question in a different way offers the patient an op-portunity to reconsider his response. A patient might say, "I've told you every-thing about my home life." Using reflection, you might respond, "Do you have other concerns about your situation after you leave the hospital?"

■ *State the implied meaning.* A patient may hint at difficulties or problems. By stating what he has left unspoken, you give him an opportunity to clarify his thoughts and accurately interpret the meaning of his statements. For example, a patient who remarks, "I'm sure my wife is glad that I'm in the hospital," may be implying several things. To clarify this statement, you might respond, "By saying your wife is glad, do you mean she has been concerned about your condition, or do you feel that you've been a burden to her at home?"

■ *Focus the discussion.* The patient may stray from the topic at hand to relate other information he feels you should know. You need to get the conversation back on track without insulting the patient or making him feel that the informa-tion isn't important. To help him refocus the conversation, you might say, "That's very interesting, but first I'd like to get back to our discussion about your last hospitalization."

■ *Ask open-ended questions.* Questions that encourage the patient to express himself elicit more information than questions that call for a one-word response. If you ask, "Do you take your medications?" the patient may respond with a sim-ple "Yes." But if you ask, "How do you take your medications?" you might dis-cover that the patient takes his antihypertensive pills sporadically because they make him feel dizzy.

Time-saving measures

■ Before the interview, fill in as much of the health history information as you can from secondary sources, such as admission forms, transfer summaries, and the medical history. This avoids duplication of effort and reduces interview time.

(continued)

Conducting the interview *(continued)*

If some of this information needs clarification, you can ask the patient to give you a fuller explanation.

■ Check your facility's policy regarding who can gather assessment data. You may be able to have a nursing assistant collect routine information, such as allergies and past hospitalizations. Remember, however, that you must review the information and verify it, as necessary.

■ Begin by asking about the patient's chief complaint and the reason for his hospitalization. Then, if the interview is interrupted, you'll have some initial information on which to base a care plan.

■ Use your facility's nursing assessment documentation form as a guide to organize information.

■ Take only brief notes during the interview to avoid interrupting the flow of conversation.

■ Document your findings using concise, specific phrases and approved abbreviations.

Techniques to avoid

■ *Don't ask judgmental or threatening questions.* A patient shouldn't have to justify his feelings or actions. Questions such as "Why did you do that?" or demanding statements such as "Explain your behavior" may be perceived as a threat or challenge. When a patient doesn't have a specific answer to this type of question, he may invent an appropriate response merely to satisfy you.

■ *Don't ask probing and persistent questions.* This style of questioning can make the patient feel manipulated and defensive, so only make one or two attempts to obtain information about a particular subject. If the patient seems to be avoiding the topic or is reluctant to answer, reevaluate the relevance of the information.

■ *Don't use inappropriate language or technical terms or jargon.* Questions such as "Do you take that med q.i.d. or p.r.n.?" can intimidate or alienate the patient and his family. It can also make the patient feel that you're unwilling to share information about his condition or to converse on his level.

■ *Don't give advice.* Giving advice implies that you know what's best for the patient. Instead, you should encourage the patient and his family to participate in health care decisions. If the patient asks for advice, inform him about available options and then help him explore his own opinions about them.

■ *Don't provide false reassurance.* Statements such as "You'll be all right" or "Everything will work out fine" tend to devalue a person's feelings. By recognizing those feelings, you can open communication channels. Saying something such as, "You seem worried or frightened" encourages the patient to speak candidly. Always try to be honest and sensitive. Even when a patient asks, "Am I going to die?" you can honestly state, "I don't know. Tell me what makes you ask that."

- condition of the lips, mucous membranes, and nail beds
- sputum color, consistency, and other characteristics, if indicated.

Cardiovascular system
After examining the cardiovascular system, document:
- heart sounds
- heart rate and rhythm
- color and temperature of the extremities
- peripheral pulses—presence and quality
- edema
- condition of neck veins
- location and characteristics of chest pain.

Eyes, ears, nose, and throat
After examining the eyes, ears, nose, and throat, document:
- ability to see objects with or without corrective lenses as appropriate
- ability to hear spoken words clearly
- characteristics and amount of discharge from the eyes, ears, nose, or gums
- condition of the teeth, gums, and mucous membranes
- location of palpable lymph nodes, if present.

GI system
After examining the GI system, document:
- type of bowel sounds in all quadrants
- presence of abdominal distention or ascites
- location and characteristics of abdomen pain or tenderness.

Genitourinary system
After examining the genitourinary system, document:
- bladder distention or incontinence
- presence of rashes, edema, or deformity of genitalia, if indicated.

(Inspection of the genitalia may be waived at the patient's request or if no dysfunction was reported during the interview.)

Musculoskeletal system
After examining the musculoskeletal system, document:
- range of motion of major joints
- swelling at the joints, contractures, muscular atrophy, or obvious deformity.

Reproductive system
After examining the reproductive system, document:
- condition of the genitalia and abnormal discharge, if indicated
- breast examination findings, if performed.

Integumentary system

After examining the integumentary system, document:
- location and characteristics of sores, lesions, scars, pressure ulcers, rashes, bruises, or petechiae, and photograph per facility policy
- condition of skin turgor.

Meeting Joint Commission requirements

The Joint Commission requires health care professionals in accredited facilities to meet certain standards for performing patient assessments, determines whether these standards have been met by reviewing the documentation of patient assessments, and requires you to obtain assessment information from the patient's family or friends when appropriate. When doing so, make sure to document the nature of the relationship and the length of time the person has known the patient.

Assessment requirements

Current Joint Commission standards mandate that each patient's initial assessment include three key categories: physical, psychological and social, and environmental factors. To make sure that your assessment meets these standards, follow these guidelines:
- Document your findings from your review of the patient's major body systems.
- Document the patient's expectations, fears, anxieties, and other concerns related to his hospitalization as well as his support system. In your documentation, include information on the patient's family structure and role and roles within that structure, work status, income level, and socioeconomic concerns.
- Document the type of dwelling the patient lives in, and whether he has adequate heat, ventilation, hot water, and bathroom facilities. Also document how many flights of stairs he has to climb, whether the layout of his home poses hazards, whether his home is convenient to stores and physicians' offices, and whether he uses equipment that isn't available in the hospital when he performs activities of daily living (ADLs) at home.
- Document the patient's food and fluid intake and his elimination patterns. Also document recent weight gain or loss. A registered dietitian should be consulted as warranted by the patient's needs or condition.
- Document how the patient's ability to perform ADLs affects his compliance with his treatment regimen before and after discharge. Assess his ability to eat, wash, dress, use the bathroom, turn in bed, get out of

bed, and get around. (Some health care facilities use a checklist to indicate whether a patient can perform these tasks independently or if he needs partial or total assistance.) Document the use of assistive devices.

■ Document your patient's knowledge of the disease process, self-care, diet, medications, recommended lifestyle changes, treatment measures, and limitations resulting from the disease or its treatment. Document any factors that may hinder his learning—such as the nature of his illness or injury, health or religious beliefs, cultural practices, educational level, sensory deficits, language barriers, stress level, age, and pain or discomfort.

■ Document the patient's discharge planning needs as soon as possible. Document where he'll go after discharge and whether follow-up care will be accessible. Also document whether community resources, such as visiting nurse services and Meals On Wheels, are available where the patient lives.

Documenting the initial assessment

Initial assessment information can be referred to by any of several names, including the "nursing admission assessment" and the "nursing database." Some facilities have adopted admission assessment forms that include information gathered from different members of the health care team. These forms may be called "integrated," "interdisciplinary," or "multidisciplinary" care team assessment forms. (See *Integrated admission database form,* pages 22 to 30.)

Documentation styles

Initial assessment findings are documented in one of three basic styles:
■ narrative notes
■ standardized open-ended style
■ standardized closed-ended style.
　　Many assessment forms use a combination of all three styles.

Narrative notes
Narrative notes consist of handwritten accounts in paragraph form that summarize information obtained by general observation, interview, and physical examination.

Advantages
■ Allow findings to be listed in order of importance
■ Are most practical for independent practitioners.

(Text continues on page 31.)

Integrated admission database form

Most health care facilities use a multidisciplinary admission form. The sample form here has spaces that can be filled in by the nurse, physician, and other health care providers.

Name *Beatrice Perry*   Admission Date *2/ 26 / 08*

Address *2 Clayton Street*   Time *1345*
          Dallas, Texas

Admitted per: _____ Ambulatory ✔ Stretcher _____ Wheelchair

T *97* P *92* R *24* BP *98/52* Ht. *5'2"* Wt. *225 lb*
          (estimated/~~actual~~)

ORIENTATION TO ROOM/UNIT POLICIES EXPLAINED

✔ Call light	_____ Living will on chart
✔ Bed operation	_____ Valuables form completed
✔ Phone	✔ Elec.
✔ Television	✔ Smoking
✔ Meals	_____ Side rails
_____ Advance directive explained	✔ ID bracelet on
_____ Living will	_____ Visiting hours

SECTION COMPLETED BY: *P. Lippman, CST*   **TIME:** *1350*

Name and phone numbers of two people to call if necessary:

Name	**Relationship**	**Phone#**
Mary Ryan	*daughter*	*665-2190*
Thomas Perry	*son*	*630-4785*

REASON FOR HOSPITALIZATION (patient quote:) *I go numb in my rt. arm and leg*

ANTICIPATED DATE OF DISCHARGE: *2/28/08*

PREVIOUS HOSPITALIZATIONS: SURGERY/ILLNESS   **DATE**
          TIA   *1/15/08*

Integrated admission database form *(continued)*

Name *Beatrice Perry*   Date *2/26/08*

HEALTH PROBLEM	Yes	No	?
Arthritis		✔	
Blood problem (anemia, sickle cell, clotting, bleeding)		✔	
Cancer		✔	
Diabetes	✔		
Eye problems (cataracts, glaucoma)		✔	
Heart problem		✔	
Liver problem		✔	
Hiatal hernia		✔	
High blood pressure	✔		
HIV/AIDS		✔	
Kidney problem		✔	
Lung problem (emphysema, asthma, bronchitis, TB, pneumonia, shortness of breath)	✔		
Stroke		✔	
Ulcers		✔	
Thyroid problem		✔	
Psychological disorder		✔	
Alcohol abuse		✔	
Drug abuse			
Drug(s)		✔	
Smoking	✔		
Other			

Comments:

ALLERGIES: ☐ no known allergies ☐ TAPE ☐ IODINE ☐ LATEX
☐ FOOD:
☑ DRUG: *Penicillin*
☐ BLOOD REACTION:
☐ OTHER:

MEDICATIONS:

HERBAL PREPARATIONS:

Information received from:
☑ Patient ☐ Relative   ☐ Friend   ☐ Other
Section completed by:
   T. Jones, RN   Date *2/26/08*   Time   *1405*

(continued)

Integrated admission database form *(continued)*

Name ___Beatrice Perry___   Date _2/26/08_

All assessment sections are to be completed by a professional nurse.

✔ _____ Clean   _____ Disheveled

SKIN INTEGRITY: Indicate the location of any of the following on the chart below using the designated letter:

a = rashes
b = lesions
c = significant bruises/abrasions
d = burns
e = pressure sores
f = recent scars
g = presence of tubes/appliances
h = other _____

Comments: ___b: ischemic Ⓡ leg ulcer (2 cm – healing)___

GENERAL PHYSICAL APPEARANCE

Integrated admission database form *(continued)*

Name: *Beatrice Perry*   Date: *2/26/08*

FALL-RISK

Impaired: _____ Sensory function   _____ Mental status
_____ Urinary/GI function   _____ General debility/weakness
_____ Mobility function
✔ History of recent falls/dizziness/blackouts
(automatically designates patient as prone-to-fall)
✔ Prone-to-fall risk (indicated on nursing Kardex ✔)

NEUROLOGICAL ASSESSMENT

_____ Dizziness   _____ Syncope   _____ Headache   _____ Blurred vision
_____ Recent seizure ✔ Numbness/tingling location: *Rt. arm and leg*
LOC: ✔ Alert   _____ Lethargic   _____ Semi-comatose   _____ Comatose
Mental Status: ✔ Oriented   _____ Confused   _____ Disoriented
Speech: ✔ Clear   _____ Slurred   _____ Garbled   _____ Aphasic

Neurological Checklist

| Right Arm | Left Arm | Right Leg | Left Leg | R. Pupil | L. Pupil | Pupil Reaction | Coma Scale | | | |
							Eyes Open	Best Verbal Response	Best Motor Response	Total
+2/+4		+2/+4		5/6		+	4	5	6	15

+1:cannot move   +3:move against gravity
+2:cannot move against gravity   +4:move strongly against gravity

Pupil Reaction
+ Reactive   > Greater than
− Nonreactive   < Less than
D Dilated   = Equal
C Constricted   S Sluggish

CODE
Pupils (mm):

1 2 3 4 5 6 7 8

GLASGOW COMA SCALE CODE

Response	1	2	3	4	5	6
EYES OPEN	Never	To Pain	To Sound	(Sponta-neously)		
VERBAL	None	Incompre-hensible Sounds	Inappro-priate Words	Confused Conversa-tion	(Oriented)	
MOTOR	None	Extension	Flexion Abnormal	Flexion Withdrawal	(Localizes Pain)	

GCS score _____ *14*

Comments: *numbness transient*

Signature *T. Jones, RN*

(continued)

Integrated admission database form *(continued)*

Name **Beatrice Perry**   Date **2/26/08**

BEHAVIORAL

Behavior: ✔ Cooperative   ____ Depressed
                 ____ Combative   ____ Unresponsive
                 ____ Uncooperative   ____ Restless
                 ✔ Anxious   ____ Other ____
Religious/Spiritual beliefs: *Lutheran*
P. request to contact minister/priest/rabbi? ✔ Y ____ N
Name *Rev. William Lacy*
Phone # *726-8039*
Comments: ____

PAIN

Pt. having pain at present? ____ Y ✔ N
Pt. had pain in last several months? ____ Y ✔ N
Rate pain on a scale of 0 to 10 (0 = no pain, 10 = severe pain) ____
Pain location ____ Quality ____
Radiation ____ Y ____ N Duration ____
What aggravates pain? ____
What alleviates pain? ____
Effects on ADLs ____
Pt. pain goals ____

CARDIOVASCULAR

Skin color: ____ Normal ____ Flushed ____ Pale ✔ Cyanotic
Apical pulse: ____ Regular ✔ Irregular
Pacemaker: Type ____ Rate ____
Peripheral pulses: ✔ Present ____ Equal ✔ Weak ____ Absent
Comments: *bilat. weak lower extremities*
Specify: R ____ radial ____ pedal L ____ radial ____ pedal
Comments: ____
Edema: ____ No ✔ Yes *+1 bilat. pretibial*
Numbness: ____ No ✔ Yes Site: *Rt. arm and leg*
Chest pain: ✔ No ____ Yes ____
Family cardiac history: ____ No ✔ Yes
Telemetry Monitor: ____ No ✔ Yes Rhythm *normal sinus*
Comments: ____

PULMONARY

Respirations: ✔ Regular ____ Irregular
              ____ Shortness of breath ____ Dyspnea on exertion
O_2 use at home? ____ Yes ✔ No
Chest expansion: ✔ Symmetrical
                 ____ Asymmetrical (explain: ____)
Breath sounds: ____ Clear ____ Crackles ____ Rhonchi ✔ Wheezing
               ____ Location *bilat upper lobe, inspiratory*
Cough: None ✔ Nonproductive ____ Productive ____ Describe ____
Comments: *pulse oximetry 98% on 2 L; sleeps with 2 pillows*

Signature *T. Jones, RN*

Integrated admission database form *(continued)*

Name *Beatrice Perry*   Date *2/26/08*

GASTROINTESTINAL

Stool:
- ✔ Formed
- Loose
- Liquid
- Mucus
- Ostomy
- Incontinent

Color:
- ✔ Brown
- Black
- Red tinged
- Bloody

Diarrhea
Constipation

Abdomen:
- ✔ Soft
- Rigid
- ✔ Nontender
- Tender
- (Location)

Bowel sounds ✔ Present
- Absent
- Hypoactive
- Hyperactive

Obese ✔
Thin
Emaciated
Nourished
*NUTRITION:
- ✔ Special Diet *1800 calorie*
- Tube feeding
- Chewing problem
- Swallowing problems
- Nausea/vomiting
- Poor appetite
- Wt. loss/gain ____ lb
*Refer to dietitian if any ✔

GENITOURINARY/REPRODUCTIVE

Color of urine: ✔ Yellow ____ Amber ____ Pink/Red tinged
____ Brown ____ Orange
____ Clear ____ Cloudy

- Ileo-conduit
- Incontinent ____ Catheter in place
- Frequency ____ Urgency
- Difficulty in initiating stream
- Pain ____ Burning
- Oliguria ____ Anuria
- Dialysis

Access site: _____ Date of last dialysis: _____
Comments: _____
Date of LMP *1983* _____ Date of last PAP *5/04*
Breast self-exam ____ Yes ✔ No
Use of contraceptives: ____ Yes (type _____) ____ No ✔ N/A
Vaginal discharge: ____ Yes (describe _____) ✔ No
Bleeding: ____ Yes (amount _____) ✔ No
Pregnancies:
Pregnant ____ Yes ____ Weeks ____ Gravida ____ Para ✔ No
Date of last prostate exam _____
Testicular self-exam ____ Yes ____ No
Comments: _____

Signature *T. Jones, RN*

(continued)

Integrated admission database form *(continued)*

Name _Beatrice Perry_   Date _2/26/08_

ACTIVITY/MOBILITY PATTERNS

_____ Ambulates independently _____ Full ROM
_____ Limited ROM (explain: _____)
✔ Ambulates with assistance (explain: _____)
✔ _____ cane _____ walker _____ crutches
_____ Gait steady/unsteady _____ Mobility in bed (ability to turn self) _____

Musculoskeletal
_____ Pain _____ Weakness _____ Contractures _____ Joint swelling
_____ Paralysis _____ Deformity _____ Joint stiffness _____ Cast
_____ Amputation
Describe: _____
Comments: _____

REST/ SLEEP PATTERNS

_____ Use of sleeping aids _____   Sleeps _6_ hr/day
Comments: _____

Additional assessment comment: _On arrival, diaphoretic and Ⓛ hand tremors. Vital signs stable. Glucose 56 mg/dl. Orange juice and lunch given to patient. 2 hr post-prandial glucose 204. Symptoms subsided with juice. Nutrition and diabetes educator consulted._ _____ _Jill O'Brien, RN_
MRI shows no cerebral lesions. Carotid doppler ultrasound pending. _____ _B. Mayer MD_

EDUCATION/DISCHARGE SECTION
Instructions: Assessment sections must be completed within 8 hours of admission. Discharge planning and summary must be completed by day of discharge.

Yes	No	
✔		Patient understands current diagnosis
✔		Family/significant other understands diagnosis
✔		Patient able to read English
✔		Patient able to write English
✔		Patient able to communicate
	✔	Patient/family understands pre-hospital medication/treatment regimen

Yes	No	**Emotional factors:**
✔		Patient appears to be coping
✔		Family appears to be coping
	✔	Any suspicion of family violence
	✔	Any suspicion of family abuse
	✔	Any suspicion of family neglect

Comments: _diabetic teaching_ _____

Language spoken, written, and read (other than English): _____
Interpreter services needed: ✔ No _____ Yes
Are there any barriers to learning (e.g., emotional, physical, cognitive)? _NO_ _____
Religious or cultural practices that may alter care or teaching needs?
_____ ✔ No Describe: _____
Is pt/family motivated to learn? ✔ Yes _____ No Describe: _____
Signature _T. Jones, RN_

Integrated admission database form *(continued)*

Name _Beatrice Perry_   Date _2/26/08_

DISCHARGE ASSESSMENT

Living arrangements/caregiver (relationship): _lives alone_

Type of dwelling:
___ Apartment ✔ House ___ Nursing home
___ More than 1 floor? ✔ Yes ___ No Describe: _____
___ Boarding home ___ Other _____

Physical barriers in home:
✔ No ___ Yes (explain: _____)

Access to follow-up medical care:
✔ Yes ___ No (explain: _____)

Ability to carry out ADLs: ___ Self-care ✔ Partial assistance ___ Total assistance

Needs help with:
✔ Bathing ___ Feeding ___ Ambulation ___ Other _____

Anticipated discharge destination:
✔ Home ___ Rehab. ___ Nursing home ___ SNF ___ Boarding home
___ Other _____

Currently receiving services from a community agency? ___ Yes ✔ No

If yes, check which one ___ Visiting nurses ___ Meals on Wheels

Concerned about returning home?
___ Being alone ___ Financial problems ___ Homemaking ___ Meal prep.
✔ Managing ADLs ___ Other _____

Assessment completed by:
T. Jones, RN   Date _2/26/08_ Time _1430_

DISCHARGE PLANNING

Resources notified	Name	Date	Time	Signature
Social worker				
Home care coordinator	M. Murphy, RN	2/28/08	0900	T. Jones, RN
Other_____				

Equipment/supplies needed: _stair chair_

Arranged for by:
M. Murphy, RN   Date _2/28/08_ Time _0930_
Comments: _Daughter to stay with pt at home_

(continued)

Integrated admission database form *(continued)*

Name _Beatrice Perry_   Date _2/26/08_

DISCHARGE SUMMARY

Alterations in patterns (If yes, explain.)	Yes	No	Explanation
Nutrition	✔		adherence to diet regimen
Elimination		✔	
Self-care		✔	
Skin integrity		✔	
Mobility	✔		needs help with stairs
Comfort pain		✔	
Mental status/behavior		✔	
Vision/hearing/speech		✔	

Discharge instructions given (specify): _standard hosp. discharge instruction sheet_

Effects of illness on employment/lifestyle: _____

Central venous line removed: _N/A_ By whom: _____

Belongings sent with patient:
   ✔ clothes   ✔ dentures   ✔ eyeglasses
   ___ hearing aid   ___ prosthesis   ___ valuables
   ✔ prescriptions   ✔ other _cane_

Follow-up medical supervision to be provided by: _Dr. Adam Schneider_
   ✔ Patient/family instructed to call for follow-up appointment

Discharge destination: _pt's home with daughter_

Section completed by:
   C. Rafferty, RN   Date _2/28/08_   Time _1130_

Disadvantages
- Mimic the medical model by focusing on a review of body systems
- Are time-consuming to write and read
- Require the nurse to remember and document all significant information in a detailed, logical sequence
- Can contain illegible handwriting that can easily lead to misinterpretation of findings.

Standardized open-ended style
The standardized open-ended style of documentation is the typical "fill-in-the blanks" assessment form that comes with preprinted headings and questions. This style may be used with a computerized system. (See *Documenting assessment on an open-ended form,* page 32.)

Advantages
- Allows information to be categorized under specific headings and questions
- Can be completed using partial phrases and approved abbreviations.

Disadvantages
- Doesn't always provide enough space or instructions to encourage thorough descriptions
- Can contain nonspecific responses that can lead to misinterpretation.

Standardized closed-ended style
Standardized closed-ended assessment forms provide preprinted headings, checklists, and questions with specific responses. You simply check off the appropriate response. (See *Documenting assessment on a closed-ended form,* page 33.)

Advantages
- Saves time
- Eliminates the problem of illegible handwriting and makes checking documented information easy
- Can be easily incorporated into most computerized systems
- Clearly establishes the type and amount of information required by the health care facility
- Uses guidelines that clearly define responses, even though closed-ended forms usually use nonspecific terminology, such as "within normal limits" or "no alteration."

Disadvantages
- May not provide a place to document relevant information that doesn't fit the preprinted choices

Documenting assessment on an open-ended form

At some health care facilities, you may use a standardized open-ended form to document initial assessment information. Below you'll find a portion of such a form.

Reason for hospitalization *"My blood sugar is high."*
Expected outcomes *By discharge, the patient and his family will understand the basic disease process of diabetes mellitus, demonstrate correct insulin administration techniques and self-testing for blood sugar, and identify signs and symptoms of hyperglycemia and hypoglycemia.*

Last hospitalization
Date *3/01/07*   Reason *high blood pressure*

Medical history *hypertension, diabetes mellitus*

Medications and allergies

Drug	Dose	Time of last dose	Patient's statement of drug's purpose
Humulin N	*30 units*	*0730*	*for sugar*
Humulin R	*5 units*	*0730*	*for sugar*
furosemide	*20 mg*	*1000*	*water pill*
atenolol	*50 mg*	*0800*	*for BP*

Allergy	Reaction
shellfish	*hives*

Signature *M. Richardson, RN*   Date *1/14/08*

■ Can be lengthy, especially when a facility's policy calls for documenting in-depth physical assessment data.

Documentation formats

Historically, nursing assessment has followed a medical format emphasizing the patient's initial symptoms and a comprehensive review of body systems. However, some facilities have adopted formats that more readily reflect the nursing process. Other documentation formats are modeled on specific conceptual frameworks based on published nursing theories and include the following systems.

Documenting assessment on a closed-ended form

At some health care facilities, you may use a standardized closed-ended form to document initial assessment information. Below you'll find a portion of such a form.

SELF-CARE ABILITY   Date _3/05/08_

Activity	1	2	3	4	5	6
Bathing		✔				
Cleaning		✔				
Climbing stairs			✔			
Cooking	✔					
Dressing and grooming		✔				
Eating and drinking	✔					
Moving in bed	✔					
Shopping					✔	
Toileting			✔			
Transferring			✔			
Walking		✔				
Other home functions			✔			

Key
1 = Independent
2 = Requires assistive device
3 = Requires personal assistance
4 = Requires personal assistance and assistive device
5 = Dependent
6 = Experienced change in last week

Assistive devices
- ☑ Bedside commode
- ☐ Brace or splint
- ☐ Cane
- ☐ Crutches
- ☐ Feeding device
- ☐ Trapeze
- ☑ Walker
- ☐ Wheelchair
- ☐ Other
- ☐ None

Activity tolerance
- ☐ Normal
- ☑ Weakness
- ☐ Dizziness
- ☑ Exertional dyspnea
- ☐ Dyspnea at rest
- ☐ Angina
- ☐ Pain at rest
- ☐ Oxygen needed
- ☐ Intermittent claudication
- ☐ Unsteady gait
- ☐ Other

Rest pattern
Sleep habits
- ☑ Less than 8 hours
- ☐ 8 hours
- ☐ More than 8 hours
- ☐ Morning nap
- ☑ Afternoon nap

Sleep difficulties
- ☐ Insomnia
- ☑ Early awakening
- ☐ Unrefreshing sleep
- ☐ Nightmares
- ☐ None

Signature _R. Smith, RN_

■ *Human response patterns.* NANDA-International (NANDA-I) has developed a classification system for nursing diagnoses based on human response patterns that relate directly to actual or potential health problems, as indicated by assessment data. Using an assessment form organized by these patterns allows you to easily establish appropriate diagnoses while you document assessment data—especially if a listing of diagnoses is included with the form.

■ *Functional health care patterns.* Developed by Marjory Gordon, this system classifies nursing data according to the patient's ability to function independently. Many nurses consider this system easier to understand and remember than human response patterns.

■ *Conceptual frameworks.* These assessment forms, which are based on nursing philosophies, reflect the individual theory's approach to nursing care. Some examples include:
– Dorothea Orem's selfcare model
– Imogene King's theory of goal attainment
– Sister Callista Roy's adaptation model.

Documenting learning needs

Most initial assessment forms have a separate section for documenting a patient's learning needs. When you reassess your patient's learning needs, document your findings in:
■ the progress notes
■ an open-ended patient education flow sheet
■ a structured patient education flow sheet designed for a specific problem such as diabetes mellitus
■ educational screens in a computerized system.

Documenting discharge planning needs

Effective discharge planning begins when you identify and document the patient's needs during the initial assessment. (See *Documenting discharge planning needs,* pages 36 and 37.) Document the patient's discharge needs on:
■ the initial assessment form (in a designated section)
■ a specially designed discharge planning form
■ the progress notes
■ a discharge planning flow sheet.

Documenting incomplete initial data

You may not always be able to obtain a complete health history during the initial assessment. When this occurs, base your initial assessment on your observations and physical examination of the patient. When documenting your findings, follow these guidelines:

■ Be sure to write an explanation such as, "Unable to obtain complete data at this time," so it doesn't appear that you failed to perform a complete assessment.

■ Obtain missing information as soon as possible, either when the patient's condition improves or when family members or other secondary sources can provide the information.

■ Document how and when you obtained the missing data.

■ When adding information to complete an initial assessment, be sure to revise your nursing care plan accordingly. Depending on your facility's policy:

– Document the information on the progress notes. This method aids in the day-to-day communication with others who read the notes, but makes it difficult to retrieve the data later.

– Return to the initial assessment form and add the new information along with the date, time, and your signature. This method makes it easy to retrieve data when needed—either during the patient's hospitalization or after discharge for quality assurance.

Ongoing assessment

Assessment of a patient is a continuous process; how often you reassess a patient depends primarily on his condition, Joint Commission requirements, and your facility's policy. (See *The Joint Commission reassessment guidelines,* page 37.)

Reassessment and effective documentation of your findings:

■ allow you to evaluate the effectiveness of nursing interventions and determine your patient's progress toward the desired outcomes

■ facilitate communication with other health care practitioners

■ allow planning for appropriate patient care.

Using flow sheets

Ongoing assessment data may be recorded on flow sheets or in narrative notes on the patient's progress report. Ideally flow sheets should be used to document all routine assessment data and routine interventions. They:

■ allow you to shorten the narrative notes to include only information regarding the patient's progress toward achieving desired outcomes as well as any unplanned assessments.

Documenting discharge planning needs

How and where you document your discharge planning will depend on the policy at the health care facility where you work. Here's one of the more common ways of documenting this information.

DISCHARGE PLANNING NEEDS

Occupation   *Retired college professor*
Language spoken   *English*
Patient lives with   *Wife*
Self-care capabilities   *Needs extensive assistance*
Assistance available
- [ ] Cooking
- [ ] Cleaning
- [x] Shopping
- [x] Dressing changes/treatments   *Irrigate ⓛ lower leg wound b.i.d. with ¹/₂ strength H_2O_2, followed by rinse with normal saline solution. Pack with ¹/₂" iodoform gauze. Apply dry sterile dressing.*

Medication administration routes
- [x] P.O.
- [ ] I.V.
- [ ] I.M.
- [ ] Subcutaneous
- [ ] Other: _____

Dwelling
- [ ] Apartment
- [x] Private home
- [ ] Single room
- [ ] Institution
- [ ] Elevator
- [x] Outside steps
  (number) *6*
- [x] Inside steps
  (number) *12*

- [x] Kitchen
  (gas stove)
  electric stove
  wood stove
- [ ] Other: _____
- [x] Bathrooms (number) *2*
  (location) *one upstairs, one downstairs*
- [x] Telephones (number) *1*
  (location) *kitchen*

Transportation
- [ ] Drives own car
- [ ] Takes public transportation
- [x] Relies on family member or friend

Documenting discharge planning needs *(continued)*

After discharge, patient will be:
- ☐ Home alone
- ☑ Home with family
- ☐ Other: _____

Patient has had help from:
- ☑ Visiting nurse
- ☑ Housekeeper
- ☑ Other: *social worker*

Anticipated needs *Nurse for dressing changes, transportation for groceries, etc.*
Social service requests *VNA*
Date contacted *2/16/08*   **Reason** *Contacted VNA for dressing changes and trans-*
portation needs.

Signature   *P. Burke, RN*

■ are a quick and consistent way to highlight trends in the patient's condition, when used to document routine assessment data.

Because flow sheets are legally accepted components of the patient's medical record, they must be documented correctly. Follow these guidelines:
- ■ Give yourself enough time to evaluate all information on the flow sheet.
- ■ Make sure that your documentation accurately reflects the patient's current clinical status.

The Joint Commisson reassessment guidelines

The following reassessment guidelines are suggested by The Joint Commission.
- ■ Reassessment occurs at regular intervals in the course of care.
- ■ Reassessment determines a patient's response to care.
- ■ Significant change in a patient's condition results in reassessment.
- ■ Significant change in a patient's diagnosis results in reassessment.

■ When documenting only the information requested on a flow sheet isn't sufficient to give a complete picture of the patient's status, document additional information in the space provided on the flow sheet. If your flow sheet doesn't have additional space and you need to document more information, use the progress notes.

■ If additional information isn't necessary, draw a line through the space. Doing so indicates that, in your judgment, further information isn't required.

Nursing diagnoses and care plans

Identify nursing diagnoses carefully. Then write a plan that not only fits your nursing diagnoses but also fits your patient. The plan should take into account the patient's needs, age, developmental level, culture, strengths and weaknesses, and willingness and ability to participate in his own care.

Formulating nursing diagnoses

Unlike a medical diagnosis, which focuses on the patient's pathophysiology or illness, a nursing diagnosis focuses on the patient's responses to illness. (See *Nursing diagnoses: Avoiding the pitfalls.*)

Types of nursing diagnoses

Depending on the policy of your health care facility, you'll either use standardized diagnoses or formulate your own diagnoses.

Benefits of using standardized diagnoses

■ By using nationally standardized diagnoses, such as NANDA-I Taxonomy II, health care facilities make communication easier and diagnoses more precise.

■ Diagnoses can be categorized according to nursing models, but other ways of categorizing diagnoses—for instance, according to Orem's self-care model—may also be used.

■ Health care facilities or units can establish their own list of nursing diagnoses, categorizing them according to medical diagnoses and surgical procedures.

Benefits of formulating your own nursing diagnoses

■ Developing your own diagnoses prevents the usage of standardized diagnoses that may be incomplete or that use overly formal or abstract language.

Nursing diagnoses: Avoiding the pitfalls

To avoid making common mistakes when formulating your nursing diagnoses, follow these guidelines.

Use nursing diagnoses
Don't use medical diagnoses or interventions. Terms such as *angioplasty* and *coronary artery disease* belong in a medical diagnosis—not in a nursing diagnosis.

Use all relevant assessment data
If you focus only on the physical assessment, for instance, you might miss psychosocial or cultural information relevant to your diagnoses.

Take your time
Take enough time to analyze the assessment data. If you rush, you might easily miss something important.

Interpret the assessment data accurately
Make sure that you follow established norms, professional standards, and interdisciplinary expectations in interpreting the assessment data. In addition, don't permit your biases to interfere with your interpretation of information.

For instance, don't assume your patient is exaggerating if he states that he feels pain during what you would consider a painless procedure. If possible, have the patient verify your interpretation.

Keep data up-to-date
Don't stop assessing and updating your diagnoses after the initial examination. As the patient's condition changes, your evaluation should be updated.

■ Developing your own diagnoses can help you characterize a problem that standardized diagnoses don't readily or specifically address.

Deciding on a diagnosis

Evaluate relevant assessment data by looking at a standardized assessment form that groups related information into categories. Looking at the data in these groupings lets you determine which patient needs require nursing intervention and associate relevant nursing diagnoses with specific assessment findings. (See *Evaluating assessment data,* page 40; see also *Relating assessment data to nursing diagnoses,* page 41.)

Evaluating assessment data

To formulate your nursing diagnoses, you must evaluate the essential assessment information. These questions will help you quickly zero in on the appropriate data.

- Which signs and symptoms does the patient have?
- Which assessment findings are abnormal for this patient?
- How do particular behaviors affect the patient's well-being?
- What strengths or weaknesses does the patient have that affect his health status?
- Does he understand his illness and treatment?
- How does the patient's environment affect his health?
- Does he want to change his state of health?
- Do I need to gather more information for my diagnoses?

Components of the diagnosis

- *The human response or problem.* The first part of the diagnosis, the human response, identifies an actual or potential problem that can be affected by nursing care.
- *Related factors.* The second part of the nursing diagnosis identifies related factors, which may precede, contribute to, or simply be associated with the human response. They make your diagnosis more closely fit the particular patient and help you choose the most effective interventions.
- *Signs and symptoms.* A complete nursing diagnosis includes the signs and symptoms that led you to the diagnosis—what NANDA-I calls the "defining characteristics."

Setting priorities

After you've determined your nursing diagnoses, rank them based on which problems require immediate attention. Maslow's hierarchy of needs is generally accepted as the basis for setting priorities. (See *Maslow's hierarchy of needs,* page 42.) When ranking diagnoses, follow these guidelines:

- The first nursing diagnosis will typically stem from the primary medical diagnosis or from the patient's chief complaint. This nursing diagnosis points out a threat to the patient's physical well-being.
- Next, rank related nursing diagnoses, those that pose less immediate threats to the patient's well-being.

Relating assessment data to nursing diagnoses

Some assessment forms group assessment information and relevant nursing diagnoses together so that you can immediately relate one to the other. This saves you from looking back through the form for assessment data when determining the nursing diagnosis. Here's a section of this type of form.

Patient *Michael Ramsey*
Age *72*
Medical diagnosis: *Heart failure*
Date *4/07/08*

ASSESSMENT FINDINGS

NURSING DIAGNOSES

Cardiopulmonary

Breath sounds
crackles, bilateral bases

Breathing pattern
☑ cough *dry*   ☐ smoker

Dyspnea
☐ on exertion   ☐ nocturnal

Sputum
color
consistency

Heart sounds
S_3 and S_4 present

Peripheral pulses
all peripheral pulses +1

Edema
☑ Extremities *ankles*
☐ Other

Cyanosis
☑ Extremities *nail beds*
☑ Other *lips*

☑ Impaired gas exchange
☐ Ineffective airway clearance
☐ Impaired spontaneous ventilation
☑ Ineffective breathing pattern
☑ Decreased cardiac output
☐ Ineffective tissue perfusion (peripheral)
☐ Ineffective tissue perfusion (cardiopulmonary)

Nutrition

Diet *2G Na, low cholesterol*

Appetite
☐ normal
☐ increased
☑ decreased
☐ vomiting
☐ nausea

Signature *B. Robinson, RN*

☑ Imbalanced nutrition: Less than body requirements
☐ Imbalanced nutrition: More than body requirements
☐ Risk for imbalanced nutrition: More than body requirements

Maslow's hierarchy of needs

Abraham Maslow's hierarchy of needs, shown below, is a system for classifying human needs that may prove useful when establishing priorities for your patient's care, especially if he has several nursing diagnoses. According to Maslow, a person's lower-level physiologic needs must be met before higher-level needs—those less crucial to survival—can be addressed. In fact, higher-level needs may not become apparent until lower-level needs are at least partially met.

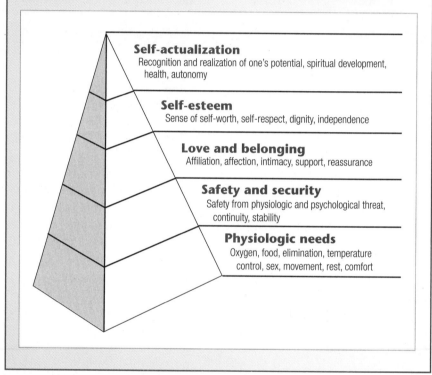

Self-actualization
Recognition and realization of one's potential, spiritual development, health, autonomy

Self-esteem
Sense of self-worth, self-respect, dignity, independence

Love and belonging
Affiliation, affection, intimacy, support, reassurance

Safety and security
Safety from physiologic and psychological threat, continuity, stability

Physiologic needs
Oxygen, food, elimination, temperature control, sex, movement, rest, comfort

■ In most cases, list nursing diagnoses that pertain to the patient's psychosocial, emotional, or spiritual needs last.
■ Keep in mind that although a nursing diagnosis may have a lower priority, you shouldn't wait to intervene until you've resolved all the higher-priority problems. Meeting a lower-priority goal may help resolve a higher-priority problem.
■ Whenever possible, include the patient in this process.

Developing expected outcomes

Based on the nursing diagnoses, expected outcomes are measurable goals that the patient should reach as a result of planned nursing interventions; they may specify an improvement in the patient's ability to function. When developing expected outcomes, remember that:
- one nursing diagnosis may require more than one expected outcome
- each outcome should expect the maximum realistic improvement for a particular patient.

Writing outcome statements

An outcome statement should include four components:
- specific behavior that will demonstrate the patient has reached his goal
- criteria for measuring the behavior
- conditions under which the behavior should occur
- time by which the behavior should occur. (See *Writing an outcome statement,* page 44.)

When you're writing outcome statements, follow these guidelines:
- Make your statements specific. Use action verbs, such as *walks, demonstrates, consumes,* and *expresses.* Clearly state which behaviors you expect the patient to exhibit and when.
- Focus on the patient and family. The outcome statement should reflect the patient's and family's behavior—not your intervention.
- Let the patient help you. A patient who takes part in developing outcome statements is more motivated to achieve his goals. His input—and the input of family members—can help you set realistic goals.
- Take medical orders into account. Don't write outcome statements that ignore or contradict medical orders.
- Adapt the outcome to the circumstances. Consider the patient's coping ability, age, educational level, cultural influences, support systems, living conditions, and socioeconomic status. Consider his anticipated length of stay when you're deciding on time limits for achieving goals, and consider the health care setting itself.
- Change your statements as necessary. Sometimes you may need to revise even the most carefully written outcome statements. If the patient has trouble reaching his goal, choose a later target date or change the goal to one the patient can reach more easily.
- Use shortcuts. Save documenting time by including only the essentials in your outcome statements. Omit the words "Patient will" from

Writing an outcome statement

An outcome statement should consist of four components:

B	M	C	T

Behavior
A desired be-havior for the patient. This behavior must be observable.

Measure
Criteria for meas-uring the behav-ior. The criteria should specify how much, how long, how far, and so on.

Condition
The conditions under which the behavior should occur.

Time
The time by which the behavior should occur.

As indicated, the two outcome statements below have these four components.

Limit sodium intake	2 g/day	using hospital menu	by 3/21/08
Eat	50% of all meals	unassisted	by 3/21/08

your outcomes because "patient" is understood. Rather than writing "Patient will demonstrate insulin self-administration by 9/18/08," simply write "Demonstrate insulin self-administration by 9/18/08." Many facilities use abbreviations for target dates, such as "HD2" for "hospital day 2" and "POD3" for "postoperative day 3."

Selecting interventions

Interventions are nursing actions that you and your patient agree will help him reach the expected outcomes. Their proper selection is important. When selecting interventions, follow these guidelines:
■ Base interventions on the second part of your nursing diagnosis, the related factors.

- Write at least one intervention for each outcome statement.
- Start by considering interventions that you or your patient have previously used successfully.
- Select interventions from standardized care plans.
- Talk and brainstorm with your colleagues about interventions they have used successfully, and check nursing journals that discuss interventions for standardized nursing diagnoses.

Writing intervention statements

Intervention statements must communicate your ideas clearly to other staff members. When writing your interventions, follow these guidelines:

- List *assessment* as an intervention. One of the first interventions in your care plan must include an assessment intervention to allow for reevaluation of the problem in the nursing diagnosis.
- Clearly state the necessary action. Include as much specific detail as possible in your interventions to allow continuity of care. Note how and when to perform the intervention as well as any special instructions.
- Tailor the intervention to the patient. Keep in mind the patient's age, condition, developmental level, environment, and value system when writing your interventions.
- Keep the patient's safety in mind. Take into account the patient's physical and mental limitations so that your interventions don't worsen existing problems or create new ones.
- Follow the rules of your health care facility. If your facility has a rule that only nurses may administer medications, don't write an intervention calling for the patient to "administer hemorrhoidal suppositories as needed."
- Take other health care activities into account. Necessary activities may interfere with interventions you want to use. Adjust your interventions accordingly.
- Include available resources. Make use of the facility's resources as well as available outside sources.

Writing your care plan

A good care plan is the blueprint for concise, meaningful documentation. If you write a good care plan, your nurses' notes will practically write themselves. A good plan consists of:

■ prioritized patient problems identified during the admission interview and hospitalization
■ realistic, measurable expected outcomes and target dates
■ specific nursing interventions that will help the patient or his family achieve these outcomes
■ an evaluation of the patient's responses to intervention and progress toward outcome achievement
■ patient teaching and discharge plans.

Types of nursing care plans

Two basic types of care plans exist: traditional and standardized. No matter which you choose, your plan should cover all nursing care from admission to discharge and should be a permanent part of the patient's medical record.

Traditional care plan

Also called the *individually developed care plan,* the traditional care plan is written from scratch for each patient. The basic form and what you must include can vary, depending on the health care facility or department. When you write a plan of this type, keep these points in mind:

■ Some forms have four main columns: one for nursing diagnoses, another for expected outcomes, a third for interventions, and a fourth for outcome evaluation. Other columns allow you to enter the date you started the care plan, the target dates for expected outcomes, and the dates for review, revisions, and resolution.
■ Some forms also have a place to sign or initial when you make an entry or a revision.
■ Some facilities require you to write only short-term outcomes that the patient should reach before discharge. However, other facilities—particularly long-term care facilities—want to include long-term outcomes that reflect the maximum functional level the patient can reach. (See *Using a traditional care plan,* pages 48 and 49.)

Standardized care plan

Developed to save documentation time and improve the quality of care, standardized care plans provide a series of standard innovations for patients with similar diagnoses. (See *Using a standardized care plan,* page 50.)

When you write a plan of this type, customize it to fit your patient's specific needs. To do this, fill in:
■ related factors and signs and symptoms for a nursing diagnosis
■ time limits for the outcomes

- frequency of interventions
- specific instructions for interventions.

Practice guidelines

Also referred to as *protocols,* practice guidelines give specific sequential instructions for treating patients with a particular problem. They're used to manage patients with specific nursing diagnoses. (See *Practice guidelines for acute pulmonary edema,* pages 52 and 53; see also *Managing ineffective breathing pattern,* page 54.)

Advantages of practice guidelines

- Because they spell out the steps to follow for a patient with a particular nursing diagnosis, practice guidelines help you provide thorough care and make sure that the patient receives consistent care from all caregivers.
- They specify what to teach the patient and what to document, and they include a reference section that lets you quickly determine how up-to-date they are.
- They spell out the roles of other health care professionals, helping all team members coordinate their efforts.
- They supply comprehensive instruction and help teach inexperienced staff members.
- They save documentation time.

Using practice guidelines

- You'll probably use some practice guidelines often, such as the generic one for pain, and other guidelines rarely.
- Note in the interventions section that you are following the guideline.
- List the practice guidelines you plan to use on a flow sheet.
- Document any modifications you'll need to make.
- After your interventions, document in your progress notes that you followed the practice guidelines, or check off the practice guidelines box on your flow sheet and initial it.
- If you find that a practice guideline doesn't exist for a patient problem, help develop a new one. Tailor it to fit your patient's needs, and document any modifications you made on the patient's care plan.
- Keep the guidelines at the nurses' station.

Patient-teaching plan

Patient-teaching plans help all the patient's educators coordinate their teaching, serve as legal proof that the patient received appropriate in-

(Text continues on page 51.)

Using a traditional care plan

Here's an example of a traditional care plan. It shows how these forms are typically organized. Remember that a traditional plan is written from scratch for each patient.

DATE	NURSING DIAGNOSIS	EXPECTED OUTCOMES	
1/8/08	Decreased cardiac output R/T reduced stroke volume secondary to fluid volume overload	Lungs clear on auscultation by 1/10/08. BP will return to baseline by 1/10/08.	

REVIEW DATES

Date	Signature
1/8/08	Karen Kramer, RN

INTERVENTIONS	OUTCOME EVALUATION (initials and date)
Monitor for signs and symptoms of hypoxemia, such as dyspnea, confusion, arrhythmias, restlessness, and cyanosis. Ensure adequate oxygenation by placing patient in semi-Fowler's position and administering supple-mental O_2 as ordered. Monitor breath sounds q 4 hr. Administer cardiac medications as ordered and document pt's response, drugs' effectiveness, and any adverse reactions. Monitor and document heart rate and rhythm, heart sounds, and BP. Note the presence or absence of peripheral pulses. ———————— ———————————————— KK	
	Initials KK

Using a standardized care plan

The standardized care plan below is for a patient with a nursing diagnosis of Impaired tissue integrity. To customize it to your patient, complete the diagnosis—including signs and symptoms—and fill in the expected outcomes. Also modify, add, or delete interventions as necessary.

Name: *Mary Jones*

Date
2/15/08

Nursing diagnosis
Impaired tissue integrity related to arterial insufficiency

Target date
2/17/08

Expected outcomes
Attains relief from immediate symptoms: *pain, ulcers, edema*
Voices intent to change aggravating behavior: *will stop smoking immediately*

Maintains collateral circulation: *palpable peripheral pulses, extremities warm and pink with good capillary refill*
Voices intent to follow specific management routines after discharge: *foot care guidelines, exercise regimen as specified by PT*

Date
2/15/08

Interventions
• Provide foot care. Administer and monitor treatments according to facility protocols.
• Encourage adherence to an exercise regimen as tolerated.
• Educate the patient about risk factors and prevention of injury. Refer the patient to a stop-smoking program.
• Maintain adequate hydration. Monitor I/O *every 8 hours*

• To increase arterial blood supply to the extremities, elevate head of bed *6" to 8"*
• Additional interventions: *inspect skin integrity every 8 hours*

Date
2/17/08

Outcomes evaluation
Attained relief of immediate symptoms: *pt. denies pain, edema decreased, ulcers unchanged*
Voiced intent to change aggravating behavior: *pt. states she will quit smoking*
Maintained collateral circulation: *all pulses palpable, capillary refill < 3 sec*
Voiced intent to follow specific management routines after discharge: *pt. states continued participation with PT and wound care*

Signature: *R. Dripps, RN*

struction, and satisfy the requirements of regulatory agencies such as The Joint Commission. When creating a patient-teaching plan, follow these guidelines:

■ Include the patient-teaching plan on your main plan, or write a separate plan, according to your facility's guidelines.

■ Document what the patient needs to learn, how he'll be taught, and what criteria will be used for evaluating his learning.

■ Adapt a multidisciplinary approach to make the plan realistic and comrehensive.

■ Include provisions for follow-up teaching at home.

■ Keep your patient-teaching plan flexible. Take into account variables that interfere with learning or teaching time.

Components of the plan

Although the scope of each teaching plan differs, all should contain the same elements:

■ Patient-learning needs, which you identify, help you decide which outcomes you should establish for your patient. When identifying these needs, consider what you, the physician, and other health care team members want the patient to learn, as well as what the patient wants to learn.

■ Expected learning outcomes should focus on the patient and be readily measurable. (See *Writing clear learning outcomes,* page 55.) They should also fall into one of three categories:

– Cognitive, relating to understanding

– Psychomotor, covering manual skills

– Affective, dealing with attitudes.

■ Teaching content, organized from the simplest concept to the most complex, includes what the patient needs to be taught to achieve the expected outcomes. Incorporate family members and other caregivers into the plan as needed to complement or enhance the patient's learning.

■ Teaching methods include one-on-one teaching, demonstration, practice, return demonstration, role playing, and self-monitoring.

■ Teaching tools—ranging from printed pamphlets to closed-circuit television programs—can familiarize the patient with a specific topic. When choosing your tools, focus on what will work best for the particular patient and keep your patient's abilities and limitations in mind.

■ Barriers to learning and the patient's readiness to learn can include physical conditions that may impede the learning process, unwillingness or inability to learn, and communication problems.

Practice guidelines for acute pulmonary edema

Practice guidelines give specific sequential instructions for treating patient with a particular problem. These guidelines demonstrate the instruction for a patient with pulmonary edema. This is an example.

Presence of predisposing factors, such as cardio-vascular diseases, persistent cough, dyspnea on exertion, possible paroxysmal nocturnal dyspnea or orthopnea	Physical findings, including restlessness; anxiety; labored, rapid respirations; frothy, bloody sputum; decreased level of consciousness; jugular vein distention; cold, clammy skin; crepitant crackles and wheezes; diastolic (S_3) gallop; tachycardia; hypotension; thready pulse	Results of chest X-ray, arterial blood gas (ABG) analysis, pulse oximetry, pulmonary artery catheterization, electrocardiography

Anxiety related to inability to breathe normally as a result of fluid accumulation

Excess fluid volume related to fluid accumulation in lungs

Thoroughly attend to patient's physical needs.

Administer prescribed diuretic.

Maintain awareness and sensitivity to patient's emotional state. → Encourage patient to verbalize feelings of anxiety.

Has anxiety decreased or abated?

Is excess fluid eliminated?

Yes

No → Stay at patient's bedside as much as possible.

Continue fluid and sodium restrictions. ← **No** **Yes**

Give clear, concise explanations of care and procedures. ← Listen attentively.

Continue to attend to physical needs.

Be prepared to administer additional medications, such as positive inotropic agents, vasopressors, arterial vasodilators, morphine, and antiarrhythmics.

Is anxiety decreased or abated now?

Yes **No**

Continue supportive care. ← Encourage a calm family member or friend (if available) to remain at patient's bedside as much as possible.

Is excess fluid eliminated now?

Obtain an order for morphine and administer as needed.

No **Yes**

Patient will experience decreased anxiety by:
- expressing that anxiety has decreased
- using available support systems
- demonstrating abated physical symptoms of anxiety.

Alert physician and anticipate changes in drug therapy.

Documenting the patient-teaching plan

Several forms are available for documenting patient-teaching plans, including some that detail the phases of the nursing process as they relate to patient education. (See *Documenting patient teaching,* pages 56

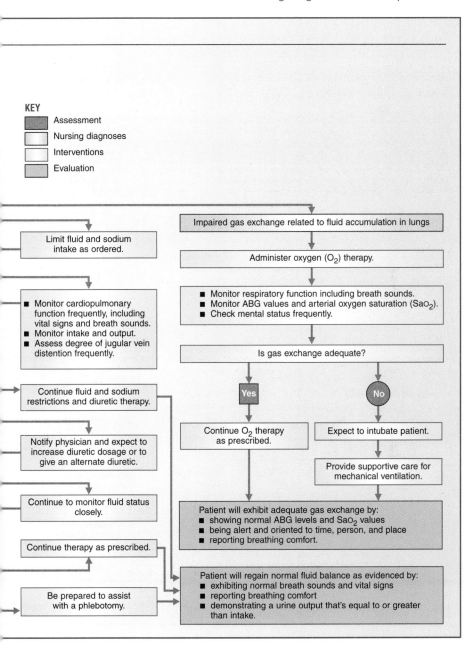

KEY

- Assessment
- Nursing diagnoses
- Interventions
- Evaluation

Limit fluid and sodium intake as ordered.

- Monitor cardiopulmonary function frequently, including vital signs and breath sounds.
- Monitor intake and output.
- Assess degree of jugular vein distention frequently.

Continue fluid and sodium restrictions and diuretic therapy.

Notify physician and expect to increase diuretic dosage or to give an alternate diuretic.

Continue to monitor fluid status closely.

Continue therapy as prescribed.

Be prepared to assist with a phlebotomy.

Impaired gas exchange related to fluid accumulation in lungs

Administer oxygen (O_2) therapy.

- Monitor respiratory function including breath sounds.
- Monitor ABG values and arterial oxygen saturation (SaO_2).
- Check mental status frequently.

Is gas exchange adequate?

Yes

No

Continue O_2 therapy as prescribed.

Expect to intubate patient.

Provide supportive care for mechanical ventilation.

Patient will exhibit adequate gas exchange by:
- showing normal ABG levels and SaO_2 values
- being alert and oriented to time, person, and place
- reporting breathing comfort.

Patient will regain normal fluid balance as evidenced by:
- exhibiting normal breath sounds and vital signs
- reporting breathing comfort
- demonstrating a urine output that's equal to or greater than intake.

and 57.) They come in two basic types that are similar to traditional and standardized care plans.

■ The traditional type begins with the nursing diagnosis statement *Deficient knowledge* and an individualized "related to" statement (for ex-

Managing ineffective breathing pattern

Below you'll find a portion of a practice guideline for a patient who has chronic obstructive pulmonary disease (COPD) and a nursing diagnosis of ineffective breathing pattern.

Nursing diagnosis and patient outcome	Implementation	Evaluation
Ineffective breathing pattern related to decreased lung compliance and air trapping By _2/10/08_ the patient will: ■ demonstrate a respiratory rate within 5 breaths/minute of baseline ■ maintain arterial blood gas (ABG) levels within acceptable ranges ■ verbalize his understanding of the disease process, including its causes and risk factors ■ demonstrate diaphragmatic pursed-lip breathing ■ take all medication as prescribed ■ use oxygen as prescribed.	■ Monitor respiratory function. Auscultate for breath sounds, noting improvement or deterioration. ■ Obtain ABG levels and pulmonary function tests as ordered. ■ Explain lung anatomy and physiology, using illustrated teaching materials, if possible. ■ Explain COPD, its physiologic effects, and its complications. ■ Review the most common signs and symptoms associated with the disease: dyspnea, especially with exertion; fatigue; cough; occasional mucus production; weight loss; rapid heart rate; irregular pulse; and use of accessory muscles to help with breathing because of limited diaphragm function. ■ Explain the purpose of diaphragmatic pursed-lip breathing for patients with COPD; demonstrate the correct technique, and have the patient perform a return demonstration. ■ If the patient smokes, provide information about smoking-cessation groups in the community. ■ Explain the importance of avoiding fumes, respiratory irritants, temperature extremes, and exposure to upper respiratory tract infections. ■ Review the patient's medications, and explain the rationale for their use, their dosages, and possible adverse effects. Advise him to report any adverse reactions to the physician immediately. ■ For the patient receiving oxygen, explain the rationale for therapy and the safe use of equipment. Explain that the oxygen flow rate should never be increased above the prescribed target.	■ Patient's respiratory rate remains within 5 breaths/minute of baseline. ■ ABG levels return to and remain within established limits. ■ Patient verbalizes an understanding of his disease. ■ Patient properly demonstrates diaphragmatic pursed-lip breathing. ■ Patient takes all medication as prescribed. ■ Patient demonstrates the appropriate use of oxygen as prescribed.

ample, *Deficient knowledge* related to low-sodium diet). This type provides the format but requires you to come up with the plan.

■ The standard type may be better for a patient who requires extensive teaching because you can check off or date steps as you complete them and add or delete information.

Traditional and standardized patient-teaching plans may include space for problems that may hinder learning, for comments and evaluations, and for dates and signatures.

Writing clear learning outcomes

The patient's learning behaviors fall into three categories: cognitive, psychomotor, and affective. With these categories in mind, you can write clear, concise, expected learning outcomes. Remember, your outcomes should clarify what you're going to teach, indicate the behavior you expect to see, and set criteria for evaluating what the patient has learned.

Review the two sets of sample learning outcomes for a patient with chronic renal failure. Notice that the outcomes in the well-phrased set start with a precise action verb, confine themselves to one task, and describe measurable and observable learning. In contrast, the poorly phrased outcomes may encompass many tasks and describe learning that's difficult or even impossible to measure.

Well-phrased learning outcomes	*Poorly phrased learning outcomes*
Cognitive domain	
The patient with chronic renal failure will be able to:	
■ state when to take each prescribed drug	■ know his medication schedule
■ describe symptoms of elevated blood pressure	■ know when his blood pressure is elevated
■ list permitted and prohibited foods on his diet.	■ know his dietary restrictions.
Psychomotor domain	
The patient with chronic renal failure will be able to:	
■ take his blood pressure accurately, using a stethoscope and a sphygmomanometer	■ take his blood pressure
■ read a thermometer correctly	■ use a thermometer
■ collect a urine specimen, using sterile technique.	■ bring in a urine specimen for laboratory studies.
Affective domain	
The patient with chronic renal failure will be able to:	
■ comply with dietary restrictions to maintain normal electrolyte values	■ appreciate the relationship of diet to renal failure
■ verbally express his feelings about adjustments to be made in the home environment	■ adjust successfully to limitations imposed by chronic renal failure
■ keep scheduled physicians' appointments.	■ understand the importance of seeing his physician.

Discharge planning

Staff nurses play a major role in preparing patients and caregivers to assume responsibility for ongoing care. If you're in charge of discharge planning for a patient, begin your planning the day the patient is admitted—or sooner, for a scheduled admission.

Components of the plan
Although discharge planning differs for each patient, the discharge plan should contain these elements:
■ Anticipated length of stay

(Text continues on page 58.)

Documenting patient teaching

Below, you'll find the first page of a patient-teaching flow sheet. Such flow sheets let you quickly and easily tailor your teaching plan to fit your patient's needs.

Name: Don Pashley   **Date:** 3/10/08

DIABETES MELLITUS

Problems affecting learning

☐ None   ☐ Communication problem

☑ Fatigue or pain   ☐ Cognitive or sensory impairment

LEARNING OUTCOMES		INITIAL TEACHING			
	Date	Time	Learner	Techniques and tools	
Basic knowledge ■ Define diabetes mellitus (DM).	3/10/08	1000	P	E,W	
■ List four symptoms of DM.	3/10/08	1000	P	E,W	
Medication ■ State the action of insulin and its effects on the body.	3/10/08	1000	P	E,W	
■ List the three major classifications of insulin. Give their onsets, peaks, and durations.	3/10/08	1000	P	E,V,W	
■ Demonstrate the ability to draw up insulin in a syringe and mix the correct amount.	3/10/08	1000	P	D	

Signature/initials Joan Martin, RN / JM

KEY
Learner

P	= patient	D1	= daughter 1	
S	= spouse	D2	= daughter 2	
M	= mother	S1	= son 1	
F	= father	S2	= son 2	
		O	= other	

Teaching techniques
D = demonstration
E = explanation
R = role-playing

☐ Physical disability
☐ Lack of motivation

☐ Other _____

Evaluation	Initials	REINFORCEMENT					
		Date	Time	Learner	Techniques and tools	Evaluation	Initials
S	JM	3/11/08	1000	P	E,W	S	JM
S	JM	3/11/08	1000	P	E,W	S	JM
S	JM						
S	JM						
Dp	JM						

Teaching tools
F = filmstrip
P = physical model
S = slide
V = videotape
W = written material

Evaluation
S = states understanding
D = demonstrates understanding
Dp = demonstrates understanding with physical coaching

Dv = demonstrates understanding with verbal coaching
T = passes written test
N = no indication of learning
NE = not evaluated

■ Teaching content, such as instructions on diet, medications, treatments, physical activity restrictions, signs and symptoms to report to the physician, follow-up medical care, equipment, and appropriate community resources
■ Instruction sheet to reinforce what the patient learns and what he needs to remember about follow-up care
■ Future care, including its setting, the patient's intended caregiver and support systems, actual or potential barriers to care, and any referrals.

Documenting the discharge plan

How you document the discharge plan will depend on the policy at your health care facility. Some facilities:
■ require an assessment of discharge needs on the initial assessment form and the discharge plan documented on a separate form
■ require the discharge plan to be included as a component of the discharge summary
■ use forms for discharge planning that allow several members of the health care team to include information.

Case management

Case management is a method of delivering health care that controls costs while still ensuring quality care. (See *How case management works.*) In this system, Medicare pays the facility based on the patient's diagnosis—not on his length of stay or the number or types of services he receives, which means that the facility loses money if the patient has a lengthy stay or develops complications. This, in turn, forces facilities to deliver cost-effective care without compromising the quality of care.

Tools for case management

Most facilities pattern their case management tools after the ones developed at the New England Medical Center. Called the *case management plan* and the *clinical pathway*, these tools allow you to direct, evaluate, and revise patient progress and outcomes.

Case management plan

The basic tool of case management systems, the case management plan spells out the standardized care that a patient with a specific diagnosis-related group should receive. The plan covers:
■ nursing-related problems
■ patient outcomes
■ intermediate patient outcomes

How case management works

When a patient is assigned a particular diagnosis-related group (DRG), he's also assigned a case manager. (In some facilities, a patient isn't assigned a DRG until after discharge—in which case, you'll make an educated guess about which DRG will be assigned to him.) Each DRG case management plan has standard outcome criteria and includes medical and nursing interventions as well as interventions from other disciplines.

The case manager discusses outcomes with the patient and family, using the established time line for the DRG. This time line should cover all the processes that must occur for the patient to reach the expected outcome—including tests, procedures, and patient teaching—and the resources the patient will need such as social services. If it doesn't, it's adapted as necessary to fit the patient's needs. If possible, all this is done before the patient is even admitted, but it must be completed within the time limit set by your facility—usually 24 hours.

After the patient is admitted, the multidisciplinary team evaluates his progress and suggests necessary revisions, keeping in mind the need for continuity of care and the best use of resources. The case manager documents variations in the time line, processes, or outcomes, along with the reasons for the changes. The case manager also keeps a lookout for duplication of services and medical orders.

An assessment of the patient's discharge needs is started at or before admission. Home health care services—including obtaining personnel and equipment—are planned well before discharge.

Types of case management systems

Several case management systems and various adaptations exist, but most facilities pattern their systems after the one developed at the New England Medical Center, one of the first centers to use case management in an acute care setting. Facilities typically adapt this system to meet their own needs and philosophy of care.

- nursing interventions
- medical interventions
- target times.

Each subsection of the plan covers a care unit to which the patient may be admitted during his illness.

Clinical pathway

Because of the length of case management plans, you probably won't use them on a daily basis. Instead, you'll turn to an abbreviated form of the plan: the clinical pathway (also known as the *health care map*), which covers only the key events that must occur for the patient to be discharged by the target date. Such events include:

- consultations
- diagnostic tests
- physical activities the patient must perform
- treatments
- diet
- medications
- discharge planning
- patient teaching. (For more details and a completed sample of a clinical pathway, see chapter 5, Documentation in acute care.)

After you have established a clinical pathway, follow these guidelines:

- Document variances from the pathway, grouping them by cause. Variances may result from the system, the caregivers, or a problem the patient develops.
- At shift report each day, review the clinical pathway with the other nurses. Document changes in the expected length of stay and point out critical events scheduled for the next shift to the nurses coming on duty. Also, discuss variances that may have occurred during your shift.

Drawbacks of case management

- It can be difficult to establish a time line for some patients.
- The expected course of treatment and length of stay will likely change for a patient with several variances.
- Documentation can become lengthy and complicated for a patient with variances.

Implementation

Documenting nursing interventions has changed dramatically over the years, mainly because of frustration with tedious traditional methods and the urgent economic need to streamline hospital operations. Narrative notes are no longer a necessity. In many cases, you can use flow sheets or refer to practice guidelines instead. (See *Performing interventions*.)

Documenting interventions

When you document your interventions, make sure that the documentation's focus is outcome-oriented by following these guidelines:

- Document that you performed an intervention, the time that you performed it, the patient's response to it, and any additional interventions that occurred based on his response.

Performing interventions

Implementing nursing interventions represents a crucial stage in the nursing process. When you carry out your interventions, you're putting your carefully constructed care plan into action.

After you've established and documented your care plan, you'll begin to implement it. You'll find that your interventions fall into two general categories: interdependent and independent. Before performing either type, you'll need to make a brief reassessment to make sure that your care plan remains appropriate.

Types of interventions

Interdependent interventions include those you perform in collaboration with other health care professionals to help achieve a patient outcome. Interdependent interventions also include activities you perform at a physician's request to help implement the medical regimen.

Independent interventions are measures you take at your own discretion, independent of other health care team members.

■ Follow your facility's policies when it comes to the exact style, format, and location of your documentation.

■ If available, use graphic records, such as a patient care flow sheet that integrates all nurses' notes for a 1-day period, integrated or separate nurses' progress notes, or other specialized documentation forms when documenting your interventions.

■ Be sure to document interventions when you give routine care, observe changes in the patient's condition, provide emergency care, and administer medications. (See chapter 2, Legal and ethical implications of documentation.)

Patient teaching

With each patient, you'll need to implement the teaching plan you've created, evaluate its effectiveness, and clearly and completely document the results. In many facilities, you'll document patient teaching on preprinted forms that become part of the clinical record. Using these forms not only makes documentation quicker but also ensures that documentation is complete.

Whether you use a preprinted form or narrative notes, follow these guidelines:

■ Check your facility's policies and procedures regarding when, where, and how to document your teaching.

■ Each shift, ask yourself, "What part of the teaching plan did I complete?" and "What other teaching have I given this patient or his family members?" Then document your answers.

■ Make sure that your documentation indicates that the patient's ongoing educations needs are being met.

■ Before discharge, document the patient's remaining learning needs.

Benefits of patient-teaching documentation

Documenting exactly what you've taught:

■ provides a permanent legal record of the extent and success of teaching

■ strengthens your defense against charges of insufficient patient care—even years later

■ helps administrators gauge the overall worth of a specific patient-education program

■ helps motivate your patient because you can show him the record of his learning successes and encourage him to continue

■ saves time by preventing duplication of patient-teaching efforts by other staff members

■ allows for communication between staff members by documenting what they've taught and how well the patient has learned

■ promotes patient and family knowledge of illness or disease, which may improve compliance with medical regimen.

Patient discharge

Joint Commission requirements specify that when preparing a patient for discharge, you must document your assessment of his continuing care needs as well as referrals for such care. To facilitate this documentation (and to save documentation time), many facilities have developed forms that combine discharge summaries and patient instructions. (See *Discharge summaries.*)

Not all facilities use these forms; some still require a narrative discharge summary. If you must write a narrative, include:

■ the patient's status on admission and discharge

■ significant highlights of the hospitalization

■ outcomes of your interventions

■ resolved and unresolved patient problems, continuing care needs for unresolved problems, and specific referrals for continuing care

■ instructions given to the patient or family member about medications, treatments, activity, diet, referrals, and follow-up appointments, as well as other special instructions.

Discharge summaries

By combining the patient's discharge summary with instructions for care after discharge (as shown below), you can fulfill two requirements with a single form. When using this documentation method, be sure to give one copy to the patient and keep one for the record.

DISCHARGE INSTRUCTIONS

1. **Recommendations**   *Lose 10–15 lb*

2. **Allergies**   *penicillin*
3. **Medications (drug, frequency, route)**   *Lopressor 25 mg every 12 hours by mouth*
   Temazepam 15 mg once daily by mouth

4. **Diet**   *Low-sodium, low-cholesterol*
5. **Activity**   *As tolerated*
6. **Discharged to**   *Home*
7. **If questions arise, contact Dr.**   *James Pritchett*
   Telephone No.   *525-1448*
8. **Special instructions**
9. **Return visit Dr.**   *James Pritchett*
   Place   *Health Care Clinic*
   On Date   *3/19/08*   **Time**   *8:45 am*

Tara Nicholas

Signature of patient for receipt of discharge instructions

JE Pritchett, RN

Signature of RN giving instructions

Evaluation

Progress notes must include an assessment of your patient's progress toward the expected outcomes you established in the care plan. This method, called *outcomes and evaluation documentation,* focuses on the patient's response to nursing care and enables the nurse to provide high-quality, cost-effective care. It also forces you to focus on patient responses and ensure that your plan is working. (See *Writing clear evaluation statements* and *Performing evaluations.*)

Writing clear evaluation statements

Below, you'll find examples of clear evaluation statements describing common outcomes. Note that they include specific details of care provided and objective evidence of the patient's response to care.

Response to p.r.n. medication within 1 hour of administration
- "Pt. states pain decreased from 8 to 4 (on a scale of 0 to 10) 10 minutes after receiving I.V. morphine."
- "Vomiting subsided 1 hr after 25 mg P.O. of prochlorperazine."

Response to patient education
- "Able to describe the signs and symptoms of a postoperative wound infection."
- "Despite repeated attempts, pt. couldn't identify signs of hypoglycemia."

Tolerance of change or increase in activity
- "Able to walk across the room, approximately 15 feet, without dyspnea."
- "Became fatigued after 5 minutes of assisted ambulation."

Ability to perform activities of daily living, particularly those that may influence discharge planning
- "Unable to wash self independently because of left-sided weakness."
- "Requires a walker to ambulate to bathroom."

Tolerance of treatments
- "Consumed full liquid lunch; pt. stated she was hungry and wanted solid food."
- "Skin became pink and less dusky 15 minutes after nasal O_2 was administered at 4 L/min."
- "Unable to tolerate having head of bed lowered from 90 degrees to 45 degrees; became dyspneic."

Performing evaluations

When you evaluate the results of your interventions, you help ensure that the care plan is working. It also gives you a chance to:
- determine if your original assessment findings still apply
- uncover complications
- analyze patterns or trends in the patient's care and his responses to it
- assess the patient's response to all aspects of care, including medications, changes in diet or activity, procedures, unusual incidents or problems, and teaching
- determine how closely care conforms to established standards
- measure how well the patient was cared for
- assess the performance of other members of the health care team
- identify opportunities to improve the quality of care.

When to perform an evaluation

If you work in an acute care setting, your facility's policy may require you to review care plans every 24 hours. If you work in a long-term care facility, the required interval between evaluations may be up to 30 days. In either case, you should evaluate and revise the care plan more often than required, if warranted.

Evaluating expected outcomes

Evaluation includes gathering reassessment data, comparing findings with the outcome criteria, determining the extent of outcome achievement (outcome met, partially met, or not met), writing evaluation statements, and revising the care plan.

Revision starts with determining whether the patient has achieved the expected outcomes. If they've been fully met and you decide that the problem is resolved, the plan can be discontinued. If the problem persists, the plan continues—with new target dates—until the desired status is achieved.

If outcomes have been partially met or unmet, you must identify interfering factors, such as misinterpreted information, and revise the plan accordingly. This may involve:
- clarifying or amending the database to reflect newly discovered information
- reexamining and correcting nursing diagnoses
- establishing outcome criteria that reflect new information and new or amended nursing strategies
- adding the revised nursing care plan to the original document
- recording the rationale for the revisions in the nurse's progress notes.

When documenting an evaluation, follow these guidelines:

- Make sure that your evaluation statements indicate whether expected outcomes were achieved. List evidence supporting this conclusion.
- Base statements on outcome criteria from the care plan.
- Use active verbs, such as demonstrate and ambulate.
- Include the patient's response to specific treatments, such as medication administration or physical therapy.
- Describe the conditions under which the response occurred or failed to occur.
- Document patient teaching and palliative or preventive care as well.
- After evaluating the outcome, be sure to document it in the patient's chart with clear statements that demonstrate the patient's progress toward meeting the expected outcomes.

2 Legal and ethical implications of documentation

The scope of your professional responsibility is set out by your state's nurse practice act and by other state and federal regulations. Documenting the nursing care that you provide in the patient's medical record is one way of accepting that responsibility. When filling out your documentation, consider that:

■ you protect your patient's interests—as well as your own—by completing your documentation in an acceptable and timely manner and in accordance with the appropriate standard of nursing care

■ the failure to document appropriately has been a pivotal issue in many malpractice cases

■ although the actual medical record, X-rays, laboratory reports, and other records belong to the facility, the information contained in them belongs to the patient, who has a right to obtain a copy of the materials.

 LEGAL LOOKOUT *In* Deford and Thompson v. Westwood Hills Health Care Center, Inc., Doctors Regional Medical Center and Barnes Hospital, St. Louis City, *Missouri Circuit Court, Case No. 922-9564 (1992), a patient died after a nurse attempted to insert a feeding tube. Seven months later, when the family requested the patient's records, Westwood Hills staff mistakenly believed they weren't authorized to release them and so refused. Copies of the records were finally released more than 1 year later. The case resulted in an $80,000 verdict against Westwood Hills on a wrongful death claim.*

Legal relevance of medical records

Accurately and completely documenting the nature and quality of nursing care is important because it:
- helps other members of the health care team confirm their impressions of the patient's condition and progress
- may signal the need for adjustments in the therapeutic regimen
- provides documentation of the RN's assessment, the care planned, and the care provided
- is used as evidence in the courtroom in malpractice suits, workers' compensation litigation, personal injury cases, and criminal cases. It's assumed that care wasn't performed if it isn't documented.

Standards of documentation

The type of nursing information that appears in the medical record is governed by standards developed by the nursing profession and state laws. Professional organizations, such as the American Nurses Association (ANA), and regulatory agencies, such as The Joint Commission and the Centers for Medicare and Medicaid Services, have established that documentation must include:
- ongoing assessment
- variations from the assessment
- nursing care
- patient's status
- relevant statements made by the patient
- allergies and allergic response the patient has experienced
- responses to therapy
- medical treatment
- patient teaching.

Timely communication

The purpose of documentation is communication, with an emphasis on timeliness. Follow these guidelines when the patient's condition deteriorates or when changes in therapy are clearly indicated:
- Document the patient's status.
- Document contact with the physician and the time the contact was made. (If the physician didn't respond in a timely manner, as set by facilty policy, or doesn't provide appropriate treatment, and the chain of command was initiated, document all actions.)

LEGAL LOOKOUT *When notification isn't documented, it's nearly impossible to prove that the physician was called in a timely manner and that all critical information was communicated. In a California case,* Malovec v. Santa Monica Hospital, Los Angeles County, *California Superior Court, Case No. SC 019-167 (1994), a woman in labor repeatedly asked the charge nurse to call the chief of obstetrics because her obstetrician refused to perform a cesarean delivery despite guarded fetal heart tracings. The charge nurse refused, and the baby was born with cerebral palsy and spastic quadriplegia. A confidential settlement was reached.*

Errors or omissions

Errors or omissions can severely undermine your credibility in court. A jury could reasonably conclude that you didn't perform a function if it wasn't documented. If you failed to document something and need to enter a late entry, follow your facility's guidelines and:

■ add the entry to the first available line and label it "late entry" to indicate that it's out of sequence

■ record the time and date of the entry and, in the body of the entry, record the time and date it should have been made.

 LEGAL LOOKOUT *In the case of* Anonymous v. Anonymous, *Suffolk Superior Court, Boston (1993), failure to document led to a $1 million settlement. A 2-year-old was admitted to Children's Hospital for correction of a congenital urinary defect. Postoperative orders required blood pressure, pulse, and temperature readings to be taken every 4 hours, and respiratory rate and reaction to analgesia every hour. However, the child's care wasn't documented for 5 hours. The child was found in cardiorespiratory arrest and died of an overdose of an opioid infusion. The responsible nurse admitted failing to assess the child strictly according to the orders; she also claimed that she had assessed the child adequately but had been "too busy" to document her observations.*

Corrections and alterations

When you make a mistake in your documentation, correct it promptly. If the chart ends up in court, the plaintiff's attorney will be looking for anything that may cast doubt on the documentation's accuracy.

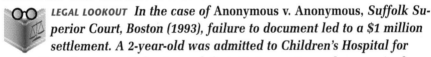 **LEGAL LOOKOUT** *Never try to make the record "better" after you learn a malpractice case has been filed. Attorneys have methods for analyzing papers and inks, and can easily detect discrepancies.*

Malpractice and documentation

Never lose sight of documentation's legal importance. Depending on how well you administer care and document your activities and observations, the documentation may or may not support a plaintiff's accusation of nursing malpractice. Legally, malpractice focuses on four elements:

■ Duty—Duty is your obligation to provide patient care and to follow appropriate standards. The courts have ruled that a nurse has a duty to provide care after a nurse–patient relationship is established.

■ Breach of duty—Breach of duty is a failure to fulfill your nursing obligations. Breach of duty can be difficult to prove because nursing responsibilities typically overlap those of physicians and other health care providers. A key question asked when a possible breach of duty is being investigated is, "How would a reasonable, prudent nurse with comparable training and experience have acted in the same or similar circumstances?"

 LEGAL LOOKOUT In judging a nurse to have breached her duty, the courts must prove that the nurse failed to provide the appropriate care—as they did in Collins v. Westlake Community Hospital, 312 N.E. 2d 614 (Ill. 1974). *A 6-year-old boy was hospitalized for a fractured leg, which was put in a cast and placed in traction. Although the physician ordered the nurse on duty to monitor the condition of the boy's toes, the medical record lacked documentation that she did so. In fact, 7 hours elapsed between documented nursing entries in the medical record. The boy's leg was later amputated, and the parents sued on behalf of their son. Because a nurse is responsible for continually assessing patients and because documentation of these assessments didn't appear in the record, the nurse was found to have breached her duty to this child.*

■ Causation—The plaintiff must prove that the breach caused the injury. For the nurse to be liable, she must have proximately caused the injury by an act or an oversight. (See *Understanding proximity.*)

■ Damages—Damages represent the amount of money the court orders the defendant to pay the plaintiff when a case is decided in the plaintiff's favor. To collect damages, the patient's attorney must prove that his client's injury was the result of malpractice. Usually, the injury must be physical, not just emotional or mental.

LEGAL LOOKOUT

Understanding proximity

The principle of proximity is important because, in a typical health care facility, many caregivers are involved in a patient's care. Even if a nurse did commit malpractice, it's conceivable that the patient's injury was caused by something other than the nursing intervention. For instance, even if a nurse gave a patient an overdose of a medication and the patient later vomited blood, the cause of the vomiting might actually be a surgical error and have nothing to do with the medication.

Policies and documentation

Although most discussions about documentation center on the patient's chart, policies and procedures contained in health care facility employee and nursing manuals are also an important aspect of documentation. When dealing with policies and procedures, keep this very important point in mind:

■ Deviation from a facility's policies and procedures suggests that an employee failed to meet the facility's standards of care.

 LEGAL LOOKOUT *In a case related to a health care facility's policies, the court was pressed to distinguish between a facility's policies and its "goals." In* H.C.A. Health Services v. National Bank, 745 S.W. 2d 120 (Ark. 1988), *three nurses were working in a nursery composed of three connecting rooms. One nurse cared for a neonate in the first (admissions) room. The other two nurses went into the second room, which housed 11 neonates (two of whom were premature and one of whom was jaundiced). There was no documentation that for 1½ hours any of the nurses went into the third room, which had six neonates. Documentation did show that when the first nurse finally entered the third room, she found that one of the neonates had stopped breathing and had no heartbeat.*

Both the facility's executive director and the nurse who found the neonate testified that, according to the facility's manual, no neonate is ever to be left alone without a member of the nursery staff present. However, they also testified that this was a goal—not a policy. Another physician testified that the neonate's problem would have been avoided if a nurse had been present. The court disagreed with the distinction between policies and goals and ruled against the facility and nurses and in favor of the plaintiff.

Risk management and documentation

To reduce injuries and accidents, minimize financial loss, and meet the guidelines of The Joint Commission and other regulatory agencies, health care facilities have instituted risk management programs. The primary objectives of a risk management program are to:

■ ensure optimal patient care
■ reduce the frequency of preventable injuries and accidents leading to liability claims by maintaining or improving quality of care
■ decrease the chance of a claim being filed by promptly identifying and following up on adverse events (incidents)
■ help control costs related to claims by identifying trouble spots early and intervening with the patient and his family. (See *Coordinating risk management and performance improvement.*)

Three important aspects of risk management include identifying sentinel events, identifying adverse events, and managing adverse events.

Identifying sentinel events

The Joint Commission requires health care facilities to identify and manage sentinel events, which are unexpected occurrences involving death or serious physical or psychological injury. When a sentinel event is identified, the facility must initiate an analysis of the situation and identify an action plan to reduce risk of the event reoccurring. The facility should also initiate an analysis whenever there's a:

■ confirmed transfusion reaction

Coordinating risk management and performance improvement

Risk management focuses on the patients' and families' perception of the care provided. Performance improvement focuses on the role and functions of the health care provider. However, rather than support two separate programs, many health care facilities coordinate their risk management and performance improvement programs to ensure that they fulfill their legal duty to provide reasonable care. In doing so, the facility may also coordinate the programs' education efforts.

Keep in mind, however, that a coordinated system usually continues its dual focus on different aspects of health care delivery.

Primary sources of information

Nurses, patient representatives, and other departments are primary sources of information for identifying adverse events as well as health care dangers or trends.

Nurses
■ Typically the first to recognize potential problems because they spend the most time with patients and their families
■ Can identify patients who are dissatisfied with their care, particularly those with complications that might result in injuries

Patient representatives
■ Keep a file of patient concerns and complaints
■ Evaluate concerns and complaints for trends
■ Can provide an early-warning signal of health care problems that need to be addressed, ranging from staffing to faulty equipment
■ Trained to recognize litigious patients
■ Maintain communication with the patient and family after an incident has occurred

Other departments
■ Can provide information about adverse events (For example, the billing department may become aware of a patient who threatens to sue after receiving his bill.)
■ Can assist with trending reports of adverse events, which can identify areas that need attention more quickly than a focused departmental review

---

■ significant adverse drug reaction
■ significant medication error.

Identifying adverse events

A key part of a risk management program involves developing a system for identifying adverse events—patient falls, for example, that would be considered an abnormal consequence of a patient's condition or treatment. These events may or may not be caused by a health care provider's breach of duty or the standard of care, which is why it's important that you have reliable sources of information and a reliable system for identifying adverse effects. (See *Primary sources of information.*) The most common "early warning systems" are as follows:

- Incident reporting—Certain criteria are used to define events that must be reported by physicians, nurses, or other health care staff, either when they're observed or shortly thereafter. All errors must be reported because it's impossible to predict which ones will require intervention.
- Occurrence screening—Adverse events are flagged through a review of all or some of the medical charts. These reviews use generic criteria, but more specific reviews may focus on specialty or service-specific criteria.

Incident reporting and occurrence screening are crucial because they:

- permit early investigation and intervention
- help minimize additional adverse consequences and legal action
- provide valuable databases for building strategies to prevent repeated incidents.

Managing adverse events

When the facility's risk manager learns of a potential or actual lawsuit:

- The risk manager notifies the chief financial officer, medical records department, the facility's insurance carrier, and the facility's attorney.
- The medical records department makes copies of the patient's chart and files the original in a secure place to prevent tampering.

A claim notice also triggers a performance improvement peer review of the medical record. This review:

- may be conducted by the chairperson of the department involved, the risk management or performance improvement department, or an external reviewer to measure the health care provider's conduct against the professional standards of conduct for the particular situation.
- helps the risk manager determine the claim's merit and helps define the facility's responsibility for care in particular situations.
- identifies areas where changes are needed, such as policy, training, staffing, or equipment.

Completing incident reports

An incident report is a formal report, written by physicians, nurses, or other staff members, that informs facility administrators about an adverse event suffered by a patient, visitor, or employee. These are continually revised, and some may be computerized. (See *Completing an incident report.*) If you're filing an incident report, follow these guidelines:

Completing an incident report

When you witness or discover a reportable event, you must fill out an incident report. Forms vary, but most include the following information.

INCIDENT REPORT

Name _Greta Manning_

DATE OF INCIDENT
_12-20-07_

Address _7 Worth Way, Boston, MA_

TIME OF INCIDENT
_1442_

Phone _(617) 555-1122_

Addressograph if patient

EXACT LOCATION OF INCIDENT
(Bldg, Floor, Room No, Area) _4-Main, Rm. 447_

TYPE OF INCIDENT (CHECK ONE ONLY)
☐ PATIENT ☐ EMPLOYEE ☑ VISITOR ☐ VOLUNTEER ☐ OTHER (specify)

DESCRIPTION OF THE INCIDENT (WHO, WHAT, WHEN, WHERE, HOW, WHY)
(Use back of form if necessary)
Patient's wife found on floor next to bed. States, "I was trying to put the siderail of the bed down to sit on it and I fell down."

Patient fall incidents	**FLOOR CONDITIONS** ☑ CLEAN & SMOOTH ☐ SLIPPERY (WET) ☐ OTHER _____
	FRAME OF BED ☐ HIGH ☑ LOW **NIGHT LIGHT** ☐ YES ☑ NO
	WERE BED RAILS PRESENT? ☐ NO ☐ 1 UP ☐ 2 UP ☐ 3 UP ☑ 4 UP
	OTHER RESTRAINTS (TYPE AND EXTENT) _N/A_
	AMBULATION PRIVILEGE ☐ UNLIMITED ☐ LIMITED WITH ASSISTANCE ☐ COMPLETE BEDREST ☐ OTHER _____
	WERE NARCOTICS, ANALGESICS, HYPNOTICS, SEDATIVES, DIURETICS, ANTIHYPERTENSIVES, OR ANTICONVULSANTS GIVEN DURING LAST 4 HOURS? ☐ YES ☑ NO DRUG AMOUNT TIME

Patient incidents	**PHYSICIAN NOTIFIED** DATE TIME COMPLETE IF APPLICABLE Name of Physician _J. Reynolds, MD_ _12-20-07_ _1445_

Employee incidents	**DEPARTMENT** JOB TITLE SOCIAL SECURITY # **MARITAL STATUS**

All incidents	**NOTIFIED** DATE TIME _C. Jones, RN_ _12-20-07_ _1500_ **LOCATION WHERE TREATMENT WAS RENDERED**
	NAME, ADDRESS, AND TELEPHONE NUMBERS OF WITNESS(ES) OR PERSONS FAMILIAR WITH INCIDENT - WITNESS OR NOT _Janet Adams (617) 555-0912 1 Main St., Boston, MA_

SIGNATURE OF PERSON PREPARING REPORT TITLE DATE OF REPORT
Connie Smith, RN   _RN_   _12-20-07_

PHYSICIAN'S REPORT — To be completed for all cases involving injury or illness
(DO NOT USE ABBREVIATIONS) (Use back if necessary)

(continued)

Completing an incident report *(continued)*

DIAGNOSIS AND TREATMENT

Received patient in Emergency Department after reported fall in husband's room. 12 cm x 12 cm ecchymotic area noted on right hip. X-rays negative for fracture. Good range of motion, no c/o pain. VAS 0/10. Ice pack applied. ———— J. Reynolds, MD

DISPOSITION

sent home, written instructions provided

PERSON NOTIFIED OTHER THAN HOSPITAL PERSONNEL

Jane Ambrose, nurse manager   Liz Sacco, house supervisor

PERSON NOTIFIED OTHER THAN HOSPITAL PERSONNEL		DATE	TIME
NAME AND ADDRESS			
R. Manning (daughter), address same as pt		*12-20-07*	*1500*

PHYSICIAN'S SIGNATURE	DATE
J. Reynolds, MD	*12-20-01*

■ Complete as soon as possible, while events are more accurately recalled.

■ Write objectively. Record the details of the incident in objective terms, describing exactly what you saw and heard.

■ Don't try to guess or explain what happened. Any nonroutine incident or accident must be recorded by the nurse who witnessed the incident.

■ Include only essential information. Document the time and place of the incident, the name of the physician who was notified, the time of the notification, and any treatment orders.

■ Avoid opinions. If you must express an opinion on how a similar incident may be avoided in the future, verbally share it with your supervisor and risk manager. Don't write it in the incident report.

■ Assign no blame. Don't admit to liability, and don't blame or point your finger at colleagues or administrators.

■ Avoid hearsay and assumptions. Don't write an incident report for an injury that occurred in another department—even if the patient who was injured is yours. The staff members in that department are responsible for documenting the details of the event.

■ File the report properly. Don't file the incident report with the medical record; instead, send it to the person designated to review it according to your facility's policy.

Documenting an incident in the medical record

When documenting an incident in the patient's medical record, keep these guidelines in mind:

■ Write a factual account of the incident, including the treatment and follow-up care provided and the patient's response. This documentation shows that the patient was closely monitored after the incident, which will help your case if it goes to court.

■ Don't document the completion of an incident report, or place one, in the medical record.

■ Document in such a way that any alterations or conditions are dated, timed, and signed, so that the original entry is still clear.

■ Include in the progress notes and in the incident report anything the patient or his family says about their role in the incident. For example, "Patient stated, 'The nurse told me to ask for help before I went to the bathroom, but I decided to go on my own.'" This kind of statement helps the defense attorney prove that the patient was guilty of contributory or comparative negligence. Contributory negligence is conduct that contributed to the patient's injuries. Comparative negligence involves determining the percentage of each party's fault.

Bioethical dilemmas and documentation

As a nurse, you routinely take part in decisions involving ethical dilemmas. Some dilemmas may be more serious than others, but they all present some kind of risk. Use these guidelines when faced with an ethical dilema:

■ The Joint Commission mandates that health care facilities address ethical issues in providing patient care by listing specific patient rights and maintaining a code of ethical behavior.

■ A few states have incorporated patient rights into their state statutes, and most have codified statutes for nursing home patients.

■ The ANA and other nursing organizations have their own ethical codes of conduct for nurses. (See *Ethical codes for nurses,* pages 78 to 80.)

Bioethical issues involving documentation include:
– informed consent (including witnessing informed consent and informed refusal)
– advance directives (also known as *living wills*)
– power of attorney (POA) or health care POA

(Text continues on page 80.)

Ethical codes for nurses

One of the most important ethical codes for registered nurses is the American Nurses Association (ANA) code. Licensed practical and vocational nurses (LPNs and LVNs) also have an ethical code, which is set forth in each state by the state's nurses association. The National Federation of Licensed Practical Nurses also has a code of ethics for its members. In addition, the International Council of Nurses, an organization based in Geneva, Switzerland, that seeks to improve the standards and status of nursing worldwide, has published a code of ethics. Summaries of these codes appear here.

ANA code of ethics

The ANA views nurses and patients as individuals who possess basic rights and responsibilities and who should command respect for their values and circumstances at all times. The ANA code provides guidance for carrying out nursing responsibilities consistent with the ethical obligations of the profession. According to the ANA code, the nurse is responsible for these actions:

- Provide services with respect for human dignity and the uniqueness of the patient unrestricted by considerations of social or economic status, personal attributes, or the nature of health problems.
- Safeguard the patient's right to privacy by judiciously protecting information of a confidential nature.
- Act to safeguard the patient and the public when health care and safety are affected by the incompetent, unethical, or illegal practice of any person.
- Assume responsibility and accountability for individual nursing judgments and actions.
- Maintain competence in nursing.
- Exercise informed judgment, and use individual competence and qualifications as criteria in seeking consultation, accepting responsibilities, and delegating nursing activities to others.
- Cooperate in activities that contribute to the ongoing development of the profession's body of knowledge.
- Participate in the profession's efforts to implement and improve standards of nursing.
- Take part in the profession's efforts to establish and maintain conditions of employment conducive to high-quality nursing care.
- Share in the profession's efforts to protect the public from misinformation and misrepresentation and to maintain the integrity of nursing.
- Collaborate with members of the health care professions and other citizens in promoting community and national efforts to meet the health needs of the public.

Ethical codes for nurses *(continued)*

Code for LPNs and LVNs

The code for LPNs and LVNs seeks to provide a motivation for establishing, maintaining, and elevating professional standards. It includes these imperatives:

■ Know the scope of maximum utilization of the LPN and LVN, as specified by the nurse practice act, and function within this scope.

■ Safeguard the confidential information acquired from any source about the patient.

■ Provide health care to all patients regardless of race, creed, cultural background, disease, or lifestyle.

■ Refuse to give endorsement to the sale and promotion of commercial products or services.

■ Uphold the highest standards in personal appearance, language, dress, and demeanor.

■ Stay informed about issues affecting the practice of nursing and delivery of health care and, where appropriate, participate in government and policy decisions.

■ Accept the responsibility for safe nursing by keeping oneself mentally and physically fit and educationally prepared to practice.

■ Accept responsibility for membership in the National Federation of Licensed Practical Nurses, and participate in its efforts to maintain the established standards of nursing practice and employment policies that lead to quality patient care.

International Council of Nurses code of ethics

According to the International Council of Nurses, the fundamental responsibility of the nurse is fourfold: to promote health, to prevent illness, to restore health, and to alleviate suffering.

The International Council of Nurses further states that inherent in nursing is respect for life, dignity, and human rights and that nursing is unrestricted by considerations of nationality, race, creed, color, age, sex, politics, or social status. Here are the key points of the code:

Nurses and people

■ The nurse's primary responsibility is to those who require nursing care.

■ The nurse, in providing care, respects the beliefs, values, and customs of the individual.

■ The nurse holds in confidence personal information and uses judgment in sharing this information.

(continued)

<hr>

Ethical codes for nurses *(continued)*

Nurses and practice
■ The nurse carries personal responsibility for nursing practice and for maintaining competence by continued learning.
■ The nurse maintains the highest standards of nursing care possible within the reality of a specific situation.
■ The nurse uses judgment in relation to individual competence when accepting and delegating responsibilities.
■ The nurse, when acting in a professional capacity, should at all times maintain standards of personal conduct that would reflect credit upon the profession.

Nurses and society
■ The nurse shares with other citizens the responsibility for initiating and supporting actions to meet the health and social needs of the public.

Nurses and coworkers
■ The nurse sustains a cooperative relationship with coworkers in nursing and other fields.
■ The nurse takes appropriate action to safeguard the individual when his care is endangered by a coworker or any other person.

Nurses and the profession
■ The nurse plays a major role in determining and implementing desirable standards of nursing practice and nursing education.
■ The nurse is active in developing a core of professional knowledge.
■ The nurse, acting through the professional organization, participates in establishing and maintaining equitable social and economic working conditions in nursing.

<hr>

– do-not-resuscitate orders
– confidentiality of the medical record.

Informed consent

Informed consent means that the patient has been presented with the component and risks of a treatment or procedure, has been given the opportunity to present questions, verbalizes understanding, and agrees to undergo the treatment or procedure by signing a consent form. Informed consent has two elements—the information and the consent. (See *The two elements of informed consent.*) Important aspects of informed consent to remember include that:
■ it's required before most treatments and procedures

The two elements of informed consent

The two elements of informed consent are the information and the consent. To be *informed,* the patient must be provided with a description of the treatment or procedure, the name and qualifications of the person who will perform it, and an explanation of risks and alternatives—all in language the patient can under-stand. Based on this, the patient may *consent* to the treatment or procedure.

The Joint Commission mandates the elements of informed consent. In addi-tion, most states have statutes that set out specific elements of informed con-sent. In a few states, the physician can explain the procedure and simply ask whether the patient has any questions. If the patient has none, the physician isn't obligated by state law to discuss alternatives and risks unless the patient re-quests the information. Although this policy is inconsistent with The Joint Com-mission's guidelines, keep in mind that those guidelines aren't the law; they're a set of requirements for licensure and accreditation.

In many cases, a patient may attempt to clarify issues with a nurse after giv-ing the physician his informed consent. If you're questioned in this way, be aware that you aren't obligated to answer the patient's questions; however, if you do, be careful to document your answers. You should also notify the physi-cian and document that you have done so, including the date and time.

 LEGAL LOOKOUT *In life-threatening emergencies, informed consent may not be required. In such cases, the law assumes that every in-dividual wants to live and allows the physician to intervene to save life without obtaining consent.*

■ the physician (or other practitioner) who will perform the procedure is legally responsible for obtaining it, even if he delegates the duty to a nurse

■ you may be asked to witness the patient's signature, depending on your facility's policy. (See *Witnessing informed consent*, page 82.)

Legal requirements

For informed consent to be legally binding, the patient must be men-tally competent and the physician must:

■ explain the patient's diagnosis as well as the nature, purpose, and likelihood of success of the treatment or procedure

■ describe the treatment or procedure and the risks and benefits asso-ciated with it

Witnessing informed consent

When you witness the patient signing an informed consent document, you're not witnessing that he received or understood the information. You're simply witnessing that the person who signed the consent form is in fact the person he says he is. For this, check the patient's armband to ensure that he is in fact the correct patient. Here's a typical form.

CONSENT FOR OPERATION AND RENDERING OF OTHER MEDICAL SERVICES

1. I hereby authorize Dr. *Mark Wesley* to perform upon *Joseph Smith* (Patient name), the following surgical and/or medical procedures: (State specific nature of the procedures to be performed) *Exploratory laparotomy*

2. I understand that the procedure(s) will be performed at Valley Medical Center by or under the supervision of Dr. *Mark Wesley*, who is authorized to utilize the services of other physicians, or members of the house staff as he or she deems necessary or advisable.

3. It has been explained to me that during the course of the operation, unforeseen conditions may be revealed that necessitate an extension of the original procedure(s) or different procedure(s) than those set forth in Paragraph 1; I therefore authorize and request that the above named physician, and his or her associates or assistants, perform such medical surgical procedures as are necessary and desirable in the exercise of professional judgment.

4. I understand the nature and purpose of the procedure(s), possible alternative methods of diagnosis or treatment, the risks involved, the possibility of complications, and the consequences of the procedure(s). I acknowledge that no guarantee or assurance has been made as to the results that may be obtained.

5. I authorize the above named physician to administer local or regional anesthesia (for all other anesthesia management, a separate consent must be signed by the patient or patient's authorized representative).

6. I understand that if it is necessary for me to receive a blood transfusion during this procedure or this hospitalization, the blood will be supplied by sources available to the hospital and tested in accordance with national and regional regulations. I understand that there are risks in transfusion, including but not limited to allergic, febrile, and hemolytic transfusion reactions, and the transmission of infectious diseases, such as hepatitis and AIDS (Acquired Immunodeficiency Syndrome). I hereby consent to blood transfusion(s) and blood derivative(s).

7. I hereby authorize representatives from Valley Medical Center to photograph or videotape me for the purpose of research or medical education. It is understood and agreed that patient confidentiality shall be preserved.

8. I authorize the physician named above and his or her associates and assistants and Valley Medical Center to preserve for scientific purposes or to dispose of any tissue, organs, or other body parts removed during surgery or other diagnostic procedures in accordance with customary medical practice.

9. I certify that I have read and fully understand the above consent statement. In addition, I have been afforded an opportunity to ask whatever questions I might have regarding the procedure(s) to be performed, and they have been answered to my satisfaction.

Joseph Smith	02/21/08	*C. Gurney, RN*
Legal Patient or Authorized Representative (State Relationship to Patient)	Date	Witness

If the patient is unable to consent on his or her own behalf, complete the following:

Patient _____ is unable to consent because _____

Legally Responsible Person _____

Physician Obtaining Consent *Mark Wesley, MD* _____

- explain the possible consequences of not undergoing the treatment or procedure
- describe alternative treatments and procedures
- inform the patient that he has the right to refuse the treatment or procedure without having other care or support withdrawn; this includes withdrawing his consent after giving it
- identify who will perform the procedure
- identify who's responsible for the patient's care
- obtain consent without coercing the patient.

Nursing responsibilities

Even if the physician obtains the informed consent himself, the nurse is usually required to witness the signature. Other responsibilities include:

- checking that the patient's record contains a signed informed consent form
- notifying the supervisor or physician if the patient appears to be concerned about the procedure or the physician's explanation of it; document your notification and the time of the notification
- notifying the physician as soon as possible if the patient wants to change his mind about undergoing the treatment or procedure. Document the patient's comments exactly, along with your notification of the physician, the time of the notification, and the physician's response.

Informed refusal

The Joint Commission requires (and federal statutes mandate) that health care facilities (acute and long-term care) inform patients soon after admission about their treatment options. The patient has the right to refuse treatment based on knowledge of the outcomes and risks. (See *Understanding informed refusal*, page 84.) When documenting a patient's informed refusal, document:

- that you informed the patient about his treatment options
- that you discussed the patient's wishes with him, which may be referred to if the patient becomes unable to participate in decision making
- drugs and treatments received in the 2 hours before refusal, and the patient's response
- that the patient refused treatment and the time and date of his refusal. (See *Witnessing refusal of treatment,* page 85.)

Understanding informed refusal

With a few exceptions, a *competent* patient has a right to refuse mechanical ventilation, tube feedings, antibiotics, fluids, and other treatments that will clearly result in his death if they're withheld. However, it's important to remember that legal competence differs from the medical or psychiatric concept of competence. The law presumes all individuals to be competent unless deemed otherwise through a court proceeding. The patient must also have *capacity*—that is, be legally considered an adult for consent purposes under state law.

Exceptions to the right to informed refusal may include pregnant women (because the life of the unborn child is at risk) and parents wishing to withhold treatment from their child.

Advance directives

The U.S. Constitution and case law have established that the patient has the right to determine what happens to his body. The Joint Commission mandates that:

■ patients have the right to participate in decisions regarding their care

■ health care facilities have a policy or procedure in place addressing how they'll implement the requirement

■ facilities address forgoing or withdrawing life-sustaining treatment and withholding resuscitative services and care at the end of life.

An advance directive (sometimes referred to as a *living will*) allows the patient to decide before he becomes terminally ill the type of care he'll be given at the end of life. The directive becomes effective only when the patient becomes terminally ill, and most state statutes require advance directives to be written. When caring for a patient with an advance directive, follow these guidelines:

■ Place a copy of the advance directive on the patient's chart and obtain physician's orders that comply with the advance directive, such as a "do-not-resuscitate (DNR)" order

■ If a competent patient says that he wants to revoke his advance directive, contact the physician and document exactly what the patient said and the time and date he said it.

 LEGAL LOOKOUT *Some state statutes have guidelines for revoking a directive, but the patient's verbal wishes will suffice until those requirements can be met.*

Witnessing refusal of treatment

If a patient refuses treatment, the physician must first explain the risks involved in making this choice. Then the physician asks the patient to sign a refusal-of-treatment release form, such as the one shown here, which you may be asked to sign as a witness. Your signature only validates the identity of the patient signing the form — not that the patient received sufficient information or understood that information.

Refusal-of-treatment release form

I, _Brenda Lyndstrom_ refuse to allow anyone to
(patient's name)

administer parenteral nutrition .
(insert treatment)

The risks attendant to my refusal have been fully explained to me, and I fully understand the benefits of this treatment. I also understand that my refusal of treatment seriously reduces my chances for regaining normal health and may endanger my life.

I hereby release _Mercy General_
(name of hospital)

its nurses and employees, together with all physicians in any way connected with me as a patient, from liability for respecting and following my express wishes and direction.

Susan Reynolds, RN   _Brenda Lyndstrom_
(witness's signature)   (patient's or legal guardian's signature)

_04/12/08_   _76_
(date)   (patient's age)

■ If the patient's request differs from what the family or physician wants, document discrepancies carefully. Use social services or the legal department for advice on how to proceed.

LEGAL LOOKOUT *If an advance directive is in effect and the nurse or other health care provider fails to honor it, any subsequent care provided may be considered unlawful touching, assault and battery, negligence, or intentional infliction of emotional, physical, and financial distress and, as such, grounds for a malpractice suit.*

LEGAL LOOKOUT

Durable power of attorney

A durable power of attorney is a legal document in which a competent person designates another person to act on his behalf if he should become incapable of managing his own affairs. Some states have created one specifically for health care. It ensures that the patient's wishes regarding treatment will be carried out if he should ever become incompetent or unable to make decisions because of illness.

Patient Self-Determination Act

The Patient Self-Determination Act of 1990 allows patients to use advance directives and to appoint a surrogate to make decisions if the patient loses the ability to do so. This act:
- mandates that on admission, each patient be informed of his right to create an advance directive
- mandates this information be documented in the medical record
- allows the patient to create an advance directive and have this document placed in the medical record and honored.

Power of attorney

Power of attorney is a legal document in which a competent person designates another to act or conduct legally binding transactions on his behalf. It may encompass all of a person's affairs, including health and financial matters, or it may be limited to one specific area. It ceases if the patient becomes incompetent or revokes the document, unless he has executed a durable power of attorney. (See *Durable power of attorney.*)

When caring for a patient with a power of attorney, follow these guidelines:
- Place a copy of the written power of attorney in a conspicuous place in the patient record.
- If a competent patient says that he wants to revoke his power of attorney, contact the physician and document exactly what he said and the time and date he said it.

Do-not-resuscitate orders

A DNR order refers to limited or withheld rescuscitation efforts in case the patient needs it. It is usually an order given per the wishes of a patient with a terminal illness. The physician writes a DNR order when it's medically indicated—that is, when a patient is terminally ill and expected to die. Despite the patient's autonomy and the requirement to honor the patient's wishes, the patient can't mandate that a facility provide futile treatment.

When caring for a patient with a DNR order, remember these points:

■ DNR orders should be reviewed as policy dictates or whenever a significant change occurs in the patient's clinical status.

■ Some facilities temporarily suspend DNR orders during surgery. Although the patient and physician aren't seeking heroic measures at the end of life, they won't allow the patient to bleed to death if he should hemorrhage during a palliative surgical procedure.

LEGAL LOOKOUT *Another exception is the concept of partial or "à la carte" resuscitation codes. These are legally precarious because the standard of care is to attempt full resuscitation through all means available, not partial resuscitation.*

■ The patient's family members or friends don't have the legal authority to write an advance directive or to advise the physician regarding a DNR order unless they have a legal power of attorney or durable power of attorney.

■ The patient is presumed to be competent and has the sole right to state what care he wishes, unless that care isn't indicated from a medical standpoint.

Confidentiality

One of your documentation responsibilities includes protecting the confidentiality of the patient's medical record. Usually, you can't reveal confidential information without the patient's permission. (See *Patient rights under HIPAA,* page 88.)

Nurse's role

Nurses assume a primary role in maintaining confidentiality and in safeguarding the privacy of medical records. Breaches in confidentiality can result from unintentional release of information, unauthorized entry into a patient's record, or even a casual conversation that's overheard by others. To prevent breaches:

Patient rights under HIPAA

The goal of the Health Insurance Portability and Accountability Act (HIPAA) is to provide safeguards against the inappropriate use and release of personal medical information, including all medical records and identifiable health information in any form (electronic, on paper, or oral).

Patients are the beneficiaries of this privacy rule, which includes these six rights:
- the right to give consent before information is released for treatment, payment, or health care operations
- the right to be educated to the provider's policy on privacy protection
- the right to access their medical records
- the right to request that their medical records be amended for accuracy
- the right to access the history of nonroutine disclosures (those disclosures that didn't occur in the course of treatment, payment, or health care operations, or those not specifically authorized by the patient)
- the right to request that the provider restrict the use and routine disclosure of information he has (providers aren't required to grant this request, especially if they think the information is important to the quality of care for the patient, such as disclosing human immunodeficiency virus status to another medical provider who's providing treatment).

Enforcement of HIPAA

Enforcement of HIPAA regulation resides with the U.S. Department of Health and Human Services (HHS) (and within the HSS, the office of Civil Rights) and is based primarily on significant financial fines. HHS can impose civil penalties up to $25,000 per year per plan for unintentional violations. With hundreds of requirements, fines could quickly add up. Criminal penalties can also be imposed for intentional violations, including fines of up to $250,000, 10 years of imprisonment, or both.

Impact on nursing practice

Keep in mind that HIPAA regulations aren't intended to prohibit health care providers from talking to one another or to patients. Instead, they exist to help ease the communication process. The regulations require organizations to make "reasonable" accommodations to protect patient privacy and to employ "reasonable" safeguards to prevent inappropriate disclosure. Changes in nursing practice will likely be needed to meet these reasonable accommodations and safeguards.

Employers must provide education to nurses regarding the policies and procedures to be followed at their individual facilities. Nurses should be aware of how infractions will be handled because they, as well as the facility, face penalties for violations.

- avoid discussing patient concerns in areas where you can be over-heard
- make sure that computer passwords are protected
- make sure that computer screens aren't in public view
- keep patient charts closed when not in use
- immediately file loose patient records
- properly dispose of unneeded patient information in accordance with the facility's procedure
- don't leave faxes and computer printouts unattended
- don't release the record without the documented consent of a competent patient; release of certain information—for example, mental health records as well as information about drug and alcohol abuse and infectious diseases—is further constrained by state statutes.

LEGAL LOOKOUT *In the case of* **Anonymous v. Chino Valley Medical Center, San Bernardino County,** *California Superior Court (1997), a 35-year-old disabled inpatient underwent a blood test for human immunodeficiency virus (HIV). He specifically told the physician that he didn't want the results to be given to anyone but him. On the day of discharge, his sister was present in the hospital room. A nurse asked the sister to come into the hall so she could tell her about the patient's diet instructions upon discharge. When in the hallway, the nurse told the sister that the patient had a positive HIV test. A few moments later, the physician approached them and also conveyed the test results. No action was filed against the physician. The nurse denied releasing the information. A trial court imposed a $5,000 statutory civil penalty against the medical center.*

In the case of **Hobbs v. Lopes, 645 N.E.2d 1261, Ohio App. 4 DST. (1994),** *a 21-year-old Ohio woman was found to be pregnant after consulting a physician for another medical problem. Options, including abortion, were discussed. The physician instructed a nurse to call the woman to find out what option she had chosen. The nurse called the woman's parents' home and disclosed the fact that their daughter was pregnant and had sought advice about an abortion. The daughter sued for medical malpractice, invasion of privacy, breach of privilege, and infliction of emotional distress.*

Remember: The law requires you to disclose confidential information in certain situations—for example, in instances of alleged child abuse, matters of public health and safety, and criminal cases.

3 Legally perilous documentation

If you're ever named in a malpractice suit that proceeds to court, your documentation may be your best defense. It provides a running record of your patient care. How and what you documented—and even what you didn't document—will heavily influence the outcome of the trial.

Credible evidence

Typically, the outcome of every malpractice trial boils down to one question: Whom will the jury believe? The answer usually depends on the credibility of the evidence. Here's what occurs in a malpractice suit:

- The plaintiff presents evidence designed to show that he was harmed or injured because care provided by the defendant (in this case, the nurse) failed to meet accepted standards of care.
- The nurse strives to present evidence demonstrating that she provided an acceptable standard of care.
- If the nurse can't offer believable evidence, the jury may have no choice but to accept the plaintiff's evidence. Even worse, if the nurse's evidence—including the medical record—is discredited, the plaintiff's attorney may convince a jury of her negligence. (See *Negligent or not.*)

By knowing how to document, what to document, when to document, and even who should document, you'll create a solid record.

Knowing how to handle legally sensitive situations, such as difficult and nonconforming patients, offers additional safeguards.

LEGAL LOOKOUT

Negligent or not

If you've actually been negligent and have truthfully documented the care given, the medical record will naturally be the plaintiff's best evidence in a malpractice case. In such instances, the case will probably be settled out of court. If you haven't been negligent, the medical record should be your best defense, providing the best evidence of quality care. If the record makes you *seem* negligent, however, the jurors may conclude that you *were* negligent because they base their decision on the evidence.

The lesson: A "bad" medical record can be used to make a good nurse look bad. A "good" medical record should defend those who wrote it.

How to document

Documentation is a craft that's refined with experience. A skilled nurse knows that she needs to document that the standard of care was delivered, keeping in mind that it isn't only what she documents but how she documents that's important.

Document objectively

The medical record should contain descriptive, objective information: what you see, hear, feel, smell, measure, and count—not what you suppose, infer, conclude, or assume. It may also contain subjective information, but only when it's supported by documented facts.

Stick to the facts

■ Document only what you see and hear. Don't document that a patient pulled out his I.V. line if you didn't witness him doing so. Instead, describe your findings—for example, "Found pt., arm board, and bed linens covered with blood. I.V. line and venipuncture device were untaped and hanging free." (See *Avoiding assumptions,* page 93.)
Here's an example of how to document a patient's fall:

2/28/08	0600	Heard pt. scream. Found pt. lying beside bed. Pt. has
		laceration 2 cm long on forehead. Side rails up. Pt.
		stated he climbed over side rails to go to the bathroom.
		BP 184/92, P 96, R 24. Pt. c/o pain in ® hip. Dr. John
		Phillips notified by telephone at 0600 and ordered
		X-ray. Pt. taken for X-ray of ® hip. — Sonia Benoit, RN

■ Describe—don't label—events and behavior. Expressions such as "appears spaced out," "exhibiting bizarre behavior," or "using obscenities," mean different things to different people. They also reflect poorly on your professionalism and force you into the uncomfortable position of having to defend your own words, which hurts your credibility and distracts the jury from the fact that you provided the standard of care to the patient.

■ Be specific. Describe facts clearly and concisely. Use only approved abbreviations and express your observations in quantifiable terms. Avoid catchall phrases such as "Pt. comfortable." Instead, describe his comfort. Is he resting, reading, or sleeping? Is he in pain?

1/18/08	1400	Dressing removed from ® mastectomy site. Incision is
		pink. No drainage. Measures 12.5 cm long and 2 cm wide.
		Slight bruising noted near center of incision. Dressing dry.
		Drain site below mastectomy incision measures 2 cm x 2 cm.
		Bloody, dime-sized drainage noted on drain dressing. No
		edema noted. New dressing applied Pt. complaining of
		mild incisional pain, 3 on a scale of 0 to 10. 2 Tylox P.O.
		given at 1330 hours. Pt. reports relief at 1355. ———
		————————————————— Joan Delaney, RN

Avoid bias

■ Document a patient's difficult or uncooperative behavior objectively. That way, the jurors will draw their own conclusions.

3/19/08	1400	Pt. refusing medication. Stated, "I've had enough pills.
		Now leave me alone." Explained the importance of the
		medication and attempted to determine why he would
		not take it. Pt. refused to talk. Dr. John Ellis notified by
		telephone at 1400 that medication was refused.
		——————————————— Anne Curry, RN

■ Don't use unprofessional adjectives, such as *obstinate, drunk, obnoxious, bizarre,* or *abusive,* that suggest a negative attitude toward the patient. This type of documentation:
– invites the plaintiff's attorney to attack your professionalism
– leads to bad feelings—and possibly more—between you and your patient.

Remember: The patient has a legal right to see his medical record. If he spots a derogatory reference, he'll be hurt, angry, and more likely to sue.

Avoiding assumptions

Always aim to record the facts about a situation—not your assumptions or conclusions. In this example, a nurse failed to document the facts and instead documented her assumptions about a patient's fall. As a result, she had to endure this damaging cross-examination by the plaintiff's attorney.

ATTORNEY: Would you read your fifth entry for January 6, please?

NURSE: Patient fell out of bed...

ATTORNEY: Thank you. Did you actually see the patient fall out of bed?

NURSE: Actually, no.

ATTORNEY: Did the patient tell you he fell out of bed?

NURSE: No.

ATTORNEY: Did anyone actually see the patient fall out of bed?

NURSE: Not that I know of.

ATTORNEY: So these notes reflect nothing more than conjecture on your part. Is that correct?

NURSE: I guess so.

ATTORNEY: Is it fair to say then, that you documented something as fact even though you didn't know it was?

NURSE: I suppose so.

ATTORNEY: Thank you.

Keep the medical record intact

The patient's medical record includes documentation about all aspects of his care. Sometimes, it can get rather big and bulky. Whatever you do, don't take this as a sign to get rid of older or less critical documents because every piece of documentation in the patient's record is important. You never know when you may have to refer back to it or rely on it during a malpractice case.

Take special care to keep the patient's record complete and intact by following these guidelines:

■ Don't discard pages from the medical record, even for innocent reasons. It's likely to raise doubt in the jury's mind about the record 's reliability. (See *Consequences of missing records,* page 94.)

■ If you replace an original sheet with a copy, cross-reference it with lines such as, "Recopied from page 4" or "Recopied on page 6," and be sure to attach the original.

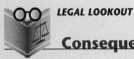

LEGAL LOOKOUT

Consequences of missing records

The case of *Keene v. Brigham and Women's Hospital 786 N.E.2d 824* (2003) underscores the significance of keeping the medical record intact.

A neonate developed respiratory distress within hours of birth. As a result of cyanosis, he was transferred to the neonatal intensive care unit. Blood tests, including a complete blood count (CBC) and a blood culture, were performed. Afterward, he was transferred back to the regular nursery for "routine care" with instructions to watch for signs and symptoms of sepsis and to withhold the antibiotic therapy pending the results of the CBC.

About 20 hours after the neonate was transferred back to the nursery, the neonate was found in septic shock. He was also having seizures. It wasn't until this time that antibiotics were administered. Subsequent testing revealed that the neonate had contracted neonatal sepsis and meningitis. The results of the blood tests revealed the presence of group B beta-hemolytic streptococcus. However, the identity of the person to whom this information was conveyed and what actions were taken or not taken couldn't be determined because about 18 hours of records, including the records relating to these events, couldn't be found.

Court's decision

Pursuant to the doctrine of spoliation, the court held the health care facility accountable for prejudice resulting from loss of evidence. Therefore, the court allowed an adverse inference to be drawn that said without evidence to the contrary, the missing records would likely contain proof that the antibiotics should have been administered sooner and that the defendant's failure to do so caused the neonate's injuries.

■ If a page is damaged, note "Reconstructed documentation," and attach the damaged page.

What to document

Juries believe that incomplete documentation suggests incomplete nursing care—which is why malpractice attorneys are fond of saying, "If it wasn't documented, it wasn't done." This isn't literally true, of course, but it's an easy conclusion for a jury to draw, which is why precise documentation is of utmost importance. (See *Documenting precisely*.) Areas of documentation that are frequently reviewed in malpractice cases include:

LEGAL LOOKOUT

Documenting precisely

Patients or their families may believe a bad outcome is due to poor care. As you know, this isn't always the case. Here's an example of how precise documentation saved the day for one nurse.

A son wanted to sue a hospital and nurse for an incident involving his elderly father, who had been hospitalized for a cholecystectomy. Several days after surgery, his father became disoriented and disorderly, fell out of bed, and broke both hips. He never walked again.

In talking with his attorney, the son claimed, "That nurse either didn't know or didn't care that Dad was confused and agitated. She did nothing to protect him from harm. I want to sue."

The son's description of the father's care sounded like nursing negligence—until the attorney reviewed the patient's record and the nurse's notes. The nurse provided a detailed account of the events preceding the fall. Clearly, she knew about the patient's problem and did everything she could to protect him. Specifically, she:

- confined him to bed with a Posey restraint in compliance with the physician's order
- assigned an aide to stay with him when he became agitated
- made sure that the side rails were always up and the bed was in the low position
- notified coworkers and asked them to watch the patient (his bed was visible from the nurses' station)
- documented all times that the patient and restraint were checked.

The record established that the nurse acted properly and showed concern for the patient. The patient's son was convinced that this unfortunate accident was just that—an accident.

Even if the case had gone to court, the nurse would have been well prepared to meet any challenge to her memory. The details were all there, in black and white.

- timely vital signs
- reporting of changes in the patient's condition
- medications given
- patient responses
- discharge teaching.

LEGAL LOOKOUT

What you don't document can hurt you

Only careful documentation can substantiate your version of events. Consider the situations here.

The case of the supposed phone call

A patient was admitted to a health care facility for surgery for epicondylitis (tennis elbow). After the surgery, a heavy cast was applied to his arm. The patient complained to the nurse of severe pain, for which the nurse repeatedly gave pain medication as ordered.

The next morning, when the surgeon visited, he split the patient's cast. By that time, the ulnar nerve was completely paralyzed and the patient was left with a permanently useless, clawed hand.

The patient subsequently sued the nurse for failing to notify the surgeon about his pain. At the deposition, the dialogue between the nurse and the plaintiff's attorney sounded like this:

ATTORNEY: Did you call the doctor?

NURSE: I must have called him.

ATTORNEY: Do you remember calling him?

NURSE: Not exactly, but I must have.

ATTORNEY: Do you have a record of making that call?

NURSE: No, I don't.

ATTORNEY: If you had made such a call, shouldn't there be a record of it?

NURSE: Yes, I guess so.

ATTORNEY: "Guess" is right; you can't really say that you made that call. You can only "guess" that you "must have."

The case of the documentation deficit

In the case of *Sweeney v. Purvis,* 665 So. 2d 926 (Ala., 1995), a 42-year-old woman was transferred to a rehabilitation facility 10 days after being admitted to another facility with a brain infarction. On her first day there, she attended therapy sessions without a problem.

The next day, after therapy, she had cramping in her left leg that wasn't relieved by analgesics. She also complained of pain in her left heel. The nursing staff called the physician, who ordered a heating pad applied to the affected leg.

The patient reported little pain that evening, but the next day her left leg appeared swollen so she stayed in bed. When she tried to get out of bed, she again had pain. The licensed practical nurse caring for her noted a positive Homans' sign, which may indicate the presence of a blood clot. The registered nurse (RN) on duty also got a positive response and reported it to her manager. Believing

What you don't document can hurt you *(continued)*

that the manager would notify the physician, the RN didn't document the positive Homans' sign or tell the next shift about it.

The next morning, a nurse practitioner and an RN examined the patient. Because her left calf appeared enlarged, the nurses were concerned about her undergoing therapy—if a clot was present, movement could cause it to move to her lung. When told about her condition, the physician told the nurses to get her up for therapy.

That afternoon at lunch, the patient shook, turned blue, and developed pinpoint pupils. Then her breathing and pulse stopped. Paramedics transported her to the hospital, where she died.

The administrator of the patient's estate sued the physician and his professional corporation for wrongful death. In court, the RN who noted the positive Homans' sign testified that she told her manager about it and the manager told her she would contact the physician. However, the RN didn't chart her actions or tell the next shift of her findings.

The nurse-manager testified that she didn't recall the RN telling her about the patient's condition and she didn't remember contacting the physician. The physician testified that he didn't recall the nurse-manager notifying him of the positive Homans' sign. Additionally, no documentation in the nurses' notes, the physician's orders, or the interdisciplinary progress notes supported the RN's claim that the physician was notified.

The jury decided in favor of the plaintiff and awarded $500,000 in damages.

The lesson? Appropriate nursing assessments aren't enough if you don't document your findings. This patient's death might have been averted if the nurse had written "positive Homans' sign" in the medical record.

Document critical and extraordinary information

The documentation of critical and extraordinary information is of utmost importance and can't be overlooked. Whenever documenting such information, follow these guidelines:

■ Whenever you encounter a critical or extraordinary situation, document the details thoroughly. Failure to document details can have serious repercussions. (See *What you don't document can hurt you;* see also *Documenting critical information: A case in point,* page 98.)

■ Never document certain things, such as conflicts among the staff. (See *Keeping the record clean,* pages 99 and 100.)

(Text continues on page 100.)

Documenting critical information: A case in point

This case illustrates the significance of documenting critical information accurately as proof that you provided the accepted standard of care.

Failure to document

Patti Bailey was admitted to the health care facility to deliver her third child. During her pregnancy, she had gained 63 lb, her blood pressure had risen from 100/70 mm Hg in her first trimester to 140/80 mm Hg at term, and an ultrasound done at 22 weeks showed possible placenta previa.

In the 4 hours after her admission, she received 10 units of oxytocin in 500 ml of dextrose 5% in lactated Ringer's solution. Documentation during this period was scant—her blood pressure was never documented, and there were only single notations of the fetal heart rate and how labor was progressing. The nurses failed to document the baby's reaction to the drug as well as the nature of the mother's contractions.

Suddenly, after complaining of nausea and epigastric pain, Mrs. Bailey suffered a generalized tonic-clonic seizure. Because her condition was so unstable, she couldn't undergo a cesarean birth, and her baby girl was delivered by low forceps. Mrs. Bailey developed disseminated intravascular coagulation and required 20 units of whole blood, platelets, and packed red blood cells within 8 hours of delivery.

Incredibly, Mrs. Bailey's nurse had documented nothing in the labor or delivery records or the progress notes.

Deficient policy and procedure manuals

When the unit's policy and procedure manuals were reviewed, no protocol for administering oxytocin and assessing the patient was included. At the very least, the manuals should have recommended using an oxytocin flow sheet to document vital signs, labor progress, fetal status, and changes in the drug administration rate.

The result

Although Mrs. Bailey recovered, her daughter has seizures and is developmentally disabled. Now age 15, the daughter can't walk or talk and has a gastrostomy tube for nutrition. The case was settled out of court for $450,000; the nurse and hospital were held responsible for one-third of the judgment and the physician paid the rest.

KNOW-HOW

Keeping the record clean

What you say and how you say it are of utmost importance in documentation. Keeping the patient's record free of negative, inappropriate information—potential legal bombshells—can be quite a challenge when you're writing detailed narrative notes. Here are some guidelines to help you sidestep documentation pitfalls and document an accurate account of your patient's care and status.

Avoid documenting staffing problems

Even though staff shortages may affect patient care or contribute to an incident, you shouldn't refer to staffing problems in a patient's record. Instead, discuss them in a forum that can help resolve the problem. Call the situation to the attention of the appropriate personnel, such as your nurse-manager, in a confidential memo or an incident report. Also, review your facility's policy and procedure manuals to determine how you're expected to handle this situation.

Keep staff conflicts and rivalries out of the record

Entries about disputes with nursing colleagues (including characterization and criticism of care provided), questions about a physician's treatment decisions, or reports of a colleague's rude or abusive behavior reflect personality clashes and don't belong in the medical record. They aren't legitimate concerns about patient care.

As with staffing problems, address concerns about a colleague's judgment or competence in the appropriate setting. After making sure that you have the facts, talk with your nurse-manager. Consult with the physician directly if an order concerns you. Share your opinions, observations, or reservations about colleagues with your nurse-manager only; avoid mentioning them in a patient's record.

If you discover personal accusations or charges of incompetence in a patient's record, discuss this with your supervisor.

Handling incident reports

An incident report is a confidential, administrative communication that's filed separately from the patient's record. Be familiar with your facility's policy so you'll know how to accurately document this.

You should always document the facts of an incident in the patient's chart. For example, "Found pt. lying on the floor at 1250 hours. No visible bleeding or trauma. Pt. returned to bed with all side rails up and bed in low position. Vital signs: BP 120/80, P 76, T 98.2°. Notified Dr. Gary Dietrich at 1253 hours, and he saw pt. at 1300 hours" is a sufficient and accurate statement of the facts.

(continued)

Keeping the record clean *(continued)*

Steer clear of words associated with errors
Terms such as *mistake, accidentally, somehow, unintentionally, miscalculated,* and *confusing* can be interpreted as admissions of wrongdoing. Instead, let the facts speak for themselves—for example, "Pt. was given Demerol 100 mg I.M. at 1300 hours for abdominal pain VAS 7/10. Dr. T. Smith was notified at 1305 and gave no new orders. Pt.'s vital signs are BP 120/82, P 80, R 20, T 98.4°."
 If the ordered drug dose was 50 mg, this entry will let other health care providers know that the patient was overmedicated.

Avoid naming names
Naming another patient in someone else's record violates confidentiality. Use the word *roommate,* initials, or a room and bed number to describe the other patient.

Never document that you informed a colleague of a situation if you only mentioned it
Telling your nurse-manager in the elevator or restroom about a patient's deteriorating condition doesn't qualify as informing her, but it *does* violate patient confidentiality. The nurse-manager is likely to forget the details and may not even realize that you expect her to intervene. You need to clearly state why you're notifying her so she can focus on the facts and take appropriate action. Otherwise, you can't say you've informed her. Document the patient's deterioration in the record, and document the time you notified your supervisor.

Here's an example showing how to document extraordinary information correctly:

1/2/08	0900	Digoxin 0.125 mg P.O. held because of nausea and vomiting. Dr. Tom Kelly notified that digoxin not given. Dr. Tom Kelly gave order for digoxin 0.125 mg I.V. Administered at 0915 hours. ———————————— Ruth Bullock, RN

Document full assessment data

Failing to document an adequate physical assessment is a key factor in many malpractice suits. When performing a physical assessment, follow these guidelines:

Using good interview techniques to improve documentation

Assessing a patient's condition adequately is part of your professional and legal responsibility. That means following up and documenting each of the patient's complaints. Documenting your data can be easier when you know how to ask questions that elicit the most information from your patient. Here's an example of an open-ended interview with a patient being assessed for abdominal pain.

NURSE: How would you describe the pain in your abdomen?

PATIENT: It's dull but constant. Actually, it doesn't bother me as much as my blurry eyesight.

NURSE: Tell me about your blurry eyesight.

PATIENT: When I work long hours at my computer, all the words and lines seem to blend together. Sometimes it also happens when I watch television. I probably should see my eye doctor, but I haven't had the time.

NURSE: We'll be sure to follow up on your blurred vision. Now, how about that abdominal pain. How does it affect your daily routine and your sleep?

A lot of things went right in this interview.

■ First, the nurse didn't dismiss the patient's vision problem. If she had and it turned out to be serious, she might have been judged negligent.

■ Second, she asked open-ended questions so that the patient could explain his answers rather than simply saying "yes" or "no."

■ Third, she didn't put words in the patient's mouth. For example, she avoided saying, "The abdominal pain bothers you when you try to sleep, doesn't it?" That would have been a leading question. And the patient, assuming the nurse knows the right answer because she's a nurse, might have answered "yes"—even if the correct answer was "no."

■ When initially assessing your patient, focus your documentation on his chief complaint, but also document all his concerns and your findings.

■ After completing the initial assessment, establish your nursing care plan. A well-written care plan provides a clear approach to the patient's problems and can assist in your defense—if it was carried out.

■ Phrase each patient problem statement clearly, and don't be afraid to modify the statement as you gather new assessment data.

■ State the care plan for solving each problem, and then identify the actions you intend to implement. (See *Using good interview techniques to improve documentation.*)

Document discharge instructions

The responsibility for giving discharge instructions is usually yours. If a patient receives improper instructions and an injury results, you could be held liable. When documenting discharge instructions, follow these guidelines:

■ Document that you distributed printed instruction sheets describing treatments and home care procedures that the patient will have to perform. Make sure that your documentation indicates which instructional materials were given and to whom, because the courts typically consider teaching materials as evidence that instruction took place.

■ Document that the instructions given were tailored to the patient's specific needs and that they included verbal or written instructions that were provided.

■ If caregivers practice procedures with the patient and family in the health care facility, document this, along with the results.

When to document

Finding the time to document can be a problem during a busy shift. But timely entries are crucial in malpractice suits. Here are some tips:

■ Document your nursing care and other relevant activity when you perform it or not long after.

■ Don't document ahead of time. Documenting before performing an intervention makes your notes inaccurate and also omits information about the patient's response to intervention. (See *Understanding the importance of timely documentation.*)

Who should document

You, and only you, should document your nursing care and observations. At times, because of understaffing or other circumstances, you may be tempted to ask another nurse to complete your portion of the medical record. However, doing so is illegal and prohibited by your state's nurse practice act.

Do your own documenting

Do your own documenting and refuse to do anyone else's. Having someone else document for you may:

Understanding the importance of timely documentation

Although you would never document care before providing it, you may wait until the end of your shift or until your dinner break to complete your nurse's notes. That's what one nurse did. Some time later she was summoned to court as a witness in a malpractice suit. She took the witness stand, answered the attorney's questions, and regularly referred to and read from the record while doing so. She relied heavily on it for her defense and, in the process, implicitly asked the jury to do the same.

The plaintiff's attorney began his cross-examination by asking the nurse to read from her entries. After a few minutes, here's what happened:

ATTORNEY: Excuse me, may I interrupt? As I listened to you read these entries, a question occurred to me. Maybe it occurred to the jury, too. Would you tell us whether you made the entries you are reading at the time of the events they describe?

NURSE: Well, no, I would have made them sometime later.

ATTORNEY: You're sure?

NURSE: Yes.

ATTORNEY: Thank you. Now, I'd like you to look at the record and tell the jury whether you noted the time that you actually gave the patient his medication.

NURSE: No, I didn't.

ATTORNEY: Now, I'd like you to look at the chart again and tell the jury whether you indicated the time that you made the entry.

NURSE: No.

ATTORNEY: Given the absence of those two pieces of information, how could you so promptly and confidently respond to my original question? How can you remember so clearly now that you made the entry sometime after the event it describes? Is it because your regular practice is to wait until the end of your shift to record each and every detail of every event that transpired over your entire shift, and that you rely solely on your memory when making all these entries?

NURSE: Well, yes, that's true.

ATTORNEY: Would you tell the jury how long a shift you worked that day?

NURSE: A 10-hour shift.

ATTORNEY: And how many patients did you see over that 10-hour period?

NURSE: About 15.

ATTORNEY: Now, each of these 15 patients was different, correct? Each had his own individualized care plan that corresponded to his particular health problems, isn't that right?

NURSE: That's right.

(continued)

Understanding the importance of
timely documentation *(continued)*

ATTORNEY: And how many different times did you see each of these different patients over the 10-hour period?

NURSE: I probably saw each one, on average, about once an hour.

ATTORNEY: In other words, you probably had 150 patient contacts on that shift alone, is that correct?

NURSE: I suppose so.

ATTORNEY: Now, during the course of your shift, do unexpected events sometimes develop? Unanticipated developments that must be attended to?

NURSE: Sometimes, yes.

ATTORNEY: And when these situations occur, do they distract you from things you had planned to do?

NURSE: Sometimes.

ATTORNEY: After working such a long shift, do you sometimes feel tired?

NURSE: Yes.

ATTORNEY: And at the end of a shift, are you sometimes in a hurry? With things to do, places to go, people to see?

NURSE: Yes.

ATTORNEY: Now, would you tell the jury the purpose of the record you keep for each patient?

NURSE: Well, we want to communicate information about the patient to others on the health care team, and we want to develop a historic account of the patient's problems, what has been done for him, and his progress.

ATTORNEY: So, other people rely on the information in this record when they make their own decisions about the patient's care?

NURSE: Yes, that's true.

ATTORNEY: So you would agree that the record must be reliable?

NURSE: Yes.

ATTORNEY: And you would agree that it must be factual and accurate in all respects?

NURSE: Yes.

ATTORNEY: And you would agree that it needs to be comprehensive and complete, wouldn't you?

NURSE: Yes, I would.

ATTORNEY: So you're trying to develop a record that's factual, accurate, and complete at a time when you're sometimes tired, sometimes in a hurry, after working 10 consecutive hours and seeing 15 different patients 10 different times, and

---

Understanding the importance of timely documentation *(continued)*

after having dealt with unexpected and distracting events. Is that the essence of your testimony?

NURSE: Well. . . yes.

ATTORNEY: Thank you. You may continue to read your entries to the jury.

By attacking the timeliness of recorded entries, the attorney undermined their reliability, accuracy, and completeness. The jurors will now probably be skeptical of the record and the nurse as well.

How to prevent untimely entries

So, how do you prevent this situation? By timely documentation. Some nurses may carry a notepad to keep working notes of events while they're fresh in their minds. This isn't recommended because during a lawsuit a plaintiff's attorney could subpoena your notes, hoping to find discrepancies between them and the record. If he succeeds, he'll use those discrepancies to discredit the record. This will also corroborate that timely documentaton doesn't exist.

- lead to disciplinary actions that range from a reprimand to the suspension of your nursing license
- harm your patient if your coworker makes an error or misinterprets information
- make you and your employer accountable for negligence because delegated documentation is illegal and may constitute fraud
- destroy the credibility and value of the medical record, leading reasonable nurses and physicians to doubt its accuracy
- diminish the record's value as legal evidence.

Remember: A judge will give little, if any, weight to a medical record that contains secondhand observations or hearsay evidence.

Countersign cautiously

Although countersigning doesn't imply that you performed the procedure, it does imply that you reviewed the entry and approved the care given. To act correctly and to protect yourself, review your employer's policy on countersigning and follow these guidelines:

- If your facility interprets countersigning to mean that the licensed practical nurse (LPN), graduate nurse, or nursing assistant performed the nursing actions in the countersigning registered nurse's presence, don't countersign unless you were there when the actions occurred.

■ If your facility acknowledges that you don't necessarily have time to witness your coworkers' actions, your countersignature implies that the LPN or nursing assistant had the authority and competence to perform the care described. In countersigning, you verify that all required patient care procedures were carried out.

■ If policy requires you to countersign a subordinate's entries, review each entry and make sure that it clearly identifies who did the procedure. If you sign off without reviewing an entry or if you overlook a problem that the entry raises, you could share liability for any patient injury that results.

■ If another nurse asks you to document her care or sign her notes, don't. Your signature will make you responsible for anything written in the notes above it.

4 *Electronic patient records*

The electronic patient record is the patient-centered product of a complex, interconnected set of clinical software applications that processes, inputs, and sends data. The computerized patient record:

- formats and categorizes information, making it readily available to provide guidance to clinicians and act as a record of the patient's care
- provides a longitudinal record of the patient's health care history in a particular facility and beyond
- includes ambulatory and inpatient records that can be accessed in many ways to fill information needs.

Whether you're a seasoned nurse or a nursing student tackling your first clinical assignment, it's up to you to learn how to incorporate the computerized patient record into your daily practice, even as its importance becomes infused with new relevance and character due to other emerging technologies, such as:

- computerized order entry
- nurse–clinician documentation systems
- real-time clinical and operational report writing
- Internet-based self-scheduling.

The move toward computerized documentation

An increase in patient mortality due to medication and other procedural errors combined with the problems created by the nursing shortage has led the health care industry to accelerate the development and implementation of computerized documentation systems. Other factors influencing this move toward increased implementation include:

- more accurate standardization of health care billing transactions, which requires far more accurate documentation to satisfy third-party payers (see *Documentation: Headed for change*)
- the increasing complexity of health care facility business functions.

The most compelling reason for the development of a proficient electronic medical record (EMR) system, however, is improved patient care.

A work in progress

Definitions and parameters for workable computerized patient records, EMRs, and other computerized patient records remain a work in progress. However, *informatics*—the merging of medical and nursing science with computer science to better manage data—continues to see its role expand in all health care environments. (See *Raising the standards and value of documentation*.) Several medical and nursing informatics organizations are working to create standards, such as:

Documentation: Headed for change

By the end of the 20th century, sky-high medical costs had broken the back of the health care system and managed care had arrived, putting the business of health care primarily in the hands of insurance companies and regulatory agencies. As a result, there are now increased demands from payers and regulators for stricter adherence to governmental and third-party payer rules and regulations. With this in mind, the government enacted the Health Insurance Portability and Accountability Act to help standardize the processes and language of the business transactions between health care providers and third-party payers. By standardizing formats and coding, all parties—third-party payers, health care facilities, and patients—will receive benefits in saved time and money. Computerized documentation will play a big role in this important transition.

Raising the standards and value of documentation

Nursing organizations and regulatory and accrediting entities are leaning toward a greater dependency on computerized documentation. The Joint Commission regularly focuses its attention on aspects of care and documentation that it views as inadequate. Nursing continues to grapple with the Nursing Minimum Data Set (NMDS) as a codified data set that will lend itself to better evaluation of patient interventions and outcomes as well as for research. Task-oriented documentation is no longer sufficient. Clinical documentation must be patient and patient-outcome supportive.

The clinical documentation system is an ideal platform for the implementation of new standards. A good example of this is The Joint Commission's initiative to improve the documentation of patient and family teaching. Before the initiative, documentation of patient teaching tended to be inconsistent. However, new computerized systems in the hands of nurses now present on-line "forms" that prompt caregivers to address the many facets of patient teaching and provide a documentation of the experience and results of the teaching in the computerized patient record. A current Joint Commission initiative is to standardize patient-teaching documentation across multidisciplinary services and departments, resulting in a multidisciplinary teaching record that's accessible and usable by everyone. Computerized documentation should help facilitate this change.

- American Medical Informatics Association
- American Nursing Informatics Association
- Healthcare Information and Management Systems Society
- NANDA-International
- Nursing Informatics Working Group.

*A*dvantages of computerized patient records

Even at this relatively early age of the computerized patient record, there are more reasons for all clinical documentation to be incorporated into a computerized patient record than not. (See *Key advantages of a computerized patient record,* page 110.) Advantages include:

- Improved standardization—Standardization of clinical data and reporting has been pushed to the forefront by the Health Insurance Portability and Accountability Act, which requires accurate and timely re-

Key advantages of a computerized patient record

This list highlights the key benefits of using a computerized patient record:

- ability for all providers to see each other's documentation
- access by different providers at different locations
- access by different providers at the same time
- access to clinical information
- access to computerized patient records at appropriate workstations
- automated reports for quality indicators
- clinical decision making easier and more accurate
- ease in auditing documentation
- ease of access—"where to look"
- increased quality of documentation
- legibility
- multidisciplinary access
- on-line clinical support information
- patient-driven care planning
- point-of-care documentation
- "real-time" diagnostic results and reports
- reduced redundant documentation
- remote access.

ports required for accrediting, regulatory, and third-party payers. This increased demand for reports requires computerization of the report writer, which, in turn, requires clinical data input.

- Improved quality of the medical record—With a properly designed and implemented clinical information system, computerized patient record documentation improves the overall caliber of clinical information. It also returns the focus of nurses to providing nursing care.
- Improved legibility—In 1999, the Institute of Medicine published a report that recommended the move toward a universal system of computerized order entry because medication errors were commonly caused by the inability to properly decipher handwritten orders. With computerized physician order entry, legibility is a nonissue, and there is no need for transcription of handwritten physician orders.
- Increased access to information—Accessing patient data is quick and painless by filing clinical information in the same location from patient to patient and department to department. Across-the-board universality also saves time and contributes to more accurate assessment

Computer-generated medication administration record

The computer-generated medication administration record, contains vital information to help guide your nursing care throughout your shift. It may be necessary to print out a new record at various times throughout your shift so new physician's orders are reflected.

```
Medical ICU-4321                    Patient Care Hospital
3/14/08      07:00                   PAGE 001
================================================================================

WILLIAMS, HENRY                     64   MWMC
MR#: 5555555         DOB 10/26/40    MICU 302
FIN#: 1010101010                    Admitted: 3/12/08
DR: Daniel Smith                    Service: Internal Medicine
================================================================================

Summary: 3/14 07:00 to 15:00

ALLERGIES AND CODE STATUS
3/12/08       MED ALLERGY: NO KNOWN DRUG ALLERGY
              NO INTUBATION

Scheduled Medications:
3/12/08       Lopressor Metoprolol Inj 5 mg, IV, q 6 hours
                 09        15
3/12/08       Heparin inj 5,000 units, SC, q 12 hours
                 09

Miscellaneous Medications:
3/13/08       Lasix Furosemide Inj 40 mg, IV, Now

PRN Medications:
3/12/08       Tylenol Acetaminophen Supp 650 mg, #1, PR, q 4 hour prn pain or
              temperature > 101 F
```

of recorded data. Mobile workstations allow access to information closer to the point of care. Most importantly, multiple caregivers and providers have access to patient information at any given time.

■ Quicker retrieval—Typically, you can retrieve information more quickly with computers than with traditional documentation systems. Most systems allow you to print a patient medication administration record each shift that contains information to guide your care. (See *Computer-generated medication administration record*.)

Disadvantages of computerized patient records

Computerized patient records are still developing. New technologies are continually emerging to expand their use. In order to take full advantage of the computer system, we must become proficient in its strengths and adapt to its weaknesses. For example:

■ Computer downtime—Unexpected downtime can occur secondary to system malfunction; however, scheduled downtime occurs more often for system updates. Follow your institution's policy and procedure for "downtime." In most cases, facilities resort to a paper system until the electronic system is functioning.

■ Unfamiliarity—There are still segments of the nursing population that aren't comfortable with computer usage. Used improperly, computerized systems can threaten a patient's right to privacy. (See *Preventing breaches in patient confidentiality.*) They can also yield inaccurate or incomplete information if multiple operating systems aren't integrated within a health care system.

Maintaining confidentiality with computerized documentation

The American Nurses Association (ANA) and the American Medical Records Association offer these guidelines for maintaining the confidentiality of computerized medical records:

■ Never share your password or computer signature. Never give your personal password or computer signature to anyone—including another nurse in the unit, a nurse serving temporarily in the unit, or a physician. Your health care facility can issue a short-term password authorizing access to certain records for infrequent users.

■ Be aware of your surroundings. Don't display confidential patient information on a monitor where it can be seen by others or leave print versions or excerpts of the patient's medical record unattended or exposed.

■ Log off if not using your terminal. Don't leave a computer terminal unattended after you've logged on. (Some computers have a timing device that shuts down a screen after a certain period of inactivity.)

■ Follow your facility's policy for correcting errors. Computer entries are part of the patient's permanent record and, as such, can't be deleted. In most cases, you can correct an entry error before storing the entry. To correct an error after storage, mark the entry "error" or "mis-

Preventing breaches in patient confidentiality

This chart provides specific measures you can take to ensure that information about your patients remains confidential.

Type of breach	How to prevent it
Computers **Displays** Displaying information on a screen that's viewed by unauthorized users (especially for handheld computers)	Make sure that display screens don't face public areas. For portable devices, install encryption software that makes information unreadable or inaccessible.
E-mail Sending confidential messages via public networks such as the Internet, where they can be read by unauthorized users	Use encryption software when sending e-mail over public networks.
Printers Sharing printers among units with differing functions and information (unauthorized people can read printouts)	Request that your unit have a separate printer not shared with another unit.
Copiers Discarded copies of patient health information in trash cans adjacent to copiers	Use secure disposal containers (similar to mailboxes) that collect paperwork for shredding.
Cordless and cellular phones Holding conversations vulnerable to eavesdropping by outsiders with scanning equipment	Use phones with built-in encryption technology.
Fax machines Faxing confidential information to unauthorized persons	Before transmission, verify the fax number and that the recipient is authorized to receive confidential information.
Voice pagers Sending confidential messages that can be overheard on the pager	Restrict use of voice pagers to nonconfidential messages.

taken entry," add the correct information, and date and electronically sign the entry.

■ Make backup files. Make sure that stored records have backup files—an important safety feature. If you inadvertently delete part of the permanent record (even though there are safeguards against this), type an explanation into the file along with the date, the time, and your initials. Submit an explanation in writing to your nurse-manager, and keep a copy for your records.

How computerized systems work

In addition to having a mainframe computer, most health care facilities have personal computers or terminals at workstations throughout the facility so departmental staff have quick access to vital information and can easily enter patient care orders. Some facilities have bedside terminals that make data even more accessible. Computer training is generally a component of orientation to the facility. If the system is just being integrated into the facility, training is provided to the employees who will be using it. Here's a quick overview of how these systems work:

■ Before entering a patient's clinical record onto a computer, you must first enter your password, which is usually your personal computer identification number. Passwords commonly specify the type of information that a particular team member can access. For example, a dietitian may be assigned a code that allows her to see dietary orders but not physical therapy orders.

■ The patient's name or account number and medical record number are entered before entering demographic data.

Bar code technology

Bar code technology is a feature that some facilities have implemented in their computer systems. With this technology, you scan a drug's bar code, scan the patient's identification bracelet, and then scan your own identification badge. As soon as the medication and patient's identification bracelet are scanned, the information immediately appears on a mobile computer screen and documents the administration. If a physician discontinues a medication, it won't show up on the screen when you scan the patient's wristband. This technology greatly reduces medication errors because it:

■ prevents situations in which medication changes come after you already administered your medications

■ connects to the order-entry system, so a discontinued medication won't show up on the patient's listed medications

■ scans the medication to ensure that the nurse hasn't inadvertently picked the wrong medication out of the medication drawer or received the wrong medication from the pharmacy.

Bar code technology improves patient safety during medication administration, streamlines documentation, and allows the nurse to immediately document a patient's refusal of medication into the computer.

■ The physician can log into the system and access the physician's order screens. When he chooses the appropriate orders, the computer system transmits the orders to the patient's nursing department and the other appropriate departments. For example, if the physician orders medications for the patient, the order is transmitted to the patient's nursing department and the pharmacy. This type of direct-order transmittal helps prevent dosing errors and decreases medication errors by eliminating order transcription errors.

■ After the physician's orders are entered, the nurse can log into the system and enter the patient's name (or choose his name from a patient census list) or account number to bring the patient's electronic chart to the screen. This will allow her to scan the record to compare data on vital signs, laboratory test results, or intake and output; enter new data on the care plan or progress notes; and sign out medications that she's administered. Bar code technology is making medication administration safer and its use is increasing. (See *Bar code technology.*)

Systems and functions

Depending on which type of computer hardware and software your health care facility has, you may access information by using a keyboard, light pen, touch-sensitive screen, mouse, or voice activation. Currently used systems include the Nursing Information System (NIS), the Nursing Minimum Data Set (NMDS), the Nursing Outcomes Classification (NOC) system, and voice-activated systems.

Nursing Information System

The NIS makes nursing documentation easier by reflecting most or all of the components of the nursing process so they can meet the standards of the ANA and The Joint Commission.

Nursing benefits

■ Each NIS provides different features and can be customized to conform to a facility's documentation forms and formats. (See *Computers and the nursing process,* pages 116 and 117.)

■ An NIS can manage information either passively or actively. Passive systems collect, transmit, organize, format, print, and display information that you can use to make a decision, but they don't suggest decisions for you. Active systems suggest nursing diagnoses based on predefined assessment data that you enter.

Computers and the nursing process

Nursing information systems (NISs) can increase efficiency and accuracy in all phases of the nursing process—assessment, nursing diagnosis, planning, implementation, and evaluation—and can help nurses meet the standards established by the American Nurses Association and The Joint Commission. In addition, an NIS can help you spend more time meeting the patient's needs. Consider the following uses of computers in the nursing process.

Assessment

Use the computer terminal to document assessment information. As data are collected, enter further information as prompted by the computer's software program. Enter data about the patient's health status, history, chief complaint, and other assessment factors. Some software programs prompt you to ask specific questions and then offer pathways to gather further information. In some systems, if you enter an assessment value that's outside the usual acceptable range, the computer will flag the entry to call your attention to it.

Nursing diagnosis

Most current programs list standard diagnoses with associated signs and symptoms as references; you must still use clinical judgment to determine a nursing diagnosis for each patient. With this information, you can rapidly obtain diagnostic information. For example, the computer can generate a list of possible diagnoses for a patient with selected signs and symptoms, or it may enable you to retrieve and review the patient's records according to the nursing diagnosis.

Planning

To help nurses begin writing a care plan, newer computer programs display recommended expected outcomes and interventions for the selected diagnoses. Computers can also track outcomes for large patient populations and general information to help you select patient outcomes. You can use computers to compare large amounts of patient data, help identify outcomes the patient is likely to achieve based on individual problems and needs, and estimate the time frame for reaching outcome goals.

Implementation

Use the computer to document actual interventions and patient-processing information, such as transfer and discharge instructions, and to communicate this information to other departments. Computer-generated progress notes automatically sort and print out patient data, such as medication administration, treatments, and vital signs, making documentation more efficient and accurate.

Computers and the nursing process *(continued)*

Evaluation

During evaluation, use the computer to document and store observations, patient responses to nursing interventions, and your own evaluation statements. You may also use information from other members of the health care team to determine future actions and discharge planning. If a desired patient outcome hasn't been achieved, document interventions taken to ensure such desired outcomes. Then reevaluate the second set of interventions.

■ More sophisticated systems provide standardized patient status and nursing intervention phrases that you can use to construct your progress notes. These systems let you change the standardized phrases, if necessary, and allow space for you to add your own documentation.

New developments

The most recent NISs are interactive, meaning they prompt you with questions and suggestions that are in accordance with the information you enter. These new systems should prove especially helpful because they:

■ require only a brief narrative, and the questioning and diagnostic suggestions that the systems provide ensure quick but thorough documentation

■ allow you to add or change information so that you can tailor your documentation to fit each patient.

Nursing Minimum Data Set

The NMDS attempts to standardize nursing information into three categories of data:

■ nursing care
■ patient demographics
■ service elements. (See *Elements of the Nursing Minimum Data Set*, page 118.)

Nursing benefits

■ The NMDS allows you to collect nursing diagnosis and intervention data and identify the nursing needs of various patient populations.

■ This system lets you track patient outcomes and describe nursing care in various settings, including the patient's home.

Elements of the Nursing Minimum Data Set

The Nursing Minimum Data Set contains three elements—nursing care, patient demographics, and service. These elements are the core data needed to support decision making in clinical nursing and to implement the computerized patient record.

Nursing care elements
- Nursing diagnoses
- Nursing interventions
- Nursing outcomes
- Nursing intensity

Patient demographic elements
- Personal identification
- Date of birth
- Gender
- Race and ethnicity
- Residence

Service elements
- Unique facility or service agency number
- Unique health record number of patient
- Unique number of principal registered nurse providers
- Episode admission or encounter date
- Discharge or termination date
- Disposition of patient
- Expected payer of medical bills

- The NMDS helps establish accurate estimates for nursing service costs and provides data about nursing care that may influence health care policy and decision making.
- The NMDS helps you provide better patient care by allowing you to compare local, regional, and national nursing trends, as well as nursing data from various clinical settings, patient populations, and geographic areas.
- The NMDS encourages more consistent nursing documentation.
- It makes documentation and information retrieval faster and easier. (Currently, NANDA-I assigns numerical codes to all nursing diagnoses so they can be used with the NMDS.)

Nursing Outcomes Classification

The NOC system provides the first comprehensive, standardized method of measuring nursing-sensitive patient outcomes.

Nursing benefits

■ The NOC system allows you to compare your patients' outcomes to the outcomes of larger groups according to age, diagnosis, or health care setting.
■ This system is essential to supporting ongoing nursing research.
■ The NOC system makes possible the inclusion of patient data-related outcomes that have been absent from computerized medical information databases in the past.

Voice-activated systems

Voice-activated systems are most useful in departments that have a high volume of structured reports such as the operating room. The software program uses a specialized knowledge base—nursing words, phrases, and report forms, combined with automated speech recognition technology—that allows the user to record, prompt, and complete nurses' notes by voice.

Nursing benefits

■ Voice-activated systems require little or no keyboard use.
■ They include information on the nursing process, nursing theory, nursing standards of practice, report forms, and a logical format.
■ These systems use trigger phrases that cue the system to display passages of report text and allow word-for-word dictation and editing.
■ Voice-activated systems increase the speed of reporting and free the nurse from paperwork so that she can spend more time at the bedside.

5 Documentation in acute care

A medical record with well-organized, completed forms will help you communicate patient information to the health care team, garner accreditation and reimbursements, and protect yourself and your employer legally. It will also allow you to spend more time providing direct patient care.

Nursing admission assessment form

Also known as a *nursing database,* the nursing admission assessment form contains your initial patient assessment data. To complete the form, you'll have to collect relevant information from various sources and analyze it to assemble a complete picture of the patient. (See *Completing the nursing admission assessment.*) Keep these points in mind when using an admission assessment form:

■ It's meant to be a record of your nursing observations, the patient's health history, and your physical examination findings.

■ It may be organized by body system or by patient responses, such as relating, choosing, exchanging, and communicating.

It may include data about:

■ patient complaint and history of current problem

– past medical and surgical history

– the patient's medications

– the patient's known allergies to foods, medications, and other substances

■ normal and abnormal assessment findings

– nursing findings related to activities of daily living (ADLs)

– the patient's current pain level

Completing the nursing admission assessment

Most health care facilities use a combined checklist and narrative admission form such as the one shown here. The nursing admission assessment becomes a part of the patient's permanent medical record.

ADMISSION DOCUMENT

Name: *Raymond Bergstrom*   Hospital I.D. No.:   *4227*

Age: *74*   Insurer: *Aetna*

Birth date: *4/15/33*   Policy No.: *605310P*

Address: *3401 Elmhurst Ave,*   Physician: *Joseph Milstein*

Jenkintown, PA 19046   Admission date: *1/28/08*

                                   Unit: *3N*

Preoperative teaching according to standard? ☑ Yes   ☐ No

Preoperative teaching completed on _____ *1/28/08*

If no, ☐ Surgery not planned   ☐ Emergency surgery

Signature *Kate McCauley, RN*

Admitted from: **Mode:**
☐ Emergency room   ☐ Ambulatory
☐ Home   ☑ Wheelchair
☑ Physician's office   ☐ Stretcher
☐ Transfer from   Accompanied by:
                                      Wife

T *101° F*   **P** *120*   **R** *24*   **Pulses:**

BP (Lying/sitting)   L: *P*   Radial *P*   DP *P*   PT

Left: R: *P*   Radial *P*   DP *P*   PT

Right: *120 / 68*   Apical pulse *120*

Height *5'7"*   ☑ Regular   ☐ Irregular

Weight *160 lb*   P = Palpable   D = Doppler   O = Absent

Pain:

⓪ 1 2 3 4 5 6 7 8 9 10   ("0" indicates no pain; "10" indicates worst pain imaginable)

Reason for visit: *Prostate surgery*

When problem started: *Unknown*

Signature *Kate McCauley, RN*

(continued)

Completing the nursing admission assessment *(continued)*

MEDICAL & SURGICAL HISTORY

Check (P) if patient or (R) if a blood relative has had any of the following. Check (H) if patient has ever been hospitalized. If it isn't appropriate to question patient because of age or gender, cross out option, e.g., ~~infertility.~~

	(H)	(P)	(R)	Interviewer comments
Addictions (e.g., alcohol, drugs)	☐	☐	☐	
Angina	☐	☐	☐	
Arthritis	☐	☐	☐	
Asthma	☐	☑	☑	
Bleeding problems	☐	☐	☐	
Blood clot	☐	☐	☐	
Cancer	☐	☐	☐	
Counseling	☐	☐	☐	
CVA	☐	☐	☐	
Depression	☐	☐	☐	
Diabetes	☐	☐	☑	
Eating disorders	☐	☐	☐	
Epilepsy	☐	☐	☐	
Eye problems (not glasses)	☐	☐	☐	
Fainting	☐	☐	☐	
Fractures	☐	☐	☐	
Genetic condition	☐	☐	☐	
Glaucoma	☐	☐	☐	
Gout	☐	☐	☐	
Headaches	☐	☐	☐	

	(H)	(P)	(R)	Interviewer comments
Hepatitis	☐	☐	☐	
High cholesterol	☐	☑	☐	
Hypertension	☐	☐	☐	
~~Infertility~~				
Kidney disease/ stones	☐	☐	☐	
Leukemia	☐	☐	☐	
Memory loss	☐	☐	☐	
Mood swings	☐	☐	☐	
Myocardial infarction	☐	☐	☐	
Prostate problems	☐	☐	☐	
Rheumatic fever	☐	☐	☐	
Sexually trans. disease	☐	☐	☐	
Thyroid problems	☐	☐	☐	
TB or positive test	☐	☐	☐	
Other	☐	☐	☐	

List any surgeries the patient has had:

Date   **Type of surgery**

Has the patient ever had a blood
transfusion: ☐ Y   ☑ N
reaction: ☐ Y   ☐ N

UNIT INTRODUCTION

Patient rights given to patient:	☑ Y	☐ N	☐ Unable
Patient verbalizes understanding:	☑ Y	☐ N	☐ Unable

☑ Patient ☑ Family oriented to:

Nurse call system/unit policies:	☑ Y	☐ N	☐ Unable
Smoking/visiting policy/intercom/ side rails/TV channels:	☑ Y	☐ N	☐ Unable

Patient valuables:

☑ Sent home
☐ Placed in safe
☐ None on admission

Patient meds:

☑ Sent home
☐ Placed in pharmacy
☐ None on admission

Signature _Kate McCauley, RN_

Completing the nursing admission assessment *(continued)*

ALLERGIES OR REACTIONS

Medications/dyes	☑ Y ☐ N	*PCN*
Anesthesia drugs	☐ Y ☑ N	
Foods	☐ Y ☑ N	
Environmental (e.g., tape, latex, bee stings, dust, pollen, animals, etc.)	☑ Y ☐ N	*Dust, pollen, cats*

ADVANCE DIRECTIVE INFORMATION

1. Does patient have an advance directive? ☑ Y ☐ N
2. Does patient have health care power of attorney? ☐ Y ☑ N

   Name: _____ Phone: _____

   If yes, request copy from patient/family and place in chart.

   Date done: _____ Init. _____

3. Educational booklet given to patient/family? ☑ Y ☐ N

MEDICATIONS

Medication (presently in use)	Dose and frequency	Last time taken
1. *Proventil*	*2 puffs q. 4 hr*	*1/21/08*
2. *ASA*	*81 mg daily*	*1/21/08*
3. *Tylenol*	*650 mg prn*	
4.		

Signature *Kate McCauley, RN*   Date *1/28/08*

– your impressions of the patient's support systems
– documentation of the patient's advance directives, if any.

   When completing the form, you may have to fill in blanks, check off boxes, or write narrative notes.

Advantages

■ Carefully completed, provides pertinent physiologic, psychosocial, and cultural information

■ Contains subjective and objective data about the patient's current health status and clues about actual or potential health problems

- Reveals the patient's expectations for treatment, his ability and potentially his willingness to comply with treatment, and details about his lifestyle, family relationships, and cultural and religious influences
- Guides you through the nursing process by helping you formulate nursing diagnoses, create patient problem lists, construct care plans, and begin discharge planning
- Identifies the patient's living arrangement, caregivers, resources, support groups, and other relevant information needed for discharge planning
- When used by The Joint Commission, quality improvement groups, and other parties to continue accreditation, justifies requests for reimbursement, and maintains or improves the standards of quality patient care
- Serves as a baseline for later comparison with the patient's progress

Disadvantages

- May be incomplete if the patient is too sick to answer questions and family members can't answer for him
- May be inconsistent if, because of time constraints, more than one nurse completes the form

Documentation style

Admission assessment forms follow a medical format, emphasizing initial symptoms and a comprehensive review of body systems or a nursing process format. (See chapter 1, Documenting from admission to discharge.) Regardless of which format you use, document admission assessments in one or more of three styles: open-ended, closed-ended, and narrative. (See *Writing a narrative admission assessment.*)

Standard open-ended style

- Is arranged categorically so you can easily document information and retrieve it
- Uses standard fill-in-the-blank pages with preprinted headings and questions
- Uses phrases and approved abbreviations

Standard closed-ended style

- Is arranged categorically with preprinted headings, checklists, and questions

(Text continues on page 128.)

Writing a narrative admission assessment

Here's an example of a nursing admission assessment form documented in narrative style.

Date: 4/02/08

Patient's name: James McGee

Address: 20 Tomlinson Road, Elgin, IL 60120

Home phone: (555) 203-0704

Work phone: (555) 389-2050

Cell phone: (555) 437-4569

Sex: Male   **Age:** 55

Birth date: 5/11/52

Marital status: Married

Dependents: 2

Emergency contact: Susan McGee (wife) (555) 203-1212 (cell)

Occupation: Teacher

Chief health complaint

States, "I've had several episodes of pain in my stomach. I also feel very tired."

Health history

Increased fatigue x 1 month. 12-lb weight loss without trying, decreased appetite. Denies nausea/vomiting. Occ dark stools—no bloody stools noted.

Past medical/surgical history: Childhood illnesses: measles, chickenpox. Immunizations up-to-date. Last tetanus—2002. Tonsillectomy—age 2. Fractured left leg—age 17. Appendectomy—age 25.

Functional health: Describes easy-going personality and good sense of humor.

Cultural and religious influence: Describes strong faith (Roman Catholic) with regular church attendance. No cultural influence.

Family relationships: Describes stable relationship with wife and 2 children. School schedule presents time restraints for family activities.

Sexuality: States no sexual problems.

Signature: *Jill Nazarene, RN*   **Date:** 4/02/08

(continued)

Writing a narrative admission assessment *(continued)*

Social support: *Strong family support. Strong friend network.*

Other:

Personal health perception and behaviors: *Smokes 1 to 2 packs cigarettes/day. Denies use of illicit drugs. Drinks 1 to 2 beers/week. Drinks 6 to 8 cups coffee/day.*

Rest and sleep: *Sleeps app 5 to 6 hours/night. Often feels tired. Occ nap.*

Exercise and activity: *No regular exercise regimen. Occ walk.*

Nutrition: *Takes vitamins daily. Skips lunch often. Frequent fast food. 24-hour recall: cereal, coffee x 5, pizza x 2, cola x 1.*

Recreation: *Likes swimming, camping. Watches TV and reads when home.*

Coping: *Describes coping by avoiding problems until they get big. Feels he copes adequately with daily stresses. Describes his job as stressful and occ feels pressure with job and family responsibilities.*

Socioeconomic: *States "adequate income." Has health insurance and retirement benefits. Wife works also.*

Environment: *Denies knowledge of environmental hazards. Works in a smoke-free facility.*

Occupational: *8 to 10 hour work day x 6 days week (most weeks).*

Family history

Father deceased at age 70—colon CA; mother deceased at age 59—breast CA. Sister age 50— healthy. Maternal grandfather deceased at age 75—stroke; maternal grandmother deceased at age 60—cause unknown; paternal grandfather deceased at age 55—heart disease; paternal grandmother deceased at age 66—cause unknown.

Signature: *Jill Nazarene, RN*   **Date:** *4/02/08*

Writing a narrative admission assessment *(continued)*

Physical status

General health and appearance: *Complains of recent stomach pain and fatigue. Had 2 URIs last winter. Recent weight loss. Denies other illnesses or complaints. Clean and neat appearance.*

Skin, hair, nails: *Pallor, no skin lesions. Hair receding, pale nails.*

Head and neck: *Occ headache—relieved by aspirin. No history of seizures. Reports no pain or limited movement.*

Nose and sinuses: *No rhinorrhea; has occ sinus infection; no history of nosebleeds.*

Mouth and throat: *Last dental exam and cleaning: 10/06. No mouth or gum soreness. Denies sore throats.*

Eyes: *Last eye exam—2/06. Wears reading glasses.*

Ears: *Denies hearing problems or ear infections. Last hearing test—childhood.*

Nervous system: *Denies numbness, tingling in extremities. Denies any confusion or difficulty with memory.*

Respiratory system: *Denies history of pneumonia, bronchitis, asthma. URI x 2 last year.*

Cardiovascular system: *Denies history of murmurs or palpitations. Denies any chest pain or leg pain.*

Breasts: *WNL for adult male.*

GI system: *c/o frequent episodes of indigestion, sometimes relieved by Mylanta. Currently c/o gnawing stomach pain—rated 5 on scale of 0 to 10. Regular bowel movements x 1 daily. Last BM this am. Occ dark stools—no frank blood noticed.*

GU system: *Denies flank pain or history of stones or UTI. No trouble with voiding. Denies STD in past. Sexually active.*

Signature: *Jill Nazarene, RN*   **Date:** *4/02/08*

(continued)

Writing a narrative admission assessment *(continued)*

Musculoskeletal system: *Denies muscle or joint pain or stiffness.*

Immune and hematologic system: *Denies unusual bleeding or lymph node swelling.*

Endocrine system: *Denies history of thyroid disease.*

Signature: *Jill Nazarene, RN*   **Date:** *4/02/08*

- Calls for you to simply check off the appropriate responses
- Eliminates the problem of illegible handwriting and makes reviewing documented information quick
- Clearly establishes the type and amount of information required by the health care facility

Narrative note style

- Is handwritten or computer-generated
- Summarizes information obtained by general observation, the health history interview, and a physical examination
- Allows you to list your findings in order of importance

KNOW-HOW *The current trend in health care facilities is to avoid writing long narrative note entries because they're time-consuming to write and to read, require you to remember and document all significant information in a detailed, logical sequence, and interfere with efficient data retrieval. If using narrative notes, make sure that you keep them concise, pertinent, and based on your evaluations.*

Documentation guidelines

- The admission assessment usually needs to be completed within a specific time frame, such as 12 or 24 hours from time of admission.
- If the patient is unable or unwilling to participate, find secondary sources (family members or past medical records, for example) to provide needed information. Document your source of information.
- During your interview, try to alleviate as much of the patient's discomfort and anxiety as possible.

■ If you're unable to complete the admission assessment, document why you couldn't obtain complete data, and complete the assessment as soon as you can.

Progress notes

Use progress notes to document the patient's status and track changes in his condition. Progress notes describe, in chronological order:
■ patient problems and needs
■ pertinent nursing observations
■ nursing reassessments and interventions
■ patient responses to interventions
■ progress toward meeting expected outcomes.

Advantages

■ Promotes effective communication among all members of the health care team and continuity of care
■ Contains a column for the date and time and a column for detailed comments (see *Keeping standard progress notes,* page 130)
■ Usually reflects the patient's problems (the nursing diagnoses)
■ Eases information retrieval
■ Contains information that doesn't fit into the space or format of other forms

Disadvantages

■ May be disorganized
■ May require reading through the entire entry to find needed information
■ May be more time consuming
■ May contain insignificant information

Documentation guidelines

■ When writing a progress note, include the date and time of the care given or your observations, what prompted the entry, and other pertinent data, such as contact with the physician or other health care provider.
■ If your facility uses progress notes designed to focus on nursing diagnoses, be sure to document each nursing diagnosis, problem, goal, or expected outcome that relates to your entry. (See *Using nursing diagnoses to write progress notes,* page 131.)

Keeping standard progress notes

Use the following example as a guide for completing your progress notes.

PROGRESS NOTES

Date	Time	Comments
2/20/08	0900	Notified Dr. T. Watts re Ⓛ lower lobe crackles and ineffective cough.
		R 40 and shallow. Skin pale. Nebulizer treatment ordered. ————
		———————————————————— Ruth Bullock, RN
2/20/08	1030	Skin slightly pink after nebulizer treatment. Lungs clear. R 24. Showed
		pt. how to do pursed-lip and abdominal breathing. — Ruth Bullock, RN
2/20/08	1400	Ⓛ leg wound 3 cm x 1 cm wide x 1 cm deep. Small amount of pink-
		yellow, non-odorous drainage noted on dressing. Surrounding skin
		reddened and tender. Wound irrigated and dressed as ordered. ——
		———————————————————— Ruth Bullock, RN
2/20/08	1930	Pt. instructed about upper GI test. Related correct understanding of test
		purpose and procedure. ———————————— Ann Barrow, RN

■ Don't repeat yourself. Avoid including information that's already on the flow sheet, unless there's a sudden change in the patient's condition or if the information needs a more detailed explanation.

■ Be specific. Avoid vague wording, such as "appears to be," "no problems," and "had a good day."

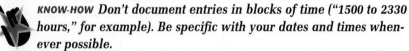

1/06/08	1000	Pt. ate 80% of breakfast and 75% of lunch; OOB to
		bathroom and walked in hallway 3 times for a distance
		of 10 feet with no shortness of breath. — K. Comerford, RN

■ Make sure that every progress note has the specific date and time of the care given or observation noted.

■ Document pertinent patient comments using quotation marks.

KNOW-HOW *Don't document entries in blocks of time ("1500 to 2330 hours," for example). Be specific with your dates and times whenever possible.*

■ Document new patient problems, resolutions of old problems, and deteriorations in the patient's condition.

Using nursing diagnoses to write progress notes

Progress notes can be written using a nursing diagnosis, as the example below shows.

Patient identification information		County Hospital, Van Nuys, CA

John Adams
111 Oak St.
Van Nuys, CA 91388
(202) 123-4560

PROGRESS NOTES

Date and time	Nursing diagnosis and related problems	Notes
1/9/08 —2300	Acute pain related to pressure ulcer on Ⓛ elbow.	Pt. rates pain an 8 on a scale of 0 to 10, with 0 being no pain and 10 being the worst pain ever experienced. Pt. frowning when pointing to wound. BP 130/84; P 96. Pain aggravated by dressing change @ 2200. Percocet ī given P.O. and pt. repositioned on Ⓡ side. ——— ———————————— *Anne Curry, RN*
1/9/08 —2330	Acute pain related to pressure ulcer on Ⓛ elbow.	States that pain is relieved (0/10 on pain scale). Will give Percocet ½ hour before next dressing change and before future dressing changes. —— ———————————— *Anne Curry, RN*

■ Document your observations of the patient's response to the care plan. If behaviors are similar to agreed-upon objectives, document that the goals are being met. If the goals aren't being met, document what the patient can or can't do to meet them.

2/9/08	1600	Dyspnea resolving. Pt. can perform ADLs and ambulate 20 feet without SOB. ——————— *Lois Cahn, RN*

2/9/08	2000	Dyspnea unrelieved. Continues to have tachypnea and tachycardia 1 hr after receiving 100% O₂ by nonrebreather mask. ABG drawn by respiratory therapist. ——————— *Carol Davis, RN*

- Outline your interventions clearly—how and when you notified the physician, what his orders were, and when you followed through with them.

2/9/08	2000	Dr. John Milstein notified of ABG results. Pt. given Lasix 40 mg I.V. ————————— *Esther Blake, RN*

1/12/08	0800	BP: 98/58. Withheld Procardia per order of Dr. Adrian Patel. ——————————————— *Dave Bevins, RN*

Kardex

The patient care Kardex (sometimes called the *nursing Kardex*) provides a quick overview of basic patient care information. It usually contains text boxes filled with information related to medications, diet, activity level, patient care activities, treatments, and tests. (See *Components of a patient care Kardex*.) It can come in various shapes, sizes, and types, or may be computer-generated. (See *Characteristics of a computer-generated Kardex*, pages 136 to 138.) A Kardex typically includes:

- patient's name, age, room number, marital status, and religion (usually on the address stamp)
- allergies
- medical diagnoses, listed by priority
- nursing diagnoses, listed by priority
- current physicians' orders for treatments, such as physical therapy, diet, I.V. therapy, diagnostic tests, and procedures, such as wound care
- do-not-resuscitate status
- consultations
- permitted activities, functional limitations, assistance needed, and safety precautions
- standing orders, such as "transfuse one unit of PRBC if Hb < 8.0"
- emergency contact numbers
- discharge plans and goals.

Advantages

- Provides quick access to data about task-oriented interventions, such as activity, I.V. therapy, and other treatments
- If combined with the care plan, provides necessary data for patient care

Components of a patient care Kardex

Here you'll find the kind of information that might be included on the cover sheet of a patient care Kardex for a medical-surgical unit. Inside the Kardex, which is folded in half horizontally, you'll find additional patient care information.

Keep in mind that the categories, words, and phrases on a Kardex are brief and intended to quickly trigger images of special circumstances, procedures, activities, or patient conditions.

Care status
Self-care ☐
Partial care with
    assistance ☐
Complete care ☑
Shower with
    assistance ☐
Tub ☐
Active exercises ☑
Passive exercises ☑

Special care
Back care ☑
Mouth care ☑
Foot care ☐
Perineal care ☑
Catheter care ☑
Tracheostomy care ☐
Other (specify): _____

Condition
Satisfactory ☐
Fair ☑
Guarded ☐
Critical ☐
No code ☑
Advance directive
    Yes ☑
    No ☐
Date: *1/18/08*

Prosthesis
Dentures
    upper ☑
    lower ☑
Contact lenses ☐
Glasses ☑
Hearing aid ☐
Other (specify): _____

Isolation
Strict ☐
Contact ☐
Airborne ☐
Neutropenic ☐
Droplet ☐
Other (specify): _____

Diet
Type: *2 gm Na*
Force fluids ☐
NPO ☐
Assist with feeding ☑
Isolation tray ☐
Calorie count ☐
Supplements: _____

Tube feedings ☐
Type: _____
Rate: _____
Route:
    NG tube ☐
    G tube ☐
    J tube ☐

Admission
Height: *6' 1"*
Weight: *161 lb (73 kg)*
BP: *118/84*
Temp: *99.6° F*
Pulse: *101*
Resp.: *21*

Frequency
BP: *q 4 hr*
TPR: *q shift*
Apical pulses: _____
Peripheral
    pulses: *q shift*
Weight: *daily*
Neuro check: _____
Monitor: _____
Strips: _____
Turn: *q 2 hr*
Cough: *q shift*
Deep breathe: *q shift*
Central venous
    pressure: _____
Other (specify): _____

(continued)

Components of a patient care Kardex *(continued)*

GI tubes
Salem sump ☐
Levin tube ☐
Feeding tube ☐
Type (specify): _____
Other (specify): _____

Activity
Bed rest ☐
Chair *t.i.d.* ☑
Dangle ☐
Commode ☐
Commode with
   assist ☑
Ambulate ☐
BRP ☐
  Low ☐
  Moderate ☐
  High ☑
Fall-risk category ☐
  Low ☐
  Moderate ☐
  High ☑
Other (specify): _____

Mode of transport
Wheelchair ☑
Stretcher ☐
With oxygen ☐

I.V. devices
Heparin lock ☐
Peripheral I.V. ☑
Central line ☐
Triple-lumen CVP ☐
Hickman ☐
Jugular ☐
Peripherally inserted ☐
Parenteral nutrition ☐
Irrigations: _____

Dressings
Type: _____
Change: _____

Allergies
_____
_____
_____
_____
_____
_____

Emergency contact
Name: _____
_____
Telephone no: _____
_____

Respiratory therapy
Pulse oximetry ☐
Oxygen ☑
  %/liters/minute *2 L/min*
Method
  Nasal cannula ☑
  Face mask ☐
  Venturi mask ☐
  Partial rebreather
    mask ☐
  Nonrebreather mask ☐
  Trach collar ☐
Nebulizer ☐
Chest PT ☑
Incentive spirometry ☑
T-piece ☐
Ventilator ☐
  Type: _____
  Settings: _____
  Other (specify): _____
_____
_____

Drains
Type: _____
Number: _____
Location: _____

Urine output
I & O ☑
Strain urine ☐
Indwelling catheter ☐
  Date inserted: _____
  Size: _____
Intermittent catheter ☐
  Frequency: _____

Side rails
Constant ☐
PRN ☐
Nights ☐

Restraints
Date: _____
Type: _____
_____

Specimens and tests
  BMG q 6 hr
24-hour collection ☐
Other (specify): _____
_____

Stools
  Occult blood X3
☐　　☐　　☐

Special notes
  Evaluate pain level q 1 hr
_____

Social services
  Consulted 1/18/08

Components of a patient care Kardex *(continued)*

The format and specific information on a Kardex will vary with the needs of the patient population. For instance, the patient care Kardex on a critical care unit would include the same basic information already shown plus information specific to the unit, including:

Monitoring
Hardwire ☑
Telemetry ☐
Arterial line ☐

Pulmonary artery
catheter ☐
Pulmonary artery
pressure:
Pulmonary artery wedge
pressure:
Other (specify): _____

Mechanical ventilation
Type: _____
Tidal volume: _____
FIo$_2$: _____
Mode: _____
Rate: _____

On an obstetrics unit, you might find this additional information on the Kardex:

Delivery
Date: _____
Time: _____
Type of delivery: _____
_____

Special procedures
Perianal rinse ☐
Sitz bath ☐
Witch hazel compress ☐
Breast binders ☐
Ice ☐
Abdominal binders ☐
Other (specify): _____

Mother
Due date: _____
Gravida: _____
Para: _____
Rh: _____
Blood type: _____
Membranes ruptured: _____
Episiotomy ☐
Lacerations ☐
RhoGAM studies?
Yes ☐ No ☐
Rubella titer?
Yes ☐ No ☐

Infant
Male ☐
Female ☐
Full term ☐
Premature ☐
Weeks: _____
Apgar score ☐
Nursing ☐
Formula ☐
Condition (specify): _____
_____
Other (specify): _____
_____

Disadvantages

- Ineffective if:
  - Not enough space for appropriate data
  - Not updated frequently
  - Not complete
  - Nurse not reading it before giving patient care
- May erroneously become the working care plan
- At most facilities, not part of the permanent record and discarded after the patient discharged

(Text continues on page 139.)

Characteristics of a computer-generated Kardex

Becoming more common, the computer-generated Kardex, as shown here, may contain information regarding medical orders, referrals, tests, diet, activity, and medications. Each facility may be different, based on the program used and information desired.

```
3/10/08      05:39                         PAGE 001
================================================================================

Stevens, James                      M 65
MR#: 000310593                      Acct#: 9400037290
DR: J. Carrio                               2/W 204-01
DX: Unstable angina                 Date:  3/10/08
Attending: Carrio, John             Location: 2W: 204A
Admitted: 3/10/08                   Printed: 3/10/08  2300
Wt: 140 lb                          Ht: 5 ft 0 in  (152.4 cm)
Kg: 63.6
DOB: 12/12/1942
Patient chief complaint: chest pain
Visit reason: Unstable angina
History/Surgeries: Arthritis, thyroid disorder

Emergency contact: Regina Stevens   Home phone: (843) 346-6859
                                    Work phone: (none)
                                    Cell phone: (842) 459-5690
================================================================================
Allergies
Medication: No known drug allergies
Food: No known food allergies
Contrast media: No known contrast allergies
Other: No known other allergies
================================================================================
Nursing orders
Order date
3/10/08          Cardiac-low fat & chol, diet
3/10/08          Activity-BRP
3/10/08          V/S per unit routine
3/10/08          Telemetry
3/10/08          Hep lock with routine care
3/10/08          O2 2l prn
3/10/08          ECG with c/o chest pain

Laboratory orders
Order date                       Service date
3/10/08          Cardiac enzymes     2000 3/10/08 Complete
3/10/08          Troponin I          2000 3/10/08 Complete
3/10/08          Cardiac enzymes     0400 3/11/08
3/10/08          Troponin I          0400 3/11/08
3/10/08          BMP                 0400 3/11/08

Ancillary orders
Order date                       Service date
3/10/08          ECG                 2000 3/10/08 Complete
3/10/08          ECG                 0400 3/10/08
```

Characteristics of a computer-generated Kardex

(continued)

```
3/10/08      05:39                          PAGE 001
==============================================================================
Stevens, James                        M 65
MR#: 000310593            Acct#: 9400037290
DR: J. Carrio                        2/W 204-01
DX: Unstable angina         Date:    3/10/08
Attending: Carrio, John     Location: 2W: 204A
Admitted: 3/10/08           Printed: 3/10/08   2300
Wt: 140 lb                  Ht: 5 ft 0 in  (152.4 cm)
Kg: 63.6
DOB: 12/12/1942
Patient chief complaint: chest pain
Visit reason: Unstable angina
History/Surgeries: Arthritis, thyroid disorder

Emergency contact: Regina Stevens   Home phone: (843) 346-6859
                                    Work phone: (none)
                                    Cell phone: (842) 459-5690
==============================================================================
Allergies
Medication: No known drug allergies
Food: No known food allergies
Contrast media: No known contrast allergies
Other: No known other allergies
==============================================================================

3/10/08       Exercise stress       0800 03/11/08
3/10/08       Chest X-ray           0500 03/11/08

Problem-focused care
Assessment                    Last performed          RN
Cardiovascular care           03/10/08 2100           JK
Pain care                     03/10/08 2100           JK
Fall risk                     03/10/08 2100           JK

Daily care                    Last performed          RN
ADLs                          03/10/08 2100           JK
Care plan review              03/10/08 2100           JK

Education/Discharge planning
Education: Interdisciplinary   03/10/08               JK
Discharge planning             ongoing

Home medications
Patient's home medication list
Medication-Strength      Dose/Route       Frequency     Reason
Synthroid                50 mcg           daily
```

(continued)

Characteristics of a computer-generated Kardex

(continued)

```
3/10/08     05:39                        PAGE 001
================================================================================

Stevens, James                       M 65
MR#: 000310593               Acct#: 9400037290
DR: J. Carrio                        2/W 204-01
DX: Unstable angina          Date:  3/10/08
Attending: Carrio, John      Location: 2W: 204A
Admitted: 3/10/08            Printed: 3/10/08  2300
Wt: 140 lb                   Ht: 5 ft 0 in  (152.4 cm)
Kg: 63.6
DOB: 12/12/1942
Patient chief complaint: chest pain
Visit reason: Unstable angina
History/Surgeries: Arthritis, thyroid disorder

Emergency contact: Regina Stevens   Home phone: (843) 346-6859
                                    Work phone: (none)
                                    Cell phone: (842) 459-5690
================================================================================
Allergies
Medication: No known drug allergies
Food: No known food allergies
Contrast media: No known contrast allergies
Other: No known other allergies
================================================================================

Current medications
Medication                   Dose        Frequency      Route      Reason

Scheduled
Synthroid                    50 mcg      Daily          PO
Nitroglycerin ointment 2%    1 inch      q6h            Topical

PRN
Nitroglycerin spray          1 spray     q5min x3       PO         chest pain
Morphine sulfate             2 mg        q1h            IV         chest pain


Monogram                     Name                       Nurse type
JK                           Jane Killian               RN

                             Last page
```

Documentation guidelines

▪ Make the Kardex more effective by tailoring the information to the needs of your particular setting.

▪ Document information that helps nurses plan daily interventions (for example, the time a particular patient prefers to bathe, his food preferences before and during chemotherapy, and which analgesics or positions are usually required to ease pain).

If you're documenting on a medication administration record (MAR)—also known as a *medication Kardex*—follow these guidelines:

▪ Be sure to document the date and time of the administration, the medication dose and route, and your initials.

▪ Indicate when you administer a stat dose and, if appropriate, the specific number of doses ordered or the stop date.

▪ Write legibly, using only standard abbreviations accepted or approved by your facility. When in doubt about how to abbreviate a term, spell it out.

▪ After giving the first dose of a medication, sign your full name, your licensure status, and your initials in the appropriate space.

▪ After withholding a medication dose, document which dose wasn't given (usually by circling the time it was scheduled or by drawing an asterisk) and the reason it was omitted (for example, withholding oral medications from a patient the morning of scheduled surgery).

▪ If your MAR doesn't have space for information, such as the parenteral administration site, the patient's response to medications given as needed, or deviations from the medication order, record this information in the progress notes.

Graphic forms

Used for 24-hour assessments, graphic forms usually have a column of data printed on the left side of the page, times and dates printed across the top, and open blocks within the side and top borders. You'll use graphic forms to plot various changes—in the patient's vital signs, weight, intake and output, blood glucose, appetite, and activity level, for instance.

Advantages

▪ Presents information at a glance
▪ Allows trending of data and quick identification of patterns
▪ Saves time because documentation easier

Using a graphic form

Plotting information on a graphic form, such as the sample shown here, helps you visualize changes in your patient's temperature, blood pressure, heart rate, weight, and intake and output.

GRAPHIC FORM

Instructions: Indicate temperature in "O" and pulse in "X"

DATE				3/5/08			3/6/08																	
POSTOP. DAY				2			3																	
	4	8	12	4	8	12	4	8	12	4	8	12	4	8	12	4	8	12	4	8	12	4	8	12

PULSE	TEMP.
150	106°
140	105°
130	104°
120	103°
110	102°
100	101°
90	100°
80	99° / 98.6°
70	98°
60	97°
50	96°
	95°

Pulse/temperature plots: X at 101° (first column), X at 102° and X at 101° (3/6/08 columns), X at 101°; O at 99°, O and O near 100°, O at 99°.

RESPIRATION	18		22	20	18																		
BLOOD PRESSURE	120/80		138/80	140/90	132/74																		

INTAKE	7-3	3-11	11-7	7-3	3-11	11-7	7-3	3-11	11-7	7-3	3-11	11-7	7-3	3-11	11-7
P.O.	480	800	600	300	250										
I.V.		100	100	50	100										
Blood/Colloid	250	900	0	0	0										
8-hour	730	1800	700	350	350										
24-hour		3230													
OUTPUT	7-3	3-11	11-7	7-3	3-11	11-7	7-3	3-11	11-7	7-3	3-11	11-7	7-3	3-11	11-7
Urine	800	550	500	450	225										
NG/Emesis	0	50	0	0	0										
Other	0	0	0	0	0										
8-hour	800	600	500	450	225										
24-hour		1900													
WEIGHT		150 lb													
STOOL	0	0	†	0	†										

Signature _____ *A. Murphy, RN* _____   Shift _7a-7p_

Disadvantages

- May be difficult to read if data placed on the graph aren't accurate, legible, or complete
- Loses value if needed information not documented
- Requires double-checking of transcription entries to ensure accuracy
- Must be combined with narrative documentation

 KNOW-HOW *Don't use the information on a graphic form alone because these forms don't present a complete picture of the patient's clinical condition.*

Documentation guidelines

- For greater accuracy, document on graphic forms at the same time each day.
- Document the patient's vital signs on both the graphic form and the progress notes when you give a medication, such as an analgesic, antihypertensive, or antipyretic. This provides a record of the patient's response to a drug that may produce a change in a particular vital sign.
- Document vital signs on both forms for events such as chest pain, chemotherapy, a seizure, or a diagnostic test to indicate the patient's condition at that time.
- Be sure to document legibly, to put data in the appropriate time line, and to make the dots on the graph large enough to be seen easily. (See *Using a graphic form.*)

Flow sheet

A flow sheet has vertical or horizontal columns for documenting dates, times, and interventions. You can insert nursing data quickly and concisely, preferably at the time you give care or observe a change in the patient's condition. Because flow sheets provide an easy-to-read record of changes in the patient's condition over time, they allow all members of the health care team to compare data and assess the patient's progress. They have several uses:

- Flow sheets are handy for documenting data related to a patient's activities of daily living, fluid balance, nutrition, pain management, and skin integrity.
- Flow sheets are useful for documenting nursing interventions.
- In response to a request by The Joint Commission, nurses are using these forms to document basic assessment findings and wound care, hygiene, and routine care interventions. (See *Using a flow sheet to document routine care,* pages 142 to 147.)

(Text continues on page 146.)

Using a flow sheet to document routine care

As this sample shows, a patient care flow sheet lets you quickly document your routine interventions.

PATIENT CARE FLOW SHEET

Date 1/22/08	2300–0700	
Respiratory		
Breath sounds	Clear 2330	
Treatments/results	———	
Cough/results	———	
O_2 therapy	Nasal cannula @ 2 L/min	
Cardiac		
Chest pain	None	
Heart sounds	S_1 and S_2	
Telemetry	N/A	
Pain		
Type and location	Dull ⓛ flank 0400	
Intervention	Meperidine 0415	
Pt. response	Improved from #9 to #3 in 1/2 hr	
Nutrition		
Type	———	
Toleration %	———	
Supplement	———	
Elimination		
Stool appearance	N/A	
Enema	N/A	
Results	———	
Bowel sounds	Normal all quadrants 2330	
Urine appearance	Clear, amber 0400	
Indwelling urinary catheter	N/A	
Catheter irrigations	———	

Signature: _D. Walters R N_

0700–1500	1500–2300
Crackles ℗L 0800	Clear 1600
Nebulizer 0830	———
Mod. amt. tenacious yellow mucus, 0900	———
Nasal cannula @2 L/min	Nasal cannula @ 2 L/min
None	None
Normal S_1 and S_2	Normal S_1 and S_2
N/A	N/A
Dull ℗ flank 1000	Dull ℗ flank 1600
Repositioned and meperidine 1010	Meperidine 1615
Improved from #8 to #2 in 45 min.	Complete relief in 1 hr
Regular	Regular
90%	80%
1 can Ensure	———
N/A	⊤ soft dark brown
N/A	N/A
———	———
Normal all quadrants 0800	Hyperactive all quadrants 1600
Clear, amber 1000	Dark yellow 1500
N/A	N/A
———	———
Signature: *S. Rayles RN*	Signature: *M. Forest RN*

(continued)

Using a flow sheet to document routine care *(continued)*

PATIENT CARE FLOW SHEET

Date 1/22/08	2300–0700	
I.V. therapy		
Tubing change	———	
Dressing change	———	
Site appearance	No edema, no redness 2330	
Wound		
Type	Ⓛ flank incision 2330	
Dressing change	Dressing dry and intact 2330	
Appearance	Wound not observed	
Tubes		
Type	N/A	
Irrigation	———	
Drainage appearance	———	
Hygiene		
Self/partial/complete	———	
Oral care	———	
Back care	0400	
Foot care	———	
Remove / reapply elastic stockings	0400	
Activity		
Type	Bed rest	
Repositioned	2330 Supine 0400 Ⓛ side	
ROM	———	
Sleep		
Sleeping	0400 0600	
Awake at intervals	2330 . 0400	
Awake most of the time	———	

Signature: *D. Walters R N*

0700–1500	1500–2300
1100	———
1100	———
No redness, no edema, no drainage 0800	No redness, no edema 1600
Ⓛ flank incision 1200	Ⓛ flank incision 2000
1200	2000
See progress note.	See progress note.
N/A	N/A
———	———
———	———
Partial 1000	Partial 2100
1000	2100
1000	2100
1000	———
1000	2100
OOB to chair X 20 min. 1000	OOB to chair X 20 min. 1800
Ⓛ side 0800 Ⓡ side 1400	Self
1000 (active) 1400 (active)	1800 (active) 2200 (active)
N/A	N/A
———	———
———	———
Signature: S. Rayles RN	Signature: M. Forest RN

(continued)

Using a flow sheet to document routine care *(continued)*

PATIENT CARE FLOW SHEET

Date 1/22/08	2300–0700	
Safety		
ID bracelet on	2330 0200 0400	
Side rails up	2330 0200 0400	
Call button in reach	2330 0200 0400	
Equipment		
Type IVAC pump	Continuous 2300	
Teaching		
Wound splinting	0400	
Deep breathing	0400	
Signature/Title	D. Walters R N	

PROGRESS SHEET

Date	Time	Comments
1/22/08	1200	① flank dressing saturated with serosang. drainage.
		opening noted at lower edge of incision. Small amount
		incision line. Sutures intact. Incision line cleansed
		Wong notified of increased amt. of drainage. ———
1/22/08	2000	Dr. Timothy Wong to see pt. ① flank drsg. removed. 2-cm
		T. Wong sutured opening with one 3-0 silk suture. No redness

> **KNOW-HOW** *If using a flow sheet to document, make sure that you don't neglect your other documentation responsibilities. Using a flow sheet doesn't exempt you from narrative documentation, patient teaching, patient responses, detailed interventions, or attending to unusual circumstances.*

0700–1500	1500–2300
0800 1200 1500	1600 2200
0800 1200 1500	1600 2200
0800 1200 1500	1600 2200
Continuous 0800	Continuous 1600
1000	————
1000	1600
S. Rayles RN	*M. Forest RN*

*Dressing removed. Wound edges well-approximated except for 2-cm
serosang. Drainage noted oozing from this area. No redness noted along
with NSS. 4" x 4" gauze pads applied and taped in place. Dr. Timothy*
—————————————————————————————————— *S. Rayles RN*

*opening noted at lower edges of incision. Otherwise, wound edges well-approximated. Dr.
or drng. noted along incision line. 4" x 4" gauze pads applied.* ——— *M. Forest RN*

Advantages

- Allows you to evaluate patient trends at a glance
- Reinforces nursing standards of care and allows precise nursing documentation
- Saves time

Disadvantages

■ Makes it difficult to document unusual events
■ Can lead to incomplete or fragmented documentation
■ May fail to reflect the needs of the patients and the documentation needs of the nurses on each unit
■ Adds bulk to the medical record, causing handling and storage problems and duplication of documentation
■ May cause legal problems if inconsistent with the progress notes

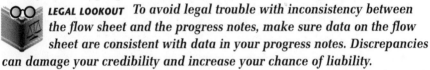 **LEGAL LOOKOUT** *To avoid legal trouble with inconsistency between the flow sheet and the progress notes, make sure data on the flow sheet are consistent with data in your progress notes. Discrepancies can damage your credibility and increase your chance of liability.*

Documentation guidelines

■ Use a flow sheet to document all routine assessment data and nursing interventions, such as the repositioning or turning of the patient, range-of-motion exercises, patient education, wound care, and medication administration.
■ Progress notes need only include the patient's progress toward achieving desired outcomes and any unplanned assessments, occurrences, or outcomes.
■ If documenting the information requested on the flow sheet isn't sufficient to give a complete picture of the patient's status, document additional information in the space provided on the flow sheet. If your flow sheet doesn't have additional space and you need to document more information, use the progress notes. If additional information isn't necessary, draw a line through this space to indicate that further information isn't required.
■ Fill out flow sheets completely, using the key symbols provided, such as a check mark, an "X," initials, circles, or the time to indicate that a parameter was observed or an intervention was carried out.
■ When necessary, use the abbreviation "N/A" (not applicable) or another abbreviation recognized by your facility.
■ Don't leave blank spaces—they imply that an intervention wasn't completed, wasn't attempted, or wasn't recognized.
■ If you have to omit something, document the reason.

Clinical pathways

A clinical pathway (also known as a *critical pathway*) integrates the principles of case management into nursing documentation. They're usually organized by categories according to the patient's diagnosis, which dictates his expected length of stay, daily care guidelines, and expected outcomes. The care guidelines specified for each day may be organized into various categories, and the structure and categories may vary from one facility to the next, depending on which are appropriate for the specific diagnosis-related group. Categories include:

- activity
- diet or nutrition
- discharge planning
- medications
- patient teaching
- treatments.

For an example of a completed clinical pathway, see *Following a clinical pathway,* pages 150 and 151.

Advantages

- Can eliminate duplicate documentation if used as a permanent documentation tool
- Allows for narrative notes to be written only when a standard on the pathway remains unmet or when the patient's condition warrants a deviation in care as planned on the pathway
- Becomes part of the patient's permanent record
- Allows nurses to advance the patient's activity level, diet, and treatment regimens without waiting for a physician's order as long as standardized orders or standing protocols have been determined and accepted
- Improves communication among all members of the health care team because everyone works from the same plan
- Improves quality of care due to the shared accountability for patient outcomes
- Improves patient teaching and discharge planning
- May decrease length of stay

(Text continues on page 152.)

Following a clinical pathway

At any point in a treatment course, a glance at the clinical pathway allows you to compare the patient's progress and your performance as a caregiver with care standards. Here is a sample pathway.

CLINICAL PATHWAY: COLON RESECTION WITHOUT COLOSTOMY

	Patient visit	Presurgery Day 1	O.R. Day	Postop Day 1
Assessments	History and physical with breast, rectal, and pelvic exam Nursing assessment	Nursing admission assessment	Nursing admission assessment on TBA patients in holding area Review of systems assessment*	Review of systems assessment*
Consults	Social service consult Physical therapy consult	Notify referring physician of impending admission	Type and screen for patients in holding area with Hgb <10	
Labs and diagnostics	Complete blood count (CBC) PT/PTT ECG Chest X-ray (CXR) Chem profile CT scan ABD w/wo contrast CT scan pelvis Urinalysis Barium enema & flexible sigmoidoscopy or colonocopy Biopsy report	Type and screen for patients with hemoglobin (Hgb) <10		CBC
Interventions	Many or all of the above labs/diagnostics will have already been done. Check all results and fax to the surgeon's office.	Admit by 8 a.m. Check for bowel prep orders Bowel prep* Antiembolism stockings Incentive spirometry Ankle exercises* I.V. access* Routine vital signs (VS)* Pneumatic inflation boots	Shave and prep in O.R. Nasogastric (NG) tube maint.* Intake and output (I/O) VS per routine* Catheter care* Incentive spirometry* Ankle exercises* I.V. site care* Head of bed (HOB) 30°* Safety measures* Wound care* Mouth care*	NG tube maintenance* I/O* VS per routine* Catheter care* Incentive spirometry* Ankle exercises* I.V. site care* HOB 30°* Safety measures* Wound care* Mouth care* Antiembolism stockings
I.V.s		I.V. fluids, $D_5\frac{1}{2}$ NSS	I.V. fluids, D_5LR	I.V. fluids, D_5LR
Medication	Prescribe GoLYTELY or Nulytely 10a—2p Neomycin @ 2p, 3p, and 10p Erythromycin @ 2p, 3p, and 10p	GoLYTELY or Nulytely 10—2p Erythromycin @ 2p, 3p, and 10p Neomycin @ 2p, 3p and 10p	Preop antibiotics (ABX) in holding area Postop ABX × 2 doses Patient-controlled analgesia (PCA) (basal rate 0.5 mg) subQ heparin	PCA (basal rate 0.5 mg) subQ heparin
Diet/GI	Clears presurgery day NPO after midnight	Clears presurgery day NPO after midnight	NPO/NG tube	NPO/NG tube
Activity			4 hours after surgery, ambulate with abdominal binder* Discontinue pneumatic inflation boots once patient ambulates	Ambulate t.i.d. with abdominal binder* May shower Physical therapy b.i.d.

KEY:
* = NSG activities
V = Variance
N = No var.
Signatures:

1.	2.	3.	1.	2.	3.	1.	2.	3.	1.	2.	3.
V	V	N	V	V	V						
N	N	N									
1. *E. Malloy, R.N.* 1/10/08			1. *M. Oconel, R.N.* 2/15/08			1. *L. Singer, R.N.* 2/16/08			1. *L. Singer, R.N.* 2/17/08		
2. _____			2. *C. Roy, R.N.* 2/15/08			2. *J. Smith, R.N.* 2/16/08			2. *J. Smith, R.N.* 2/17/08		
3. _____			3. *J. Kim, RN* 2/15/08			3. *D. Joseph, R.N.* 2/16/08			3. *D. Joseph, R.N.* 2/17/08		

Following a clinical pathway (continued)

CLINICAL PATHWAY: COLON RESECTION WITHOUT COLOSTOMY

	Postop Day 2	Postop Day 3	Postop Day 4	Postop Day 5
Assessments	Review of systems assessment*	Review of systems assessment*	Review of systems assessment*	Review of systems assessment*
Consults		Dietary consult		Oncology consult if indicated (or to be done as outpatient)
Labs and diagnostics	Electrolyte 7 (EL-7) CXR	CBC EL-7	Pathology results on chart	CBC EL-7
Interventions	Discontinue NG tube if possible* (per guidelines) I/O* VS per routine* Discontinue catheter* Ambulating* Incentive spirometry* Ankle exercises* I.V. site care* HOB 30°* Safety measures* Wound care* Mouth care* Antiembolism stockings	I/O* VS per routine* Incentive spirometry* Ankle exercises* I.V. site care* Safety measures* Wound care* Antiembolism stockings	I/O* VS per routine* Incentive spirometry* Ankle exercises* I.V. site care* Safety measures* Wound care* Antiembolism stockings	Consider staple removal Replace with Steri-Strips Assess that patient has met discharge criteria*
I.V.s	I.V. fluids $D_5\frac{1}{2}$ NSS+ MVI	I.V. convert to Heplock	Heplock	Discontinue Heplock
Medication	PCA (0.5 mg basal rate)	Discontinue PCA P.O. analgesia Resume routine home meds	P.O. analgesia Preoperative meds	P.O. analgesia Preoperative meds
Diet/GI	Discontinue NG tube per guidelines: (Clamp tube at 8 a.m. if no N/V and residual <200 ml, Discontinue tube @ 12 noon)* (Check with physician first)	Clears if pt. has BM/flatus Advance to postop diet if tolerating clears (at least one tray of clears)*	Regular	Regular
Activity	Ambulate q.i.d. with abdominal binder* May shower Physical therapy b.i.d.	Ambulate at least q.i.d. with abdominal binder* May shower Physical therapy b.i.d.	Ambulate at least q.i.d. with abdominal binder* May shower Physical therapy b.i.d.	Ambulate ad lib with abdominal binder
Teaching	Reinforce preop teaching* Patient and family education p.r.n.* re: family screening	Reinforce preop teaching* Patient and family education p.r.n.* re: family screening Begin discharge teaching	Reinforce preop teaching* Patient and family education p.r.n.* Discharge teaching re: reportable s/s, F/U and wound care*	Review all discharge instructions and Rx including* follow-up appointments: with surgeon within 3 weeks, with oncologist within 1 month if indicated
KEY: * = NSG activities V = Variance N = No var. **Signatures:**	1. 2. 3. V V V Ⓝ Ⓝ Ⓝ 1. *H. McCarthy, RN* 2/16/08 2. *R. Mayer, RN* 2/18/08 3. *P. Drake, RN* 2/18/08	1. 2. 3. V V V Ⓝ Ⓝ Ⓝ 1. *H. McCarthy, RN* 2/19/08 2. *R. Mayer, RN* 2/19/08 3. *P. Drake, RN* 2/19/08	1. 2. 3. V V V Ⓝ Ⓝ Ⓝ 1. *L. Singer, RN* 2/20/08 2. *J. Smith, RN* 2/20/08 3. *D. Joseph, RN* 2/20/08	1. 2. 3. V V V Ⓝ Ⓝ Ⓝ 1. *L. Singer, RN* 2/21/08 2. *J. Smith, RN* 2/21/08 3. *D. Joseph, RN* 2/21/08

KNOW-HOW *If your facility uses clinical pathways, check its policy to see if it allows certain adapted clinical pathways to be distributed to patients. Some facilities find that many patients feel less anxiety and cooperate more with therapy when they know what to expect.*

Disadvantages

■ Most effective for a patient who has only one diagnosis; less effective for a patient with several diagnoses or one who experiences complications (because of the difficulty establishing a time line for such a patient)
■ Lengthy, fragmented documentation possible (if the care plan is likely to change)

Documentation guidelines

■ When writing a clinical pathway, collaborate with the physician and other members of the health care team. Standardized orders for the clinical pathway require the physician's signature on admission of the patient.
■ To ensure consistent documentation from shift to shift, review the clinical pathway during the change-of-shift report with the nurse who's taking over. Point out critical events, note changes in the patient's expected length of stay, and discuss variances that may have occurred during your shift.
■ If an objective for a particular day remains unmet, document this fact on the appropriate form as justifiable or unjustifiable.
■ When developing a clinical pathway to distribute to patients, use simple vocabulary, keep your instructions short, and avoid unapproved abbreviations and complex medical terminology. Explain the diagnosis, review tests and care the patient can expect, and inform him about activity restrictions, diet, medications, and home health care services.

Patient-teaching plans

Standard-setting and reimbursing agencies require health care facilities to instruct patients about their condition and treatment regimen. Teaching plans must meet your patient's particular needs. (See *Filing a teaching plan,* pages 154 and 155.) When constructing a teaching plan, follow these steps:

- Assess the patient's cognitive level, any barriers to learning (such as language, hearing loss, illiteracy, cultural beliefs, or others), and what he already knows about the topic.
- Compile learning outcomes or objectives—a list of topics and strategies that the patient needs to know or perform to attain his maximum level of health and selfcare.
- Use available teaching activities, methods, and tools (such as brochures, one-on-one discussions, and videotapes) to convey and reinforce the information.

The instructive elements and activities should:
- define the patient's condition
- identify risk factors associated with the patient's condition
- explain what causes the patient's condition and variations of the patient's condition
- point out the importance of therapy, emphasizing, if necessary, the consequences of untreated disease
- explain the goals of treatment and identify the components of the treatment plan
- define the patient's anticipated learning outcomes and provide a time frame
- evaluate patient understanding through verbalization of topics discussed and demonstration of skills learned, if indicated.

Advantages

- Becomes part of the patient's care plan, which is part of the medical record
- Communicates to other health care team members what the patient has been taught and what teaching is still necessary
- Shows performance-improvement measures in progress and meets professional and accrediting requirements

Disadvantages

- May fail to be specific enough for unusual teaching circumstances
- May cause legal problems if incomplete

Filing a teaching plan

Your teaching plan should include your assessment findings; projected learning outcomes, methods, and tools to accomplish the outcomes; and the techniques you'll use to evaluate the effectiveness of teaching.

This teaching plan was structured for a patient who has heart failure.

Patient *Harold Harmon*   Date: *1/13/08*

Assessment findings	Expected learning outcomes
Learning need: heart failure	*H. Harmon will:*
	—explain how to identify fluid increase
	—discuss behaviors that increase incidence of
	heart failure.
Learning need: medication information	*H. Harmon will:*
(digoxin)	*—explain the reason for digoxin*
	—state when to take digoxin
	—state possible adverse effects.
Learning need: how to obtain a pulse	*H. Harmon will:*
	—demonstrate how to obtain his pulse.
Learning need: coping skills for anxiety	*H. Harmon will:*
	—describe two techniques that will help him
	relax.

Documentation guidelines

- When writing the teaching plan, be sure to follow the nursing process.
- Keep the plan succinct and precise.

Teaching methods	Teaching tools	Evaluation methods
Discussion	Patient teaching guide with information regarding heart failure	Discussion/question and answer
Discussion	Printed material describing digoxin and possible adverse effects	Discussion/question and answer
Demonstration Supervised practice sessions Discussion	Demonstration	Demonstration
Discussion	Printed material regarding relaxation techniques for suggestion Discussion	Demonstration Discussion

■ Talk with the patient and his family about the patient-teaching plan and agree on realistic learning outcomes. Encourage participation in the plan. Doing so usually increases his cooperation and your effectiveness.

Patient-teaching forms

Although patient-teaching forms vary according to the health care facility, most contain general information about the patient's learning abilities, goals to be met, and skills to be acquired by the time of discharge. You can document information by filling in blanks, checking boxes, or writing brief narrative notes. (See *Documenting your teaching.*)

Advantages

- Makes documenting patient teaching quicker and easier by creating a record of a patient's outcomes, responses, and level of learning
- Provides a legal defense against charges of inadequate patient care
- Prevents duplication of patient-teaching efforts by other staff members and other disciplines
- Provides a tool for performance improvement

Disadvantages

- If not used by all disciplines, may provide incomplete, inconsistent, or scattered documentation
- May fail to be specific enough for unusual teaching circumstances

Documentation guidelines

- When filling out patient-teaching forms, include the patient's learning ability, his response to teaching, and the outcomes.
- Check your facility's policies and procedures regarding when, where, and how to document your teaching. If your facility doesn't have a preprinted form, talk to your supervisor about developing one. In the meantime, document your patient teaching in accurate, detailed progress notes.
- Each shift, ask yourself these questions: What part of the teaching plan did I complete? What other instruction did I give the patient or his family? Document your answers.
- Document that the patient's ongoing educational needs are being met.
- Before discharge, document the patient's remaining learning needs and note whether you provided him with printed or other patient-teaching aids.

(Text continues on page 162.)

Documenting your teaching

Use the model patient-teaching form here—for a patient with diabetes mellitus—as a guideline for documenting your teaching sessions clearly and completely.

PATIENT TEACHING
Instructions for Diabetic Patients
County Hospital, Waltham, MA

> Bernard Miller
> 7 Main St.
> Waltham, MA 04872

Admission date: 1/3/08   **Anticipated discharge:** 1/8/08
Diagnosis: TIA/type 2 diabetes

Educational assessment
Comprehension level
Ability to grasp concepts
☑ High
☐ Average
☐ Needs improvement
Comments: _____

Motivational level
☑ Asks questions
☐ Eager to learn
☐ Anxious
☐ Uncooperative
☐ Disinterested
☐ Denies need to learn
Comments: _____

Knowledge and skill levels
Understanding of health condition and how to manage it
☐ High (>75% working knowledge)
☐ Adequate (50% to 75% working knowledge)

☑ Needs improvement (25% to 50% working knowledge)
☐ Low (< 25% working knowledge)
Comments: _____

Learning barriers
☑ None
☐ Language (specify: foreign, impairment, laryngectomy, other): _____

☐ Vision (specify: blind, legally blind, other): _____
☐ Hearing (impaired, deaf)
☐ Memory
  ☐ Change in long-term memory (specify): _____

  ☐ Change in short-term memory (specify): _____

☐ Other (specify): _____

Anticipated outcomes
Patient will be prepared to perform self-care at the following level:
☑ High (total self-care)
☐ Moderate (self-care with minor assistance)
☐ Minimal (self-care with more than 50% assistance)

(continued)

Documenting your teaching *(continued)*

Key

P	=	patient taught	N/A	=	not applicable
F	=	caregiver or family taught	A	=	asked questions
R	=	reinforced	B	=	nonattentive, poor concentration

	1/4/08	1/5/08	1/5/08	
Date				
Time	1900	0800	1330	
Assessed educational needs				
Assessment of patient's (or caregiver's) current knowledge of disease (include medical, family, and social histories)	A/CW			
Assessment of learner's reaction to diagnosis (verbal and nonverbal responses)	A/CW			
General diabetic education goals The patient (or caregiver) will:				
▪ define diabetes mellitus.	P/A/CW	R/EG	D/ME	
▪ state hormone produced in the pancreas.	P/A/CW	R/EG	D/ME	
▪ identify three signs and symptoms of diabetes.	P/CW	R/EG	D/ME	
▪ discuss risk factors associated with the disease.	P/CW	R/EG	D/ME	
▪ differentiate between type 1 and type 2 diabetes.	P/A/CW	R/EG	D/ME	
Survival skill goals The patient (or caregiver) will:				
▪ identify the name, purpose, dose, and time of administration of medication ordered.		P/EG	R/ME	
▪ properly administer insulin.	N/A			
–draw up insulin properly.	N/A			
–discuss and demonstrate site selection and rotation.	N/A			
–demonstrate proper injection technique with needle angled appropriately.	N/A			
–explain correct way to store insulin.	N/A			
–demonstrate correct disposal of syringes.	N/A			
▪ distinguish among types of insulin.	N/A			
–species (pork, beef, recombinant DNA)	N/A			
– regular	N/A			
– NPH/Ultralente (longer acting)	N/A			
▪ Properly administer mixed insulins.	N/A			
–demonstrate injecting air into vials.	N/A			
–draw up mixed insulin properly (regular before NPH).	N/A			
▪ demonstrate knowledge of oral antidiabetic agents.				
–identify name of medication, dose, and time of administration.		P/EG	A/ME	
–identify purpose of medication.		P/EG	A/ME	
–state possible adverse effects.		P/EG	A/ME	

C = expressed denial, resistance
D = verbalized recall
E = demonstrated ability

| 1/5/08 | 1/6/08 | 1/7/08 | 1/7/08 | 1/8/08 |
1830	1000	0800	1830	0800
				D/EG
				D/EG
				D/EG
				D/EG
				D/EG
D/LT				D/EG
	D/EG	F/EG	R/LT	D/EG
	D/EG	F/EG	R/LT	D/EG
	D/EG	F/EG	R/LT	D/EG

(continued)

Documenting your teaching *(continued)*

Date	1/4/08	1/5/08	1/5/08
Time	1900	0800	1330
▪ list signs and symptoms, causes, implications, and treatments of hyperglycemia and hypoglycemia.		P/EG	A/ME
▪ monitor blood glucose levels satisfactorily.			
– demonstrate proper use of blood glucose monitoring device.			
– perform fingerstick.			
– obtain accurate blood glucose reading.			
Healthful living goals The patient (or caregiver) will:			
▪ consult with the nutritionist about meal planning.			P/ME
▪ follow the diet recommended by the American Diabetes Association.			P/ME
▪ state importance of adhering to diet.			P/ME
▪ give verbal feedback on 1-day meal plan.			P/ME
▪ state the effects of stress, illness, and exercise on blood glucose levels.			P/ME
▪ state when to test urine for ketones and how to address results.			P/ME
▪ identify self-care measures for periods when illness occurs.			P/ME
▪ list precautions to take while exercising.			P/ME
▪ explain what steps to take when patient doesn't want to eat or drink on proper schedule.			P/ME
▪ agree to wear medical identification (for example, a MedicAlert bracelet).			P/ME
Safety goals The patient (or caregiver) will:			
▪ state the possible complications of diabetes.	P/CW	R/EG	
▪ explain the importance of careful, regular skin care.	P/CW	R/EG	
▪ demonstrate healthful foot care.	P/CW	R/EG	
▪ discuss the importance of regular eye care and examinations.	P/CW	R/EG	
▪ state the importance of oral hygiene.	P/CW	R/EG	
Individual goals			

Initial	Signature			
CW	Carol Witt, R.N, B.S.N			
EG	Ellie Grimes, RN, MSN			
ME	Marianne Evans, RN			
LT	Lynn Tata, RN, BSN			

| 1/5/08 | 1/6/08 | 1/7/08 | 1/7/08 | 1/8/08 |
1830	1000	0800	1830	0800
		F/EG		D/EG
P/LT	E/EG	E/EG	R/LT	E/EG
P/LT	E/EG	E/EG	R/LT	E/EG
P/LT	E/EG	E/EG	R/LT	E/EG
R/LT	A/EG			D/EG
R/LT	A/EG			D/EG
R/LT	A/EG			D/EG
D/LT	A/EG			D/EG
D/LT	A/EG			D/EG
D/LT	A/EG			D/EG
D/LT	A/EG			D/EG
D/LT	A/EG			D/EG
D/LT	A/EG			D/EG
A/LT				D/EG
D/LT		F/EG		D/EG
D/LT		F/EG		D/EG
D/LT		F/EG		D/EG
D/LT				
D/LT				

Evaluating your teaching: The checklist method

A checklist is a simple, quick way of obtaining information, evaluating your teaching, and gauging your patient's progress at various learning stages. It clearly shows you and your patient which goals he has achieved and which goals remain. A checklist should follow these tips:

■ The list is concise but wide-ranging enough to cover all aspects of the skill or activity being evaluated.

■ The items on the checklist are limited to a group of related activities, such as the steps in tracheostomy care or the segments of a cardiac rehabilitation plan.

■ The items are arranged in a logical order—sequentially, chronologically, or in order of importance.

■ The essential steps of the activities or behavior to evaluate are identified.

■ The items on the list are related to the patient's learning goal and to the teaching methods.

■ Only one idea or concept is used for each item.

■ Each item is phrased succinctly and accurately.

   The sample checklist here might be used for evaluating how well a diabetic patient has learned to draw up insulin.

	DRAWING UP INSULIN	
Yes	**No**	
☐	☐	Disinfects top of vial thoroughly
☐	☐	Inserts needle into vial without contamination
☐	☐	Withdraws proper amount of insulin
☐	☐	Expels air from syringe
☐	☐	Retains exact dose of insulin in syringe
☐	☐	Replaces cap on needle without contamination

■ Evaluate your teaching. One way is by using a checklist. (See *Evaluating your teaching: The checklist method.*)

Discharge summary–patient instruction form

To comply with Joint Commission requirements related to discharge planning, you must document your assessment of a patient's continuing care needs as well as any referrals for such care. To facilitate this kind of documentation, many health care facilities combine discharge summaries and patient instructions in one form. On such forms, a narrative style coexists with open- and closed-ended styles.

Another form summarizes the discharge plans made by the different services on one page, emphasizing and documenting a team approach to discharge planning. This form is started at admission, updated during the hospital stay, and completed as discharge arrangements are finalized. (See *Using a discharge document,* pages 164 and 165.)

Advantages

- Provides useful information about additional teaching needs
- Documents physician discharge orders for home care, activity, diet, medications
- Provides information regarding follow-up care
- Establishes compliance with Joint Commission requirements
- Helps safeguard the nurse from malpractice accusations

Disadvantages

- Usually completed by the nurse without multidisciplinary input
- May not provide for unusual circumstances related to discharge

Documentation guidelines

- On discharge, give your patient a copy of his discharge instructions and document his receipt of them and that the instructions were reviewed.
- Document a final physical assessment, including vital signs.
- Document the date, time, location, and mode of discharge.
- Outline the patient's care, provide useful information for further teaching and evaluation, and document that the patient has the information he needs to care for himself or to get further help.

(Text continues on page 166.)

Using a discharge document

Many health care facilities use a discharge form. This sample form has spaces that can be filled in by the nurse, physician, and other health care providers.

ADMISSION/DISCHARGE DOCUMENT

Patient name: _Mary Mayer_

Address: _312 Woodlake Drive_

Philadelphia, PA 19111

Birth date: _4/12/41_

Patient no.: _34719284_

Physician: _Dr. Michael Bloom_

Date of admission: _2/1/08_

HMO no.: _43217575_

Discharge date: _2/9/08_   Unit: _SN_

Discharged to:	Discharged by:	Accompanied by:
☑ Home	☐ Ambulatory	_husband_
☐ Transfer to:	☑ Wheelchair	
	☐ Stretcher	

Valuables w/patient ☑ Y ☐ N

Meds w/patient   ☑ Y ☐ N

I.V. access DC'd   ☑ Y ☐ N

Discharge planning

1. Name _Frank Mayer_

Phone (H) _555-492-7342_

2. Name _Rose Hayes_

Phone (H) _555-492-1965_

3. Name _____

Phone (H) _____

4. Name _____

Phone (H) _____

5. Name _____

Phone (H) _____

Family/Friend contacts

Relationship _Husband_

(W) _____

Relationship _Sister_

(W) _____

Relationship _____

(W) _____

Relationship _____

(W) _____

Relationship _____

(W) _____

Health team referrals

Date	Discipline contacted	Reason	Signature
2/1/08	Nutritional services	Dietary compliance	C. Weir, RN
2/5/08	Respiratory therapy	Treatments	P. Cummins, RT
2/7/08	Physical therapy	Weight bearing	L. Doyle, RN

Supplies/Equipment needed at home

Date	Item	Provider	Signature
2/8/08	Walker	DME R US	B. Frank, MSW
2/8/08	O₂ supplies	DME R US	B. Frank, MSW

Using a discharge document *(continued)*

Community resources — Resource information provided (list resources)

Date		Signature
2/9/08	1. Meals On Wheels	B. Frank, MSW
	2.	
	3.	
	4.	

Education needs — Teaching topic completed
(refer from 24-hour document)

Date		Signature
2/1/08	1. Medication: Digoxin	C. Weir, RN
2/2/08	2. Low-salt diet restrictions	D. Brown, NT
2/4/08	3. Taking a pulse	C. Weir, RN
2/6/08	4. Diagnosis: Heart failure	C. Weir, RN
	5.	
	6.	
	7.	
	8.	

Medications on discharge

1. Digoxin 0.125 mg daily p.o.
2.

Follow-up

1. Appt. with Dr. Michael Bloom on 2/20/08 @ 10 AM
2.

Learning ability — Knowledge assessment of discharge needs

Date		Patient	Caregiver (Indicate relationship)		Signature
2/9/08	States diagnosis/disease	☑Y ☐N	☑Y ☐N	husband	C. Weir, RN
2/9/08	States prognosis	☑Y ☐N	☑Y ☐N		C. Weir, RN
2/9/08	States medication regimen	☑Y ☐N	☑Y ☐N		C. Weir, RN
2/9/08	States complications	☑Y ☐N	☑Y ☐N		C. Weir, RN
2/9/08	Asks pertinent questions	☑Y ☐N	☑Y ☐N		C. Weir, RN
2/9/08	Other	☐Y ☑N	☐Y ☑N		C. Weir, RN

Dictated documentation

In some situations, nurses dictate from a nursing unit or clinical setting, and clerical personnel transcribe the information for the written clinical record. This occurs commonly among visiting nurses who may dictate into a recorder or a cell phone between patient visits.

Advantages

- Convenient and highly accurate
- Can be performed without the distractions and interruptions encountered in a clinical setting
- Allows the nurse more time for patient care
- Can be done at any time of day or night
- Complies with accreditation and regulatory standards such as Joint Commission standards
- May actually improve the quality of documentation

Disadvantages

- If delayed, can prevent necessary documentation from being made readily available to physicians and other health care team members
- More costly than handwritten documentation
- May require an adjustment period for staff unaccustomed to this type of documentation

Documentation guidelines

- Refer to your health care facility's policy and procedures manual for dictation guidelines, and consult the transcriptionist if you have related questions.
- Before dictating a report, familiarize yourself with the recording equipment. Then review the existing records and the notations you made during contact with your patient.
- Prepare a brief outline of your report so that it illustrates the nursing process.
- At the beginning of your dictation, name the patient and state his identification number.
- Tell the transcriptionist when the report begins and ends. Be sure to provide the date of the report and the date of the visit with the patient. Instruct the transcriptionist to provide the date of transcription. At the end of the report, include a summary, evaluation, and recommendations. Discuss your plans for the next time you'll see the patient.

■ Use a checklist as you dictate to make sure that you include all the necessary information. For example, state the purpose of your time with the patient, list assessments performed and findings, discuss any new or changing patient problems, list interventions and patient responses, identify future care needs, explain patient teaching provided, and describe the patient's response.

■ Try to dictate the information as near to the time that you provided care as possible so that your activities and observations are fresh in your mind.

■ Speak clearly and slowly, avoiding unnecessary medical terminology or uncommon abbreviations.

■ If you need to add information or change something you've said, give the transcriptionist clear and specific directions.

Patient self-documentation

Although self-documentation obviously isn't feasible or desirable for every patient, it can be effective for those who must perform considerable self-care (patients with diabetes, for example) or for patients trying to discover what precipitates a problem (such as those with chronic headaches). (See *Teaching self-documentation skills,* pages 168 and 169.)

Advantages

■ Can be used in inpatient and outpatient care settings
■ May become a permanent part of the medical record, depending on health care facility policy
■ Aids in teaching the patient about his problem and its causes, symptoms, and treatment
■ Provides needed clues to the problem's precipitators and suggests solutions to the problem
■ Improves therapeutic compliance by making the patient an active participant in his treatment and providing him with some control
■ May be more accurate than data interpreted by someone else

Disadvantages

■ Takes time, patience, planning, motivation, and perseverance—by both the nurse and the patient

Teaching self-documentation skills

For some patients, self-documentation has wide-ranging benefits. By learning to keep a log or a journal, for example, a patient may find out what triggers certain health problems (such as headaches, asthma attacks, or hypoglycemic episodes). When the trigger emerges, the patient and caregiver can implement preventive strategies.

To help a patient learn self-documentation skills, some health care facilities use individual self-documentation forms such as the sample headache log shown at right.

Reviewing instructions

Give the patient instructions and review them with him. Tell him to complete the headache log daily. Inform him that doing so may help him to identify what triggers his headaches (for example, environmental factors, foods, or stress). Explain that information collected in the log may also help him discover effective ways to relieve a headache after it starts.

Instruct the patient to describe the details of each headache in a diary, log, or small notebook.

HEADACHE LOG

Date and time headache began
2/25/08 – 5:00 p.m.

Warning signs
- ☑ Flashing lights
- ☐ Blind spots
- ☐ Colors
- ☐ Zigzag patterns
- ☐ None
- ☐ Other

Intensity
- ☐ Mild
- ☑ Moderate
- ☐ Severe
- ☐ Disabling

Duration
- ☑ Less than 4 hours
- ☐ 4 to 7.5 hours
- ☐ 8 to 11.5 hours
- ☐ 12 to 24 hours
- ☐ More than 1 day
- ☐ More than 2 days

Associated signs and symptoms
- ☐ Upset stomach
- ☑ Nausea or vomiting
- ☐ Dizziness
- ☑ Sensitivity to light
- ☐ Sensory, motor, or speech disturbances
- ☐ Other

Measures for relief
- ☑ Medication
- ☐ Rest
- ☑ Sleep
- ☐ Biofeedback
- ☐ Ice pack
- ☐ Relaxation exercises

Extent of relief
- ☐ None
- ☑ Mild
- ☐ Moderate
- ☐ Marked
- ☐ Complete

Possible triggers
Caffeine and sugar

Checking the boxes
Review these steps with the patient:
- Using the log page at right as a guide, document the date and time of the headache and any warning signs.
- Put a check mark in the appropriate box to indicate the headache's intensity.
- Next, check the box to mark how long you've had the headache.
- Check the appropriate box for other signs or symptoms that accompany your headache, such as nausea, vomiting, or sensitivity to light.

<u>**Teaching self-documentation skills**</u> *(continued)*

■ Continue by checking the steps you took to relieve the headache (for example, medication, biofeedback, rest) as well as the effectiveness of these measures.

Completing the log
Urge the patient to think carefully about the events that occurred before the headache. For instance, was his headache triggered by emotional stress, by drinking a cup of coffee, or by something else? Tell him to write down the details of such potential triggers in his log.

■ Necessity of understanding how to keep careful documentation, what's important to document, and when to document; otherwise rendering the documentation useless and possibly adversely affecting the patient's treatment and recovery

Documentation guidelines

■ Help the patient become comfortable with the documentation system he'll be using. If he's to use preprinted forms, take the time to review each aspect of a form with him. If he's to use a chart or a graph, show him how to use them. If he's to keep journal-style documentation, tell him exactly how you want him to document and, if possible, show him examples of self-documentation. (See *Keeping a record of monitored activity,* page 170.)

■ Identify the person whom the patient can contact if he has questions.

■ Emphasize the benefits of self-documentation to the patient (increased knowledge about his condition and increased control of his treatment, for example). By doing so, you may help boost his interest in keeping his records updated.

■ Finally, show him the results of his self-documentation, pointing out how or what the data contribute to his treatment.

Keeping a record of monitored activity

In many situations, your patient can provide more information more accurately than a member of the health care team can. For example, a patient who wears a Holter monitor to evaluate the effect of medication on his heart and his daily activities is better aquainted with his status than a health care provider is.

Keeping this in mind, some health care facilities prepare patient instructional materials in conjunction with a diary-like chart (such as the example shown here), which the patient refers to and completes for the medical record.

Date	Time	Activity	Feelings
1/15/08	10:30 a.m.	Rode home from hospital in cab	Legs tired, felt short of breath
	11:30 a.m.	Watched TV in living room	Comfortable
	12:15 p.m.	Ate lunch, took propranolol	Indigestion
	1:30 p.m.	Walked next door to see neighbor	Felt short of breath
	2:45 p.m.	Walked home	Very tired, legs hurt
	3:00 to 4:00 p.m.	Urinated, took nap	Comfortable
	5:30 p.m.	Ate dinner slowly	Comfortable
	7:20 p.m.	Had bowel movement	Felt short of breath
	9:00 p.m.	Watched TV, drank one beer	Heart beating fast for about 1 minute, no pain
	11:00 p.m.	Took propranolol, urinated, and went to bed	Tired
1/16/08	8:15 a.m.	Woke up, urinated, washed face and arms	Very tired, rapid heartbeat for about 30 seconds
	10:30 a.m.	Returned to hospital	Felt better

Miscellaneous forms

Individual facilities or units may have specific forms that they require for documentation of specific incidents or interventions. The respiratory care department may have flow sheets where they chart ventilator settings and checks. The emergency department uses triage forms to initially evaluate patients as they come in to the department. The rapid response team (qualified health care providers who respond to critical situations for evaluation and rapid treatment) may use a specific form to document emergent interventions. (See *Rapid response documentation.*)

Rapid response documentation

The rapid response team is a group of select health care providers (such as a critical care nurse, respiratory therapist, and nursing supervisor) who respond to critical situations for rapid evaluation and treatment. The purpose of this team is to avoid code situations and to improve patient outcomes with a rapid response to potentially life-threatening situations. Here is an example of a computerized documentation of a rapid response situation.

RAPID RESPONSE DOCUMENTATION

1/13/08   0922   VXW

Date called: 1/13/08
Time called: 0800
Time arrived: 0803
End time: 0900
Responders: V. Wate, M. Brown, B. Grach
Situation: Decreased LOC

Background: Admitted 2 days ago for high blood sugars. Has insulin pump which he is taking care of himself.
Physician notification: Paul Sugarman   **Date:** 1/13/08   **Time:** 0830

Primary RN: J. Dachel
Assessment: Lethargic, diaphoretic. Capillary blood sugar—42, HR 106, BP 100/60, RR 20
Medications reviewed: Yes
Labs reviewed: Yes
Interventions: Given ½ amp 50% dextrose.

Outcome: Repeat blood sugar—75. Pt more alert. Remains on unit.

Monogram initials: VXW   **Name:** Virginia Wate

Advantages

■ Specialized documentation forms that meet the specific needs of individual departments
■ Quicker retrieval of specific information, such as ventilator settings

Disadvantages

■ Increased amount of paperwork based on the number of forms the department requires for documentation
■ Different documentation requirements at each facility; if you work in multiple places (as with agency nurses), documentation may be incomplete due to lack of knowledge of specific forms to complete

Documentation guidelines

■ Follow the guidelines for each form per department or facility.

Part two

Charting examples

A

Abuse, suspected

Abuse may be suspected in any age group, cultural setting, or environment. The patient may readily report being abused or may fear reporting the abuser. Types of suspected abuse include neglect and physical, sexual, emotional, and psychological abuse.

In most states, a nurse is required by law to report signs of abuse in children, the elderly, and the disabled. (See *Common signs of neglect and abuse*.) Use appropriate channels for your facility and report your suspicions to the appropriate administrator and agency. Document suspicions on the appropriate form for your facility and in your nurse's notes. If the patient is a child, interview the child alone and try to interview caregivers separately to note inconsistencies with histories. An injunction can be obtained to separate the abuser and the abused, ensuring the patient's safety until the circumstances can be investigated. If necessary, call local police officials for assistance.

Remember, certain cultural practices that produce bruises or burns, such as coin rubbing in Vietnamese groups, may be mistaken for child maltreatment. Regardless of cultural practices, the judgment of child maltreatment is decided by the department of child or adult welfare and the health care team. (See *Your role in reporting abuse*, page 177.)

Essential documentation

When documenting, record only the facts and not personal opinions and judgments. Record the date and time of the entry. Provide a comprehensive history, noting inconsistencies in histories, evasive answers, delays in treatment, medical attention sought at other hospitals,

Common signs of neglect and abuse

If your assessment reveals any of the following signs, consider neglect or abuse as a possible cause and document your findings. Be sure to notify the charge nurse or nurse-manager, appropriate agencies, and risk management, per facility policy.

Neglect
- Failure to thrive in infants
- Malnutrition
- Dehydration
- Poor personal hygiene
- Inadequate clothing
- Severe diaper rash
- Injuries
- Failure of wounds to heal
- Periodontal disease
- Infestations, such as scabies, lice, or maggots in a wound

Abuse
- Recurrent injuries
- Multiple injuries or fractures in various stages of healing
- Unexplained bruises, abrasions, burns, bites, damaged or missing teeth, strap or rope marks
- Head injuries or bald spots from pulling out hair
- Bleeding from body orifices
- Genital trauma
- Sexually transmitted diseases in children
- Pregnancy in young girls or women with physical or mental handicaps
- Verbalized accounts of being beaten, slapped, kicked, or involved in sexual activities
- Precocious sexual behaviors
- Exposure to inappropriately harsh discipline
- Exposure to verbal abuse and belittlement
- Extreme fear or anxiety

Additional signs
- Mistrust of others
- Blunted or flat affect
- Depression or mood changes
- Social withdrawal
- Lack of appropriate peer relationships

(continued)

Common signs of neglect and abuse *(continued)*

■ Sudden school difficulties, such as poor grades, truancy, or fighting with peers
■ Nonspecific headaches, stomachaches, or eating and sleeping problems
■ Clinging behavior directed toward health care providers
■ Aggressive speech or behavior toward adults
■ Abusive behavior toward younger children, older adults, and pets
■ Runaway behavior

---

and the person caring for the individual during the incident. Document your physical assessment findings using illustrations and photographs as necessary (per police department and social service guidelines). Describe the patient's response to treatments given. Record the names and titles of people notified within the facility. Provide the names of people notified in outside agencies, such as social services, the police department, and welfare agencies. Record any visits or evaluations by these agencies. Include any teaching or support given.

1/8/08	1700	Circular burns 2 cm in diameter noted on lower ® and ⓛ
		scapulae in various stages of healing while auscultating breath
		sounds. Pt. states these injuries occurred while playing with
		cigarettes he found at his babysitter's home. When parents
		were questioned separately as to the cause of injuries on
		child's back, mother stated the child told her he fell off a
		swing and received a rope burn. Father stated he had no
		idea of the child's injuries. Parents stated the child is being
		watched after school until they get home by the teenager
		next door, Sally Johnson. Parents stated that their son
		doesn't like being watched by her anymore, but they don't
		know why. Parents state they're looking into alternative care
		suggestions. Dr. John Gordon notified of injuries and examined
		pt. at 1645. Social worker, Nancy Stiller, and nursing supervisor,
		Nancy Taylor, RN, notified at 1650. ———— Joanne M. Allen, RN

Activities of daily living

Activities of daily living (ADLs) checklists are standard forms completed on each shift by the nursing staff and, in some cases, the patient performing the activities. After completion, you review and sign them. These forms tell the health care team members about the patient's abilities, degree of independence, and special needs so they can determine the type of assistance each patient requires. Tools that are useful in as-

LEGAL LOOKOUT

Your role in reporting abuse

As a health care provider, you play a crucial role in recognizing and reporting incidents of suspected abuse. While caring for patients, you're in a position to readily note evidence of abuse. If you do, you're required to pass along the information to the appropriate authorities. In many states, failure to report actual or suspected abuse constitutes a crime.

The Child Abuse Prevention and Treatment Act protects you against liability if you file a report. If your report is bona fide (that is, if you file it in good faith), the law protects you from any suit filed by an alleged abuser.

sessing and documenting ADLs include the Katz index, Lawton scale, and Barthel index and scale. If your facility does not use these checklists, document patient activity on the flow sheet or in your nurse's note.

Essential documentation

Be sure to include the patient's name, the date and time of the evaluation, and your name and credentials.

On the Katz index, rank your patient's ability in six areas:
- bathing
- dressing
- toileting
- moving from wheelchair to bed and returning
- continence
- feeding.

Rate your patient's ability to perform these tasks using a point system, with one point given for independence with the task and zero points for dependence. (See *Katz index*, page 178.)

The Lawton scale evaluates your patient's ability to perform complex personal care activities necessary for independent living, such as:
- using the telephone
- cooking or preparing meals
- shopping
- doing laundry
- managing finances
- taking medications
- doing housework.

Katz index

Below you'll find a sample of the Katz index, which is used to assess six basic activities of daily living.

Evaluation Form   Name *Harold Kaufmann*   Date *4/1/08*

For each area of functioning listed below, check the description that applies. Give one point for independence, zero for dependence.

Activities	Indicates independence	Indicates dependence
Bathing: Sponge bath, tub bath, or shower.	☑ Receives no assistance; gets into and out of tub, if tub is usual means of bathing.	☐ Receives assistance in bathing more than one part of the body or can't bathe.
Dressing: Gets outer garments and underwear from closets and drawers and uses fasteners, including suspenders, if worn.	☑ Gets clothes and gets completely dressed without assistance.	☐ Receives assistance in getting clothes or in getting dressed or stays partly or completely undressed.
Toileting: Goes to the room termed "toilet" for bowel movement and urination, cleans self afterward, and arranges clothes.	☑ Goes to toilet room, cleans self, and arranges clothes without assistance. May use object for support, such as cane, walker, or wheelchair, and may manage night bedpan or commode, emptying it in the morning.	☐ Doesn't go to toilet room for the elimination process.
Transfer: Gets in and out of bed to the chair.	☑ Moves into and out of bed and chair without assistance. May use object, such as cane or walker, for support.	☐ Doesn't get out of bed.
Continence: Controls elimination.	☑ Controls urination and bowel movement completely by self.	☐ Supervision helps keep control of urination or bowel movement, or catheter is used, or is incontinent.
Feeding: Provides self with nutrition.	☑ Feeds self without assistance.	☐ Receives assistance in feeding or is fed partly or completely through tubes or by I.V. fluids.

Evaluator: *Holly Sebastain, RN*

Overall score: *6*

6 = High – patient independent
0 = Low – patient dependent

Rate your patient's ability to perform these activities using a three-point scale: (1) completely unable to perform task, (2) needs some help, or (3) performs activity without help. (See *Lawton scale.*)

The Barthel index and scale (see *Barthel index,* pages 180 and 181) is used to evaluate:

- feeding

Lawton scale

The Lawton scale evaluates more sophisticated functions—known as instrumental activities of daily living—than the Katz index. Patients or caregivers can complete the form in a few minutes. The first answer in each case—except for 7a—indicates independence; the second indicates capability with assistance; and the third, dependence. In this version, the maximum score is 18, although scores have meaning only for a particular patient, as when declining scores over time reveal deterioration. Questions 4 to 6 may be gender specific; modify them as necessary.

Name *Martha Lutz*   **Rated by** *Nancy Kline, RN*   **Date** *2/13/08*

1. Can you use the telephone?
   Without help . . . .(2)
   With some help 1
   Completely unable .0

2. Can you get to places beyond walking distance?
   Without help . . . .(2)
   With some help 1
   Completely unable .0

3. Can you go shopping for groceries?
   Without help . . . .(2)
   With some help 1
   Completely unable .0

4. Can you prepare your own meals?
   Without help 2
   With some help . . . .(1)
   Completely unable .0

5. Can you do your own housework?
   Without help 2
   With some help . . . .(1)
   Completely unable .0

6. Can you do your own laundry?
   Without help . . . .(2)
   With some help 1
   Completely unable .0

7a. Do you take medicines or use any medications?
   Yes (If yes, answer Question 7b.) . . . .(Yes)
   No (If no, answer Question 7c.) . . . . .No

7b. Do you take your own medicine?
   Without help (in the right doses at the
   right times) . . . .(2)
   With some help (if someone prepares it for you
   and reminds you to take it) 1
   Completely unable .0

7c. If you had to take medicine, could you do it?
   Without help (in the right doses at the
   right times) 2
   With some help (if someone prepares it for you
   and reminds you to take it) 1
   Completely unable .0

8. Can you manage your own money?
   Without help . . . .(2)
   With some help 1
   Completely unable .0

Total Score *14*

Adapted with permission from Lawton, M.P., and Brody, E.M. "Assessment of Older People: Self-Maintaining and Instrumental Activities of Daily Living," *The Gerontologist* 9(3):179-186, Autumn 1969.

- moving from bed to chair and returning
- performing personal hygiene
- getting on and off the toilet
- bathing

(Text continues on page 182.)

Barthel index

The Barthel index, shown below, is used to assess the patient's ability to perform 10 activities of daily living, document findings for other health care team members, and reveal improvement or decline.

Date _____ 1/14/2008 _____

Patient's name _____ Joseph Amity _____

Evaluator _____ John Kaiser, RN _____

Action	Unable	With help	Independent
Feeding (if food needs to be cut = help)	0	5	⑩
Moving from chair to bed and return (includes sitting up in bed)	0	5 to ⑩	15
Personal grooming (wash face, comb hair, shave, clean teeth)	0	0	⑤
Getting on and off toilet (handling clothes, wipe, flush)	0	⑤	10
Bathing self	0	0	⑤
Walking on level surface (or, if unable to walk, use wheelchair)	0	5	⑩ or 15
Ascending and descending stairs	0	⑤	10
Dressing (includes tying shoes, fastening fasteners)	0	⑤	10
Controlling bowels	0	5	⑩
Controlling bladder	0	⑤	10

Definition and Discussion of Scoring

A person scoring 100 is continent, feeds himself, dresses himself, gets up out of bed and chairs, bathes himself, walks at least one block, and can ascend and descend stairs. This doesn't mean that he's able to live alone; he may not be able to cook, keep house, or meet the public, but he's able to get along without attendant care.

Feeding

10 = Independent. The person can feed himself a meal from a tray or table when someone puts the food within his reach. He must be able to put on an assistive device, if needed, cut the food, use salt and pepper, spread butter, and so forth. Also, he must accomplish these tasks in a reasonable time.

5 = The person needs some help with cutting food and other tasks, as listed above.

0 = Unable to do.

Moving from wheelchair to bed and return

15 = The person operates independently in all phases of this activity. He can safely approach the bed in his wheelchair, lock brakes, lift footrests, move safely from bed, lie down, come to a sitting position on the side of the bed, change the position of the wheelchair, if necessary, to transfer back into it safely, and return to the wheelchair.

10 = Either the person needs some minimal help in some step of this activity, or needs to be reminded or supervised for safety in one or more parts of this activity.

5 = The person can come to a sitting position without the help of a second person but needs to be lifted out of bed, or needs a great deal of help with transfers.

0 = Immobile.

Handling personal grooming

5 = The person can wash hands and face, comb hair, clean teeth, and shave. He may use any kind of razor but he must be able to get it from the drawer or cabinet and plug it in or put in a blade without help. A woman must put on her own makeup, if she uses any, but need not braid or style her hair.

0 = The person needs help with personal grooming.

Barthel index *(continued)*

Getting on and off toilet

10 = The person is able to get on and off the toilet, unfasten and refasten clothes, prevent soiling of clothes, and use toilet paper without help. He may use a wall bar or other stable object for support, if needed. If he needs to use a bed pan instead of toilet, he must be able to place it on a chair, use it competently, and empty and clean it.

5 = The person needs help to overcome imbalance, handle clothes, or use toilet paper.

0 = The person is dependent on other for toileting activity.

Bathing self

5 = The person may use a bath tub or shower or give himself a complete sponge bath. Regardless of method, he must be able to complete all the steps involved without another person's presence.

0 = The person is unable to bathe self.

Walking on a level surface

15 = The person can walk at least 50 yards without help or supervision. He may wear braces or prostheses and use crutches, canes, or a walkerette, but not a rolling walker. He must be able to lock and unlock braces, if used, get the necessary mechanical aids into position for use, stand up and sit down, and dispose of the aids when he sits. (Putting on, fastening, and taking off braces is scored under Dressing).

5 = If the person can't ambulate but can propel a wheelchair independently, he must be able to go around corners, turn around, maneuver the chair to table, bed, toilet, and other locations. He must be able to push a chair at least 150' (45.7 m). Don't score this item if the person receives a score for walking.

0 = Unable to walk.

Ascending and descending stairs

10 = The person can go up and down a flight of stairs safely without help or supervision. He may and should use handrails, canes, or crutches when needed, and he must be able to carry canes or crutches as he ascends or descends.

5 = The person needs help with or supervision of any one of the above items.

0 = Unable to climb stairs.

Dressing and undressing

10 = The person can put on, fasten, and remove all clothing (including any prescribed corset or braces) and tie shoe laces (unless he requires adaptations for this). Such special clothing as suspenders, loafers, and dresses that open down the front may be used when necessary.

5 = The person needs help in putting on, fastening, or removing any clothing. He must do at least half the work himself and must accomplish the task in a reasonable time. Women need not be scored on use of a brassiere or girdle unless these are prescribed garments.

0 = Dependent on others for dressing or undressing.

Controlling bowels

10 = The person can control his bowels without accidents. He can use a suppository or take an enema when necessary (as in spinal cord injury patients who have had bowel training).

5 = The person needs help in using a suppository or taking an enema or has occasional accidents.

0 = Incontinent.

Controlling bladder

10 = The person can control his bladder day and night. Spinal cord injury patients who wear an external device and leg bag must put them on independently, clean and empty the bag, and stay dry, day and night.

5 = The person has occasional accidents, can't wait for the bed pan or get to the toilet in time, or needs help with an external device.

0 = Incontinent.

The total score is less significant or meaningful than the individual items because these indicate where the deficiencies lie. Any applicant to a long-term care facility who scores 100 should be evaluated carefully before admission to see whether admission is indicated. Discharged patients with scores of 100 shouldn't require further physical therapy but may benefit from a home visit to see whether any environmental adjustments are needed.

Adapted with permission from Mahoney, F.I. and Barthel, D.W. "Functional Evaluation: The Barthel Index," *Maryland State Medical Journal* 14:61-65, 1965.

- walking on a level surface or use of a wheelchair
- going up and down stairs
- dressing and undressing
- maintaining bowel continence
- maintaining bladder continence.

Score each ADL according to the amount of assistance the patient needs. Over time, results reveal improvement or decline. Another scale, the Barthel self-care rating scale, evaluates function in more detail.

2/12/08	1000	Assisted pt. with breakfast and morning care. Pt. unable to shower
		on own, assisted with bed bath and dressing. Pt. showing difficulty
		with movement due to arthritis pain in wrist and knees. Dr. Kevin
		Devine aware. Occupational and physical therapy consulted. ———
		———————————————————————— P. Maurer, RN

Advance directive

An advance directive is a legal document used as a guideline for life-sustaining medical care of a patient with an advanced disease or disability who is no longer able to indicate his own wishes. Advance directives also include living wills (which instruct the physician regarding life-sustaining treatment) and durable powers of attorney for health care (which names another person to act on the patient's behalf for medical decisions in the event that the patient can't act for himself).

Because laws vary from state to state, be sure to find out how your state's laws apply to your practice and to the medical record.

If a patient has previously executed an advance directive, request a copy for the chart and make sure the physician is aware of it. Some health care facilities routinely make this request a part of admission procedures. If the patient does not have an advance directive, facilities will provide information on initiating one. (See *Advance directive checklist.*)

Essential documentation

Document the existence of an advance directive, and notify the physician. Include the name, address, and telephone number of the person entrusted with decision-making power. Obtain a copy of the advance

Advance directive checklist

The Joint Commission requires that information on advance directives be charted on the admission assessment form. However, many facilities also use checklists like the one shown below.

ADVANCE DIRECTIVE CHECKLIST

I. DISTRIBUTION OF ADVANCE DIRECTIVE INFORMATION

A. Advance directive information was presented to the patient: . . . . ☑
   1. At the time of preadmission testing . . . . ☑
   2. Upon inpatient admission . . . . ☐
   3. Interpretive services contacted . . . . ☐
   4. Information was read to the patient . . . . ☐
B. Advance directive information was presented to the next of kin as
  the patient is incapacitated . . . . ☐
C. Advance directive information wasn't distributed as the patient is
  incapacitated and no relative or next of kin was available . . . . ☐

Susan Long, RN   4/01/08
    RN   Date

	Upon admission		Upon transfer to Critical Care Unit	
II. ASSESSMENT OF ADVANCE DIRECTIVE UPON ADMISSION	**YES**	**NO**	**YES**	**NO**
A. Does the patient have an advance directive?	☑	☐	☐	☐
If yes, was the attending physician notified?	☑		☐	
B. If he has no advance directive, does the patient want to execute an advance directive?	☐	☐	☐	☐
If yes, was the attending physician notified?	☐		☐	
Was the patient referred to resources?	☐		☐	

Susan Long, RN
  RN   RN
4/01/08
  Date   Date

III. RECEIPT OF AN ADVANCE DIRECTIVE AFTER ADMISSION

A. The patient has presented an advance directive after admission
  and the attending physician has been notified.

    RN   Date

directive and place it on the patient's chart. Forward it to risk management for review if required by your facility. If the patient's wishes differ from those of his family or physician, make sure that the discrepancies are thoroughly documented in the chart.

If a patient doesn't have an advance directive, document that he was given written information concerning his rights under state law to make decisions regarding his health care. If the patient refuses information regarding an advance directive, document this refusal. Document conversations with the patient regarding his decision making. If appropriate, document that proof of competence was obtained (usually the responsibility of the medical, legal, social services, or risk management department).

3/28/08	1000	*Pt. admitted with an advance directive. Dr. Charles Wellington*
		notified at 0950 about advance directive in chart. Copy
		of advance directive read and placed in medical record,
		and copy forwarded to Melissa Edwards in Risk Manage-
		ment. Mary Gordon, pt.'s daughter, has durable power of
		attorney for health care (123 Livingston Drive, Newton,
		VT, phone: 123-456-7890). ———— Carol Edwards, RN

*A*gainst medical advice, discharge

There are many reasons why a patient leaves a health care facility against medical advice (AMA). It may be because he doesn't understand his condition or agree with his treatment, or he may have pressing personal or financial problems, want to exert control over his health care, or has religious or cultural objections to his care.

Although a patient can choose to leave a health care facility AMA at any time, the law requires clear evidence that he's mentally competent to make that choice. In most facilities, an AMA form (also known as a *responsibility release form*) serves as a legal document to protect the nurse, the physicians, and the facility if any problems arise from a patient's unapproved discharge. (See *Patient discharge against medical advice.*)

If possible, notify the attending physician of the patient's decision before the patient leaves. Provide routine discharge care, if the patient permits it. Even though your patient is leaving AMA, his rights to discharge planning and care are the same as those of a patient who's dis-

LEGAL LOOKOUT

Patient discharge against medical advice

The patient's bill of rights and the laws and regulations based on it give a competent adult the right to refuse treatment for any reason without being punished or having his liberty restricted. Some states have turned these rights into law, and the courts have cited the bills of rights in their decisions. The right to refuse treatment includes the right to leave the hospital against medical advice (AMA) any time, for any reason. All you can do is try to talk the patient out of it.

If your patient still insists on leaving AMA and your hospital has a policy on managing the patient who wants to leave, follow it exactly. Adhering to policy will help to protect the hospital, your coworkers, and you from charges of unlawful restraint or false imprisonment.

charged with medical advice. If the patient agrees, escort him to the door (in a wheelchair, if necessary), arrange for medical or nursing follow-up care, and offer other routine health care measures.

Essential documentation

Have the patient sign the AMA form, and in your notes clearly document:

- patient's reason for leaving AMA, using patient's own words if possible
- that the patient knows he's leaving AMA
- names of individuals notified of the patient's decision and the dates and times of the notifications
- notification of the physician, physician's visit, and any instructions or orders given
- explanation of the risks and consequences of the AMA discharge, as told to the patient, including the name of the person who provided the explanation
- discharge teaching and prepared materials offered to the patient
- instructions regarding alternative sources of follow-up care given to the patient
- list of those accompanying the patient at discharge and the instructions given to them

Responsibility release form

An against medical advice (AMA) form is a medical record as well as a legal document. It's designed to protect the nurse, the physician, and your institution from liability resulting from the patient's unapproved discharge.

RESPONSIBILITY RELEASE

This is to certify that I, _____ Robert Brown _____

a patient in _____ Jefferson Memorial Hospital _____

am being discharged against the advice of my doctor and the hospital administration. I acknowledge that I have been informed of the risk involved and hereby release my doctor and the hospital from all responsibility for any ill effects that may result from such a discharge. I also understand that I may return to the hospital at any time and have treatment resumed.

Robert Brown	1/4/08
[Patient's signature]	[Date]
Carl Giordano, RN	1/4/08
[Witness' signature]	[Date]

RE: _____ Robert Brown _____   Patient identification # _____ 123456 _____
[Name of patient]

- patient's destination after discharge, if known. (See *Responsibility release form.*)

Document any statements and actions reflecting the patient's mental state at the time he chose to leave the facility. This will help protect you, the physicians, and the facility against a charge of negligence. The patient may later claim that his discharge occurred while he was mentally incompetent and that he was improperly supervised while he was in that state.

Check your facility's policy regarding incident reports. If the patient leaves without anyone's knowledge or if he refuses to sign the AMA form, you may be required to complete an incident report.

If a patient refuses to sign the AMA form, document this refusal on the AMA form, and enter it in his chart. Use the patient's own words regarding his refusal.

3/4/08	1500	Pt. found in room packing his clothes. When asked why
		he was dressed and packing, he stated, "I'm tired of all
		these tests. They keep doing tests, but they still don't
		know what's wrong with me. I can't take anymore. I'm
		going home." Dr. Tom Giordano notified and came to speak
		with pt. Doctor told pt. of possible risks and consequences
		of his leaving the hospital with headaches and hyper-
		tension. Pt. agrees to see Dr. Giordano in his office in
		2 days. Prescriptions given to pt. Pt.'s wife notified, and
		she came to the hospital. She was unable to persuade
		husband to stay. Pt. signed AMA form. Discussed low Na
		diet, meds, and appt. with pt. and wife. Gave pt. drug
		information sheets. Pt. states he's going home after
		discharge. Accompanied pt. in wheelchair to main lobby
		with wife. Pt. left at 1445. —————— Lynn Nakashima, RN

Arrhythmias

Arrhythmias occur when abnormal electrical conduction or automaticity changes heart rate or rhythm, or both. Arrhythmias vary in severity from mild, asymptomatic disturbances requiring no treatment to life-threatening ventricular fibrillation, which requires immediate resuscitation. Arrhythmias are classified according to their origin (ventricular or supraventricular). Their clinical significance depends on their effect on cardiac output and blood pressure. Prompt detection and response to a patient's arrhythmia can affect his outcome.

Essential documentation

Record the date, time, and type of the arrhythmia. Place a rhythm strip or ECG on the patient's chart that confirms the arrhythmia. Document the patient's vital signs and symptoms. Record the findings of your physical assessment, such as pallor, cold and clammy skin, shortness of breath, palpitations, weakness, chest pain, dizziness, syncope, and decreased urine output. Include the activity level of the patient. Note the name of the physician notified and time of notification. If ordered, obtain a 12-lead ECG and report the results. Document your interventions and the patient's response. Include any emotional support and education given. Note any emergency measures initiated, as well as the patient's outcomes. (See *Responding to an arrhythmia,* pages 188 and 189.)

(Text continues on page 190.)

CASE CLIP

Responding to an arrhythmia

Mr. L. is a 73-year-old male who was admitted to the medical-surgical unit of the hospital for prostate surgery. His past medical history includes arthritis and heart failure. His home medications include:

- Lasix 40 mg by mouth (P.O.) daily
- Tylenol extra strength 1,000 mg P.O. as needed
- K-Lor 10 mEq P.O. daily.

His vital signs on admission were:

- temperature: 98.4° F (36.9° C)
- heart rate (HR): 100 beats/minute
- respiratory rate (RR): 25 breaths/minute
- blood pressure (BP): 139/88 mm Hg
- pulse oximetry: 93%.

On his admission assessment, it was noted that he had basilar crackles and had slight dyspnea on exertion. He was given Lasix 40 mg P.O. × 1.

His admitting laboratory work showed a potassium (K) level of 3.2 mEq/L, blood urea nitrogen level of 18 mg/dl and creatinine level of 1 mg/dl. Mr. L. admitted to already taking his K-Lor medication before he came into the hospital.

Mr. L. was placed on oxygen at 2 L/minute and his pulse oximetry increased to 96%. He appeared comfortable while sitting up in the chair. His surgery was scheduled for 0700 the next morning.

Two hours after admission, Mr. L. called the nurse and stated that he felt "strange beats" in his chest. He also reported that he felt a little dizzy. Vital signs at that time were:

- temperature: 98.7° F (37° C)
- HR: 68 beats/minute
- RR: 26 breaths/minute
- BP: 88/50 mm Hg
- pulse oximetry: 95%.

Mr. L.'s apical pulse was irregular. Cardiac monitoring was initiated and his rhythm was determined to be normal sinus rhythm with frequent premature ventricular contractions (PVCs). Within 10 minutes after initiating cardiac monitoring, Mr. L.'s rhythm showed short runs of ventricular tachycardia (3 to 4 beats). He then related to the nurse that he was having some chest pressure, which he rated a 5 on a scale of 0 to 10. His skin was diaphoretic.

The rapid response team (RRT) was notified. They reported to Mr. L.'s room within 3 minutes.

Responding to an arrhythmia *(continued)*

After a quick assessment of Mr. L.'s history, laboratory results, and medications, the RRT obtained an electrocardiogram that showed continued short runs of V-tach. An I.V. access was obtained and normal saline solution started at 100 ml/hour. A 20 mEq K rider was started and was to run over 4 hours. Cardiac monitoring was continued. Vital signs after 5 minutes were:

- HR: 88 beats/minute
- RR: 20 breaths/minute
- BP: 100/60 mm Hg
- pulse oximetry: 95%.

Mr. L. continued to complain of chest pressure at a rate of 4. He was given morphine 2 mg I.V. Cardiac enzymes and troponin levels were drawn and sent to the laboratory. After speaking with his attending physician, Mr. L. was transferred to the intermediate unit for closer monitoring. His chest pain was relieved after the morphine administration. Vital signs after transfer were:

- HR: 90 beats/minute
- RR: 16 breaths/minute
- BP: 106/80 mm Hg
- pulse oximetry: 97%.

After transfer, Mr. L.'s cardiac monitor showed occasional PVCs. After the completion of the K rider, his K level increased to 3.6 mEq/L. Mr. L. also received K-Lor 20 mEq P.O. that evening, per his physician's orders. His cardiac enzymes and troponin levels were negative.

Mr. L.'s surgery proceeded as scheduled the next morning.

3/24/08	1700	While assisting pt. with ambulation in the hallway at 1640,
		pt. c/o feeling weak and dizzy. Pt. said he was "feeling my
		heart hammering in my chest." Pt. stated he never felt like
		this before. Apical rate 170, BP 90/50, RR 24, peripheral
		pulses weak, skin cool, clammy, and diaphoretic. Denies chest
		pain or SOB. Breath sounds clear bilaterally. Pt. placed in
		wheelchair and assisted back to bed without incident. O₂ via
		NC started at 2 L/min. Dr. Janine Brown notified at 1645 and
		orders noted. Lab called to draw stat serum electrolyte and
		digoxin levels. Stat ECG revealed PSVT at a rate of 180.
		I.V. infusion of D₅W started in Ⓛ hand at 30 ml/hr with
		18G cannula. Placed pt. on continuous cardiac monitoring
		with portable monitor from crash cart. At 1650 apical rate
		180, BP 92/52, and pulses weakened all 4 extremities, lungs
		clear, skin cool and clammy. Still c/o weakness and dizziness.
		Patient transferred to telemetry unit. Report given to
		Nancy Powell, RN. Nursing supervisor, Carol Jones, RN,
		notified. ————————————— — Cathy Doll, RN

Arterial catheter insertion

An arterial catheter permits continuous measurement of systolic, diastolic, and mean pressures as well as arterial blood sampling.

After obtaining informed consent, the practitioner anesthetizes the insertion site. Under sterile technique, he then inserts the catheter into the artery and attaches it to prepared pressure tubing that is attached to a monitor via a cable.

Arterial blood pressure monitoring is indicated when highly accurate or frequent blood pressure measurements are required, when blood pressure medications are being titrated, or when frequent blood sampling is necessary.

Essential documentation

When assisting with the insertion of an arterial catheter, record the practitioner's name; date and time of insertion; insertion site; type, gauge, and length of the catheter; whether the catheter is sutured in place, and the type of dressing applied. Document systolic, diastolic, and mean pressure readings upon insertion, and then as ordered or per unit policy. Place a monitor strip of the waveform in the chart on insertion. Record circulation in the extremity distal to the insertion site by assessing color, pulses, and sensation. Include the amount of flush solution infused every shift. Document emotional support, patient teaching, and patient's understanding of the teaching. Write the date and time on the flush solution and pressure tubing. Make sure that the date of insertion and dressing application is also written on the dressing.

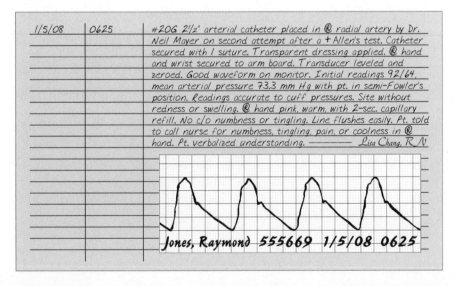

| 1/5/08 | 0625 | #20G 2½" arterial catheter placed in ® radial artery by Dr. Neil Mayer on second attempt after a + Allen's test. Catheter secured with 1 suture. Transparent dressing applied. ® hand and wrist secured to arm board. Transducer leveled and zeroed. Good waveform on monitor. Initial readings 92/64, mean arterial pressure 73.3 mm Hg with pt. in semi-Fowler's position. Readings accurate to cuff pressures. Site without redness or swelling. ® hand pink, warm, with 2-sec. capillary refill. No c/o numbness or tingling. Line flushes easily. Pt. told to call nurse for numbness, tingling, pain, or coolness in ® hand. Pt. verbalized understanding. ———— Lisa Chang, R.N |

Jones, Raymond 555669 1/5/08 0625

Arterial catheter removal

An arterial catheter is removed when it's no longer necessary, the insertion site needs to be changed, or the catheter is no longer functional. Consult your facility's policy and procedures to determine whether registered nurses with specialized training are permitted to perform this procedure. Explain the procedure to the patient, and assemble the necessary equipment. Observe standard precautions, turn off the monitor alarms, and disconnect the cable from the monitor. Carefully remove the dressing and sutures, if present. Withdraw the catheter using a gentle, steady motion. Apply pressure to the removal site for at least 10 minutes, and cover the site with an appropriate dressing.

Essential documentation

When an arterial catheter is removed, record the date and time, name of the person removing the catheter, length of the catheter, condition of the insertion site, and the reason why the catheter is being removed. Be sure to document whether a catheter specimen was obtained for culture. Record how long pressure was maintained on the site to control bleeding. Include the type of dressing applied. Document circulation in the extremity distal to the insertion site, including color, pulses, and sensation, and compare findings to those of the opposite extremity. Continue to document circulation in the distal extremity per facility policy.

3/7/08	1200	Arterial catheter removed from ℞ radial site. Insertion
		site without bruising, swelling, or hematoma. No drainage
		noted on dressing. BP 102/74, P 84, RR 16, oral T 99.7° F.
		Catheter tip sent to laboratory for culture and sensitivity.
		Pressure applied for 10 min. Sterile gauze dressing with
		povidone-iodine ointment applied. ℞ and ℄ hands warm,
		pink. Radial pulse strong. No c/o numbness, tingling, or
		pain in ℞ or ℄ hand. Will continue to check circulation to
		℞ hand according to orders. ————————Lisa Chang, RN

Arterial pressure monitoring

Used for direct arterial blood pressure monitoring, an arterial catheter permits continuous measurement of systolic, diastolic, and mean pressures. It also permits arterial blood sampling.

Direct arterial blood pressure monitoring is indicated when highly accurate or frequent blood pressure measurements are required, such as for patients with low cardiac output and high systemic vascular resistance or patients who receive titrated vasoactive drugs. Patients who need frequent blood sampling may also benefit from arterial line insertion.

Essential documentation

Document systolic, diastolic, and mean arterial blood pressure readings as indicated for the patient's condition or per unit protocol. Some facilities may use a frequent vital signs assessment sheet for this purpose. Describe the appearance of the waveform, and include a monitor strip documenting the waveform. Document a comparison with a manual blood pressure reading.

Record circulation in the extremity distal to the site by assessing and noting color, warmth, capillary refill, pulses, pain, movement, and sensation. Describe the appearance of the insertion site, noting any evidence of infection or bleeding. Document change of the tubing or flush solution, a dressing change and site care, or recalibration of the equipment. Infused flush solution is recorded on the intake and output record.

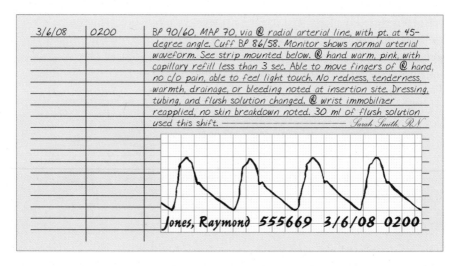

3/6/08	0200	BP 90/60, MAP 70, via ℞ radial arterial line, with pt. at 45–
		degree angle. Cuff BP 86/58. Monitor shows normal arterial
		waveform. See strip mounted below. ℞ hand warm, pink, with
		capillary refill less than 3 sec. Able to move fingers of ℞ hand,
		no c/o pain, able to feel light touch. No redness, tenderness,
		warmth, drainage, or bleeding noted at insertion site. Dressing,
		tubing, and flush solution changed. ℞ wrist immobilizer
		reapplied, no skin breakdown noted. 30 ml of flush solution
		used this shift. ———————————— *Sarah Smith, RN*

Jones, Raymond 555669 3/6/08 0200

B

Bladder irrigation, continuous

Continuous bladder irrigation can help prevent urinary tract obstruction by flushing out small blood clots that form after prostate or bladder surgery. It may also be used to treat an irritated, inflamed, or infected bladder lining.

This procedure requires placement of a triple-lumen indwelling urinary catheter. The first lumen allows balloon inflation, the second allows irrigant inflow, and the third allows irrigant outflow. The continuous flow of irrigating solution through the bladder also creates a mild tamponade that may help prevent venous hemorrhage. The catheter may be inserted in the operating room after prostate or bladder surgery, or at the bedside.

The irrigating solution typically is provided in 3-L bags (of normal saline solution) and is connected with a special bifurcated tubing that allows two bags of solution to be connected—one that is infusing, and the other on "stand-by" for a quick switch when required. Medication may be added to the irrigation solution if ordered.

Essential documentation

Each time you finish a container of solution, record the date, time, and type and amount of fluid given on the intake and output record. Include any medications added to the solution. Also record the time and amount of fluid each time you empty the drainage bag. True urine output should be calculated at the end of each shift. Note the appearance

Documenting bladder irrigation

As this sample shows, you can monitor your patient's fluid balance by using an intake and output record.

Name: Joseph Klein   Rm # 204A

Identification #: 49731

Admission date: 3/9/08

INTAKE AND OUTPUT RECORD

	INTAKE						OUTPUT				
	Oral	Tube feeding	Instilled	I.V. and IVPB	TPN	Total	Urine	Emesis	NG	Other	Total
Date 3/11/08			NSS Bladder irr.								
0700–1500	250		3000	1000		2050	3700				3700
1500–2300	200		3000	1000		2000	3850				3850
2300–0700	100		3000	1000		1900	3900				3900
24hr total	550		9000	3000		5950	11450			True o/p 2450	11450
Date											
24hr total											
Date											
24hr total											
Date											
24hr total											

Key: IVPB = I.V. piggyback   TPN = total parenteral nutrition   NG = nasogastric

Standard measures

Styrofoam cup	240 ml	Water (large)	600 ml	Milk (large)	600 ml	Ice cream, sherbet,	
Juice	120 ml	Water pitcher	750 ml	Coffee	240 ml	or gelatin	120 ml
Water (small)	120 ml	Milk (small)	120 ml	Soup	180 ml		

of the drainage and any complaints by the patient. Document any changes in the patient's condition (such as a distended bladder, clots, or bright red outflow), the name of the physician notified, date and time of notification, and actions taken. (See *Documenting bladder irrigation*.)

4/11/08	2300	3000 ml NSS irrigating solution hung at 2250, infusing
		through intake flow port at 100 gtt/min. Drainage bag
		emptied for 2500 ml of pink-tinged fluid with few small
		clots. No c/o abdominal discomfort. No bladder distention
		palpated. See I/O record for totals. ——— James Black, RN

Blood transfusion

A blood transfusion provides whole blood or a blood component, such as packed cells, plasma, platelets, or cryoprecipitates, to replace losses from surgery, trauma, or disease. With every blood product you administer, you must use proper identification and crossmatching procedures to make sure that the correct patient receives the correct blood product for transfusion to prevent a life-threatening transfusion reaction secondary to red blood cell hemolysis.

Essential documentation

Before administering any blood transfusion, verify that a physician's order has been written and that a consent form has been signed. Match the blood product to the order. Next, along with another health care provider or an automated identification system such as bar coding, clearly document that you matched the label on the blood bag to the:
- patient's name
- patient's identification number
- patient's blood group or type
- patient's and donor's Rh factor
- crossmatch data
- blood bank identification number
- expiration date of the product.

This verification must take place at the patient's bedside. When you have determined that all the information is accurate and the patient's vital signs are within acceptable parameters per your facility's policy, you may administer the transfusion. The transfusion record should contain:

■ date and time that the transfusion was started and completed
■ signature of the health care professionals who verified the information
■ total amount of the transfusion
■ patient's vital signs before the transfusion, 15 minutes after the transfusion is initiated, and after the transfusion is completed, according to facility policy
■ patient's response to the transfusion.

A copy of the transfusion record should remain with the patient's chart and another copy is sent to the laboratory for their records.

Additional documentation in the nurse's notes regarding the transfusion should include:

■ type and gauge of the I.V. catheter
■ infusion devices used (if any)
■ use of blood warmer unit
■ amount of normal saline infused
■ patient response to transfusion
■ blood count results obtained after transfusion.

If the patient receives his own blood, document the amount of autologous blood retrieved and reinfused in the intake and output records. Also monitor and document laboratory data during and after the transfusion, such as coagulation profile, hematocrit and hemoglobin, arterial blood gas, and calcium levels. Note the patient's pretransfusion and posttransfusion vital signs.

2/16/08	1015	Pt. to be transfused with 1 unit of PRBCs over 4 hr,
		according to written orders of Dr. Robert Mays. Label on
		the blood bag checked by me and Nancy Gallager, RN, who
		verified the following information on the blood slip:
		1 unit PRBCs for George Andrews, #123456, pt. and
		donor O+, Rh+ compatible crossmatch, blood bank #54321,
		expiration date 2/23/08. ———— Maryann Belinsky, RN
2/16/08	1030	Infusion of 1 unit of PRBCs started at 1025 through
		18G catheter in ① forearm at 15 ml/hr using blood
		transfusion tubing. P 82, BP 132/84, RR 16, oral T 98.2° F.
		Remained with pt. for 1st 15 min. and increased rate to
		60 ml/hr. ———— Maryann Belinsky, RN
2/16/08	1045	No c/o itching, chills, wheezing, or headache. No evidence
		of vomiting, swelling, laryngeal edema, or fever noted.
		PRBCs increased to 63 ml/hr. P 84, BP 128/82, RR 17,
		oral T 97.9° F. ———— Maryann Belinsky, RN
2/16/08	1430	Transfusion of 1 unit PRBCs complete. P 78, BP 130/78,
		RR 16, oral T 98.0° F. No c/o itching, chills, wheezing, or
		headache. No evidence of vomiting, swelling, laryngeal
		edema, or fever noted. ———— Maryann Belinsky, RN

Blood transfusion reaction

During transfusion of blood products, the patient is at risk for developing a transfusion reaction. If he develops a reaction, immediately take the following steps:

- Stop the transfusion.
- Take down the blood tubing.
- Hang new tubing with normal saline solution running to maintain vein patency.
- Notify the physician and follow facility policy for a blood transfusion reaction.
- Notify the blood bank and laboratory.
- Handle remaining blood products according to facility policy. (See *Responding to a transfusion reaction,* pages 198 and 199.)

Essential documentation

Be sure to document the date and time of the reaction, type and amount of infused blood or blood products, time you started the transfusion, and time you stopped it. Also record clinical signs of the reaction in order of occurrence, the patient's vital signs, urine specimen or blood samples sent to the laboratory for analysis, physician notification, treatment given, and the patient's response to treatment. Indicate that you sent the blood transfusion equipment (discontinued bag of

CASE CLIP

Responding to a transfusion reaction

Mrs. M. is a 59-year-old female at 2 days post–abdominal hysterectomy. She has a history of renal insufficiency and chronic anemia. Her morning laboratory results revealed a hemoglobin level of 6.2 g/dl and hematocrit of 22%. She was ordered to receive 2 units of packed red blood cells (PRBCs) to infuse over 3 hours each.

Mrs. M. was typed and screened before her surgery. She had also signed a consent for blood products at that time.

The first infusion of PRBCs was infused without incident. The nurse obtained the second unit of PRBCs and started the infusion at 1315. Vital signs at the start of the infusion were:

- temperature: 98.6° F (37° C)
- heart rate (HR): 90 beats/minute
- respiratory rate (RR): 16 breaths/minute
- blood pressure (BP): 110/76 mm Hg
- pulse oximetry: 98%.

At 1325, Mrs. M. started to complain of "feeling funny" and reported that she felt slightly short of breath with slight difficulty swallowing. Lung sounds revealed bibasilar crackles. Vital signs at this time were:

- temperature: 101.1° F (38.4° C)
- HR: 118 beats/minute
- RR: 28 breaths/minute
- BP: 118/80 mm Hg
- pulse oximetry: 92%.

The nurse noted that Mrs. M. had slight facial swelling and her voice was becoming hoarse. Within 5 minutes, Mrs. M. displayed signs of increasing respiratory difficulty, using accessory muscles to breathe, with pulse oximetry dropping to 89%.

The rapid response team (RRT) was called and responded within 3 minutes. The blood transfusion was stopped and disconnected. The I.V. line was flushed with normal saline solution (NSS) and an infusion of NSS was started at 10 ml/hour. The respiratory therapist drew arterial blood gases (ABGs). Oxygen was started via Venturi mask at 50% FIO_2. A portable chest X-ray was obtained. Mrs. M. continued to show signs of respiratory distress.

Test results

- ABG analysis: pH: 7.28; O_2: 85 mm Hg; CO_2: 32 mm Hg; HCO_3^-: 24 mEq/L; Sao_2: 87%
- Chest X-ray: pulmonary congestion

Responding to a transfusion reaction *(continued)*

It was undecided if Mrs. M.'s symptoms were due to a transfusion reaction or fluid overload. She was given 25 mg diphenhydramine I.V. and 40 mg furosemide I.V. The blood bank was notified and the unused portion of blood was returned to the lab along with a blood sample and urine specimen. The blood label was checked by the RRT who found the labeling to have the correct patient information. Her attending physician was notified. Mrs. M. was transferred to the intermediate care unit for closer monitoring.

After 1 hour, vital signs were:
- temperature: 98.1° F (36.7° C)
- HR: 90 beats/minute
- RR: 20 breaths/minute
- BP: 114/76 mm Hg
- pulse oximetry: 99%.

Mrs. M. diuresed 1,000 ml and reported that her breathing was easier. Facial swelling and hoarseness resolved within 2 hours.

blood, administration set, attached I.V. solutions, and all related forms and labels) to the blood bank. Some health care facilities require the completion of a transfusion reaction report that must be sent to the blood bank. An incident report may also be required according to facility policy. (See *Transfusion reaction report,* pages 200 and 201.) Document your follow-up care.

2/13/08	1400	Pt. reports chills. Cyanosis of lips noted at 1350. Transfusion of packed RBCs stopped. Approximately 100 ml of blood infused. Transfusion started 1215, stopped at 1350. Tubing changed. I.V. of 1000 ml NSS infusing at 30 ml/hr rate in ® forearm. Notified Dr. Will Cahill and blood bank. BP 168/88, P 104, RR 25, rectal T 97.6° F. Blood sample taken from PRBCs. Two red-top tubes of blood drawn from pt. sent to lab. Urine specimen obtained from catheter and sent to lab for U/A. Administered diphenhydramine 50 mg I.M. per order of Dr. Cahill. Two blankets placed on pt. Blood transfusion equipment sent to blood bank. Transfusion reaction report completed and sent to lab. ———————— Maryann Belinsky, R N
	1415	Pt. reports he's getting warmer. BP 148/80, P 96, RR 20, T 97.6° F. ———————————— Maryann Belinsky, R N
	1430	Pt. no longer complaining of chills. I.V. of 1000 ml NSS infusing at 125 ml/hr in ® arm. BP 138/76, P 80, RR 18, T 98.4° F. ——— ———————————— Maryann Belinsky, R N

(Text continues on page 202.)

Transfusion reaction report

If your facility requires a transfusion reaction report, you'll include the following types of information.

TRANSFUSION REACTION REPORT

Nursing report

1. Stop transfusion immediately. Keep I.V. line open with saline infusion.
2. Notify responsible physician.
3. Check all identifying names and numbers on the patient's wristband, unit, and paperwork for discrepancies.
4. Record patient's posttransfusion vital signs.
5. Draw posttransfusion blood samples (clotted and anticoagulated) avoiding mechanical hemolysis.
6. Collect posttransfusion urine specimen from patient.
7. Record information as indicated below.
8. Send discontinued bag of blood, administration set, attached I.V. solutions, and all related forms and labels to the blood bank with this form completed.

Clerical errors
☑ None detected
☐ Detected

Vital signs

	Pre-TXN	Post-TXN
Temp.	98.4°F (36.9°C)	97.6°F (36.4°C)
B.P.	120/60	160/88
Pulse	88	104

☐ Urticaria ☐ Nausea ☐ Shock ☐ Hemoglobinuria
☐ Fever ☐ Flushing ☐ Oozing
☑ Chills ☐ Dyspnea ☐ Back pain ☐ Oliguria or anuria
☐ Chest pain ☐ Headache ☐ Infusion site pain
☐ Hypotension ☐ Perspiration ☐ Cyanosis of lips noted

Reaction occurred

During administration? *Yes*
After administration? _____
How long? _____
Medications added? *No*
Previous I.V. fluids? *NSS at 30 ml/hr*
Blood warmed? *No*

Specimen collection

Blood: Difficulty collecting? *No*
Urine: Voided *Yes — sent to lab*   Catheterized _____

Comments:
Given diphenhydramine 50 mg IM

Signature *Maryann Belinsky, RN*   Date *2/13/08*

BLOOD BANK REPORT

Unit #	1. Clerical errors
22FM80507	☑ None detected
Component Returned	☐ Detected
Yes	
Volume Returned	Comments:
185 ml	

2. Hemolysis

Note: If hemolysis is present in the posttransfusion sample, a posttransfusion urine sample must be tested for free hemoglobin immediately.

	None	Slight	Moderate	Marked
Patient pre-TXN sample	☑ None	☐ Slight	☐ Moderate	☐ Marked
Patient post-TXN sample	☑ None	☐ Slight	☐ Moderate	☐ Marked
Blood Bag	☑ None	☐ Slight	☐ Moderate	☐ Marked
Urine HGB (centrifuged)	☐ None	☐ Slight	☑ Moderate	☐ Marked

(continued)

Transfusion reaction report *(continued)*

BLOOD BANK REPORT *(continued)*

3. Direct antiglobulin test

Pretransfusion _____ Posttransfusion _____

If No. 2 and No. 3 are negative, steps 4 through 6 aren't required. Report results to the blood bank physician. Steps 7 and 8 or further testing will be done as ordered by blood bank physician.

4. ABO and Rh Groups

Repeat testing	Cell reaction with							Serum reaction with		ABO/Rh
	Anti-A	Anti-B	Anti-A,B	Anti-D	Cont.	Du	Cont.	CCC	A1 cells	B cells
Pretransfusion										
Posttransfusion										
Unit #										
Unit #										

5. Red cell antibody screen

		Saline/AB				INT
Pretransfusion	Cell	RT	37° C	AHG	CCC	
Date of sample	I					
	II					
By:	Auto					

		Saline/AB				INT
Posttransfusion	Cell	RT	37° C	AHG	CCC	
Date of sample	I					
	II					
By:	Auto					

Specificity of antibody detected:

6. Crossmatch compatibility testing

Use patient pre-TXN and post-TXN serum and the suspected unit red cells obtained from inside the container or from a segment still attached to bag. Observe appearance of blood in bag and administration tubing.

		Albumin			INT
Pretransfusion	RT	37° C	AHG	CCC	
Unit #					
Unit #					

		Albumin			INT
Posttransfusion	RT	37° C	AHG	CCC	
Unit #					
Unit #					

All units on hold for future transfusion must be recross-matched with the posttransfusion sample.

7. Bacteriologic testing

Pretransfusion _____ Posttransfusion _____

8. Other testing results

Total bilirubin   **Coagulation studies**   **Urine output studies**

Patient pre-TXN _____ mg/dl

Patient 6 hrs. post-TXN _____ mg/dl

Pathologist's conclusions:

Signature _____ Date _____

Brain death

Brain death is commonly defined as the irreversible cessation of all brain function, including the brain stem. The Uniform Determination of Death Act (1980) established the standards for diagnosing brain death. The American Academy of Neurology (AAN) used these standards to develop practice guidelines in 1995. Other organizations have also published guidelines for diagnosing brain death. That's why it's important to know your state's laws regarding the definition of brain death as well as your facility's policy. (See *Know your state's laws concerning brain death.*)

The current AAN guidelines recommend that a physician confirm the presence of the three cardinal signs of brain death:

■ coma or unresponsiveness
■ absence of brain stem function
■ apnea (lack of spontaneous breathing).

To make this determination, the physician should test the patient for responsiveness or movement, brain stem reflexes (pupillary, corneal, gag/cough, oculocephalic, and oculovestibular), and apnea. He should also evaluate laboratory and diagnostic test results to eliminate other causes of coma. Although standards may vary by state or facility, the AAN recommends that the physician perform the examination twice, at least 6 hours apart.

Essential documentation

Your nurse's note for a patient undergoing evaluation for brain death should include:

LEGAL LOOKOUT
Know your state's laws concerning brain death

In states without laws defining death or without judicial precedents, the common law definition of death (cessation of circulation and respiration) is still used. In these states, doctors are understandably reluctant to discontinue artificial life support for brain-dead patients. If you're likely to be involved with patients on life-support equipment, protect yourself by finding out how your state defines death.

- date and time of the examination
- the name of the person performing the test
- the patient's response and any action taken (If you notified anyone about the test and results, include the date and time of notification, the name of the person notified, the person's response, and any action taken.)
- time of brain and cardiopulmonary death (include any evidence such as electrocardiograph strips)
- family teaching and emotional support given.

In addition, individuals performing the tests, such as a respiratory therapist, will need to complete their documentation in appropriate sections of the chart.

4/1/08	0800	Dr. Richard Malone in to speak with pt.'s son, Mark Newton, who has health care POA, about pt.'s condition. The son verbalized understanding about probable brain death due to subarachnoid hemorrhage and agreed to tests to determine brain death. When offered, stated he didn't want a visit by clergy or social worker. ——— Dawn Silfies, RN
	0815	Dr. Malone performed clinical exam. See Physical Progress Notes for full report. Son present for exam and results explained by Dr. Malone. Son understands that another dr. not involved with his father's care will repeat the exam in 6 hours. ——————————— Dawn Silfies, RN
	0830	ABG results obtained by Michael Burke, RPT, with pt. on ventilator. Results pH 7.40, PO_2 100, PCO_2 40. Pt. taken off ventilator by respiratory therapist and placed on 100% O_2 via T-piece. Dr. Malone in attendance. Cardiac monitor showing NSR at a rate of 70, O_2 sat. via continuous pulse oximetry 99%. Within 1 minute of testing, heart rate 150 with PVCs, and O_2 sat. dropped to 91%. Pt. without spontaneous respirations. ABGs drawn by respiratory therapist showed pH 7.32, PO_2 60, PCO_2 65. Pt. placed back on ventilator. Son verbalized understanding of the results showing apnea. Son states he will stay with his dad until exam at 1430 with Dr. Sam Porter. Dr. Malone will meet with son at 1500 to discuss results and plan. ————————— Dawn Silfies, RN

C

Cardiac monitoring

Because it allows continuous observation of the heart's electrical activity, cardiac monitoring is useful not only for assessing cardiac rhythm but also for evaluating a patient's response to drug therapy and detecting complications associated with diagnostic and therapeutic procedures. Like other forms of electrocardiography, cardiac monitoring uses electrodes placed on the patient's chest to transmit electrical signals that are converted into a tracing of cardiac rhythm on an oscilloscope. Cardiac monitoring may be hardwire monitoring, in which the patient is connected to a monitor at the bedside, or telemetry, in which a small transmitter connected to the patient sends an electrical signal to a central monitor screen for display.

Essential documentation

In your note, document the date and time that monitoring began and the monitoring leads used. Attach a rhythm strip to the record every shift or with any rhythm change. Be sure to label the rhythm strip with the patient's name, his room number, and the date and time. Measure and document the PR interval, QRS duration, and QT interval along with an interpretation of the rhythm.

If cardiac monitoring for rhythm evaluation is to be done after the patient's discharge (such as with Holter monitoring), provide teaching on monitor care, equipment malfunction, and event recording, and document.

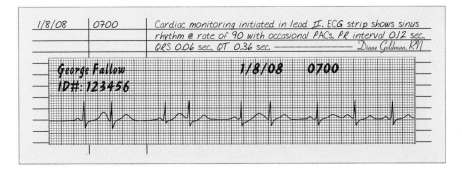

| 1/8/08 | 0700 | Cardiac monitoring initiated in lead II. ECG strip shows sinus rhythm @ rate of 90 with occasional PACs. PR interval 0.12 sec., QRS 0.06 sec., QT 0.36 sec. ———————— Diane Goldman, RN |

George Fallow
ID#: 123456   1/8/08   0700

Cardiac tamponade

With cardiac tamponade, a rapid, unchecked rise in intrapericardial pressure impairs diastolic filling of the heart. The rise in pressure usually results from blood or fluid accumulation in the pericardial sac. If fluid accumulates rapidly, the patient requires emergency lifesaving measures.

Cardiac tamponade may be idiopathic (Dressler's syndrome) or may result from effusion, hemorrhage from trauma or nontraumatic causes, pericarditis, acute myocardial infarction, chronic renal failure during dialysis, drug reaction, or connective tissue disorders.

If you suspect cardiac tamponade in your patient, notify the physician immediately and prepare for pericardiocentesis (needle aspiration of the peritoneal cavity), emergency surgery (usually a pericardial window), or both. Anticipate the need for I.V. fluids, inotropic drug infusion, and blood products to maintain blood pressure until treatment is performed.

Essential documentation

Note the date and time that you detect signs of cardiac tamponade. Document your assessment findings, such as neck vein distention, decreased blood pressure, pulsus paradoxus, narrow pulse pressure, muffled heart sounds, acute pain, dyspnea, diaphoresis, anxiety, restlessness, pallor or cyanosis, rapid and weak pulses, and hepatomegaly. Record the date and time when the physician was notified, and document which physician was notified. Document treatments, procedures, and the patient's response. Note any patient teaching provided. Document vital signs and medicated I.V. infusions on appropriate flow sheets.

4/5/08	1320	BP at 1300 90/40 via cuff on ℝ arm. Last BP at 1245 was 120/60. Drop of 17 mm Hg in systolic BP noted during inspiration. P 132 and regular, RR 34, oral T 97.2° F. See frequent vital sign sheet for q15min VS. Neck veins distended with pt. in semi-Fowler's at 45-degrees, heart sounds muffled, peripheral pulses weak. Pt. anxious and dyspneic, skin pale and diaphoretic. Pt. c/o chest soreness. Slight ecchymosis visible across chest. Pt. awake, alert, and oriented to time, place, and person. Dr. Regina Hoffmann notified at 1305. Stat portable CXR shows slightly widened mediastinum and enlargement of the cardiac silhouette. ECG shows sinus tachycardia with rate of 130. 200-ml bolus of NSS given. Dopamine 400 mg in 250 D₅W started via distal port of ℝ subclavian TLC at 4 mcg/kg. Urine output is 25 ml for last hr. Awaiting Dr. John Brown's arrival for pericardiocentesis. Explained the procedure to pt. and wife and answered their questions. ——————— Cindy Rogers, RN

Cardiopulmonary arrest and resuscitation

Guidelines established by the American Heart Association direct you to keep a written, chronological account of a patient's condition throughout cardiopulmonary resuscitation (CPR). If you're the designated recorder, document therapeutic interventions and the patient's responses as they occur. Don't rely on your memory later. (See *Responding to a code*.)

Writing "recorder" after your name indicates that you documented the event but didn't participate in the code.

The form used to chart a code is the code record. It incorporates detailed information about your observations and interventions as well as drugs given to the patient. Remember, the code response should follow advanced cardiac life support guidelines.

Some facilities use a resuscitation critique form to identify actual or potential problems with the resuscitation process. This form tracks personnel responses and response times as well as the availability of appropriate drugs and functioning equipment. A brief nurse's note also needs to be included in the patient's record.

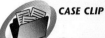 **CASE CLIP**

Responding to a code

Mrs. D. is a 41-year-old female admitted to the hospital after experiencing a seizure. Her past medical history includes type 2 diabetes mellitus. She was being treated with phenytoin while being evaluated for the cause of the seizure. She was awaiting results of an EEG. The nurse went to Mrs. D.'s room to provide care and found Mrs. D. in the midst of a seizure. The seizure ended and Mrs. D.'s vital signs were:

- temperature: 97° F (36.1° C)
- heart rate (HR): 64 beats/minute
- respiratory rate (RR): 12 breaths/minute
- blood pressure (BP): 120/46 mm Hg
- pulse oximetry: 94%.

Mrs. D. was somnolent but appeared to be breathing regularly and was uninjured. Within 5 minutes, another seizure started. Mrs. D. at this time was also making gurgling noises. The nurse called the rapid response team (RRT) who arrived within 3 minutes. The seizure was just resolving. Mrs. D. was unresponsive and her respirations were infrequent—8 breaths/minute. Other vital signs were:

- HR: 110 beats/minute
- BP: 100/50 mm Hg
- pulse oximetry: 80% on room air.

The RRT placed Mrs. D. on a cardiac monitor and started oxygen at 100% via a nonrebreather mask. Mrs. D then stopped breathing. A code was called and the code team arrived within 3 minutes. Mrs. D. was intubated and placed on a mechanical ventilator. The attending physician was notified and Mrs. D. was transferred to the intensive care unit.

Essential documentation

The code record is a precise, quick, and chronological recording of the events of the code. (See *The code record,* page 208.) Document the date and time the code was called. You'll also need to record the patient's name, location of the code, person who discovered the patient, the patient's condition, and whether the arrest was witnessed or not witnessed. Record the name of the physician who attended the code and

The code record

Here's an example of the completed resuscitation record for inclusion in your patient's chart.

CODE RECORD

Pg. _1_ of _1_

Arrest Date: _1/9/08_
Arrest Time: _0631_
Rm/Location: _431-2_
Discovered by:
C. Brown
☑ RN ☐ MD
☐ Other

Methods of alert:
☐ Witnessed, monitored: rhythm
☐ Witnessed, unwitnessed
☑ Unwitnessed, unmonitored
☐ Unwitnessed, monitored; rhythm _____
Diagnosis: _Post anterior wall MI_

Condition when found:
☑ Unresponsive
☐ Apneic
☐ Pulseless
☐ Hemorrhage
☐ Seizure

Ventilation management:
Time: _0635_
Method: _oral ET tube_
Precordial thump: _____
CPR initiated at: _0631_

Previous airway:
☐ ET tube
☐ Trach
☑ Natural

Addressograph

CPR PROGRESS NOTES

Time	Pulse CPR	Resp. rate Spont; bag	Blood pressure	Rhythm	Defib (joules)	Atropine	Epinephrine	Amiodarone	Responses to therapy, procedures, labs drawn/results
0631	No pulse CPR	Bag	0	V fib	200				No change.
0632		Bag	0	V fib	300				No change
0633	No pulse CPR	Bag	0	Asystole	360		1 mg		No change
0635	40	Bag	60 palp	SB PVCs					Oral intubation by Dr. David Hart
0645	60	Bag	80/40	SB PVCs					ABGs drawn. ℞ fem pressure applied.

I.V. PUSH: Atropine, Epinephrine — INFUSIONS: Amiodarone — ACTIONS/PATIENT RESPONSE

ABGs & Lab Data

Time Spec Sent	pH	PCO	Po₂	HCO₃⁻	Sat%	Fio₂	Other
0653	7.1	76	43	14	80%		

Resuscitation outcome

☑ Successful ☑ Transferred to _CCU_ at _0700_
☐ Unsuccessful — Expired at _____
Pronounced by: _____ MD
Family notified by: _S. Quinn, RN_
Time: _0645_
Attending notified by: _S. Quinn, RN_ Time _0645_
Code Recorder _S. Quinn, RN_
Code Team Nurse _B. Mullen, RN_
Anesthesia Rep. _J. Hanna, RN_
Other Personnel _Dr. Hart_
B. Russo, RT
Signature _Connie Brown, R N_ Recorder

when the attending physician was notified. List other health care professionals who participated in the code. Record the exact time for each code intervention, and include vital signs, heart rhythm, laboratory results (such as arterial blood gas or electrolyte levels), type of treatment (such as CPR, defibrillation, or cardioversion), drugs (name, dosage, and route), procedures (such as intubation, temporary or transvenous pacemaker, and central line insertion), and patient response. Record the time that the family was notified. At the end of the code, indicate the patient's status and the time that the code ended. Some facilities require that the physician leading the code and the nurse recording the code review the code sheet and sign it.

In your nurse's note, record why the code was called, who initiated CPR, and other interventions performed before the code team arrived. Include the patient's response to interventions. Indicate in your note that a code record was used to document the events of the code.

2/9/08	0650	Found by CNA (J. Ross) unresponsive in bed without
		respirations or pulse. Code called at 0630. Initiated
		CPR with Ann Barrow, RN. Code team arrived at 0632
		and continued resuscitative efforts. (See code record.)
		Dr. Richard Mallon notified. Family notified. Pt. transferred
		to ICU with code team ———————— Connie Brown, RN

Cardioversion, synchronized

Used to treat tachyarrhythmias, cardioversion delivers an electrical charge to the myocardium at the peak of the R wave. This causes immediate depolarization, interrupting reentry circuits and allowing the sinoatrial node to resume control. Synchronizing the electrical charge with the R wave ensures that the current won't be delivered on the vulnerable T wave and thus disrupt repolarization.

Indications for cardioversion include stable paroxysmal atrial tachycardia, unstable paroxysmal supraventricular tachycardia, atrial fibrillation, atrial flutter, and ventricular tachycardia. Cardioversion may be an elective or urgent procedure, depending on how well the patient tolerates the arrhythmia. (See *Responding to the need for cardioversion,* pages 210 and 211.)

CASE CLIP

Responding to the need for cardioversion

Mr. R. is a 68-year-old male who presented to the emergency department (ED) complaining of bilateral arm pain and chest pain. He related that he had been doing yard work at home, which involved raking and replacing mulch. After dinner, his pain started in his arms and then extended to his chest. The pain wasn't relieved by rest. He rated the pain as a 6 on a scale of 0 to 10. He stated that he had never experienced chest pain in the past.

Past medical history includes hypertension and high cholesterol. Home medications are:

- hydrochlorothiazide (HydroDIURIL) 50 mg by mouth (P.O.) daily
- atorvastatin (Lipitor) 20 mg P.O. daily.

Vital signs on admission were:

- temperature: 98° F (36.7° C)
- heart rate (HR): 58 beats/minute
- respiratory rate (RR): 20 breaths/minute
- blood pressure (BP): 110/70 mm Hg
- pulse oximetry: 97% on oxygen at 2 L/minute.

Mr. R. was given nitroglycerin spray × 2, which relieved his chest pain, and was started on a nitroglycerin infusion at 20 mcg/minute. Mr. R.'s cardiac rhythm was sinus bradycardia. Cardiac workup revealed that Mr. R. suffered a non–Q wave myocardial infarction. He was admitted to the cardiac care unit (CCU) for observation.

At 0300, Mr. R.'s cardiac monitor alarm went off for an HR of 160 beats/minute. The rhythm was interpreted as rapid atrial fibrillation. Within minutes, the heart rate increased to 175 and Mr. R. complained of chest pressure, feeling anxious, and shortness of breath.

Vital signs at this time were:

- HR: 175 beats/minute
- RR: 30 breaths/minute
- BP: 88/42 mm Hg
- pulse oximetry: 94% on 2 L/minute oxygen.

The rapid response team (RRT) was notified and arrived within 3 minutes. After a quick assessment of the patient's history and medications, the RRT obtained an electrocardiogram (ECG), which confirmed rapid atrial fibrillation.

Vital signs at this time were:

- HR: 180 beats/minute
- RR: 30 breaths/minute
- BP: 72/38 mm Hg
- pulse oximetry: 94%.

Responding to the need for cardioversion *(continued)*

Normal saline solution was started at 500 ml/hour. Electrodes were placed on Mr. R., and he was connected to the defibrillator monitor. Defibrillation pads were then placed on Mr. R.'s chest. The ED physician was notified and came to Mr. R.'s room to oversee synchronized cardioversion. Mr. R. was given 1 mg midazolam (Versed) I.V. The defibrillator was charged to 100 joules, synchronized. After the shock was delivered, Mr. R.'s cardiac rhythm showed normal sinus rhythm.

Vital signs at this time were:
- HR: 90 beats/minute
- RR: 22 breaths/minute
- BP: 104/66 mm Hg
- pulse oximetry: 95%.

Mr. R. related relief of chest pain. An ECG was done. The attending physician was updated on the events. Mr. R. remained in the CCU for 2 additional days before being transferred to the telemetry unit before discharge to home.

Essential documentation

Document the date and time of the cardioversion. Verify a signed consent form and any patient teaching provided. Include any preprocedure activities, such as withholding food and fluids, withholding drugs, removing dentures, giving a sedative, and obtaining a 12-lead ECG. Document vital signs, obtain a rhythm strip, and take a "time out" to verify the patient's identity and procedure to be performed before starting. Note that the cardioverter was on the synchronized setting, how many times the patient was cardioverted, and the voltage used each time. After the procedure, obtain vital signs, place a rhythm strip in the chart, and record that a 12-lead ECG was obtained. Assess and document the patient's level of consciousness, airway patency, respiratory rate and depth, and use of supplemental oxygen until he's awake.

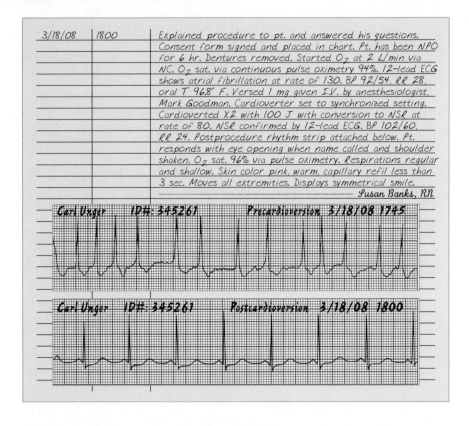

3/18/08	1800	Explained procedure to pt. and answered his questions.
		Consent form signed and placed in chart. Pt. has been NPO
		for 6 hr. Dentures removed. Started O_2 at 2 L/min via
		NC. O_2 sat. via continuous pulse oximetry 94%. 12-lead ECG
		shows atrial fibrillation at rate of 130. BP 92/54, RR 28,
		oral T 96.8° F. Versed 1 mg given I.V. by anesthesiologist,
		Mark Goodman. Cardioverter set to synchronized setting.
		Cardioverted X2 with 100 J with conversion to NSR at
		rate of 80. NSR confirmed by 12-lead ECG. BP 102/60,
		RR 24. Postprocedure rhythm strip attached below. Pt.
		responds with eye opening when name called and shoulder
		shaken. O_2 sat. 96% via pulse oximetry. Respirations regular
		and shallow. Skin color pink, warm, capillary refil less than
		3 sec. Moves all extremities. Displays symmetrical smile.
		—————————————————— Susan Banks, RN

Central venous catheter insertion

A central venous (CV) line is a sterile catheter that's inserted through a major vein, such as the subclavian vein or the jugular vein. A CV catheter provides access for CV pressure monitoring, which indicates blood volume or pump efficiency, permits aspiration of blood samples for diagnostic tests, and allows administration of I.V. fluids and medication. A CV line is needed when prolonged I.V. therapy or disease reduces the number of accessible peripheral veins, when solutions must be diluted (for large volumes or for irritating or hypertonic fluids such as total parenteral nutrition solutions), and when long-term access is needed to the patient's venous system. A peripherally inserted central catheter (PICC) is inserted in a peripheral vein, such as the basilic vein, and used for infusion and blood sampling only. Specially trained nurses may insert a PICC line, but a CV catheter must be inserted by a physician or specially trained practitioner.

Essential documentation

When you assist the physician who inserts a CV line, verify that a signed consent form is on the chart, document the date and time of insertion; type, length, and location of the catheter; solution infused; the physician's name; and the patient's response to the procedure. If the ports aren't being used, document that they have needle-free injection caps and include any orders related to maintaining patency. Also document the time that the X-ray was performed to confirm placement, the X-ray report, and your notification of the physician. Note whether the catheter was sutured in place and the type of dressing applied. For a PICC, record the length of the external catheter. Write the date the PICC was inserted and dressing applied directly on the dressing.

2/24/08	1100	Procedure explained to pt. and written consent obtained by Dr. Julian
		Chavez. Pt. in Trendelenburg's position and 20.3 cm TLC placed
		by Dr. Chavez on first attempt in ® subclavian vein. Cath sutured
		in place with 3-0 silk, and sterile dressing applied per protocol.
		Needle-free injection caps placed on all lines. Lines flushed with
		NSS – 10 ml. Portable CXR obtained to confirm line placement.
		Results pending. P 110, BP 90/58, RR 24, oral T 97.9° F. Pt.
		sitting in semi-Fowler's position and breathing easily, with equal
		breath sounds. Chest expansion symmetrical. — Louise Flynn, RN
	1130	Chest X-ray confirms proper placement of CV line in superior vena cava.
		Dr. Julian Chavez notified by phone of report. ———— Joyce Williams, RN

Central venous catheter occlusion

A central venous (CV) catheter may become occluded because of kinks in the tubing, closed clamps, the presence of a blood clot or fibrin sheath, or crystalline adherence. Signs of occlusion include the inability to draw blood, infuse a solution, or flush the catheter. If you suspect CV catheter occlusion, check the tubing for kinks. You may need to remove the dressing to check for kinks under it. Check the infusion pump system, and ensure that all clamps are open. Ask the patient to cough or change position. Attempt to withdraw blood or gently flush with normal saline solution. Don't force the flush through the catheter because this may dislodge a clot. For a multilumen catheter, label the occluded lumen "Occluded: Do not use." Depending on the catheter, a thrombolytic may be used to lyse a clot or dissolve a fibrin sheath. Follow the physician's orders and facility policy. A new CV line may be inserted, if necessary.

Essential documentation

Document the date and time of the occlusion. Record evidence of catheter occlusion. Describe your actions and the results. Include the name of the physician notified, the time of notification, and any orders given. Depending on your facility's policy, you may also need to document the occlusion on the I.V. therapy flow sheet.

3/4/08	1220	Unable to aspirate blood from distal port of TLC. Unable to
		flush line with NSS. Pt. changed from supine to Ⓡ and Ⓛ lateral
		position and asked to cough; still unable to obtain blood return
		or flush with NSS. Distal port labeled "occluded." Dr. Joe Brown
		notified of the occlusion at 1210. ———— Ruth Clark, RN

Central venous catheter removal

A central venous (CV) line may be removed when it's no longer necessary, is nonfunctional, is displaced, or has reached the recommended number of insertion days, or if the patient shows signs of infection. A physician or a specially trained nurse may remove the CV line. Verify your facility's policy and protocols related to CV line removal by a registered nurse. It may be ordered that the tip of the catheter be sent for culture after removal.

Essential documentation

After assisting with a CV line's removal or performing the CV line removal yourself, record the name of the person discontinuing the line, the date and time of the removal, the length of time that pressure was held to the site, and the type of dressing applied. Note the length of the catheter and the condition of the insertion site. When assessing the dressing, note any bleeding. Also document the collection of any catheter specimens for culture or other analysis.

2/24/08	1100	20.3 cm CV catheter removed by Dr. Maria Romero at 1045 and
		pressure held for 5 min. Catheter tip present, sent to laboratory for
		culture. Povidone-iodine applied to insertion site and covered with
		gauze pad and transparent semipermeable dressing. No drainage,
		redness, or swelling noted at insertion site. ———— *Louise Flynn, RN*

Central venous catheter site care

Central venous (CV) catheter site care and frequency of care vary according to the type of catheter and facility policy. Frequency of site care varies from daily to every 48 hours for gauze dressings to every 3 to 7 days for transparent dressings. Dressings should always be changed when they become soiled or lose integrity.

Site care is performed using aseptic technique. After the catheter is inserted, use normal saline solution to clean the site. Don't apply ointment to the insertion site.

The insertion site should be visually inspected and palpated daily through an intact transparent dressing. When the dressing is removed, inspect the site for signs and symptoms of infection, such as discharge, inflammation, and tenderness. Many facilities have preassembled care kits. Chlorhexidine is replacing povidone-iodine and alcohol as the antiseptic of choice for site care because of its increased efficacy.

Essential documentation

After you've completed the dressing change, label the dressing with the date, time, and your initials. In your documentation, record the date and time of site care. Depending on facility policy, this documentation may be in the nurse's notes, I.V. therapy flow sheet, or nurse's flow sheet. Note the marking indicating catheter length, appearance of the insertion site, method of cleaning site, and type of dressing applied. Describe any drainage on the dressing. If complications are noted, record the name of the physician notified, the time of notification, and any orders given.

4/25/08	1220	® subclavian TLC care done. Suture intact, insertion site
		without redness or drainage, catheter marking at 12 cm. Pt.
		denies tenderness. Using sterile technique, area and insertion
		site cleaned with chlorhexidine. Catheter secured with tape
		and covered with transparent semipermeable membrane
		dressing. ————————————————— *Nick Cerone, RN*

Central venous pressure monitoring

Central venous pressure (CVP) can be monitored via a catheter inserted through a vein and advanced until the tip lies in or near the right atrium. CVP is an index of right ventricular function and monitoring helps assess cardiac function, evaluate venous return to the heart, and indirectly gauge how well the heart is pumping. CVP monitoring may be done with a water manometer or pressure monitoring system with readings recorded intermittently or continuously.

Essential documentation

Record CVP readings on a flow sheet or in your nurse's note, according to your facility's policy. When writing your note, record the date and time of assessment. Record the CVP reading, the patient's position, and whether the transducer was at the zero reference point. Describe the appearance of the waveform and your evaluation. Place a printout of recordings, if available, in the patient's chart. Include any relevant assessments of the patient. Document the name of the physician notified of abnormal readings, the time of notification, and whether any actions were taken.

1/5/08	0500	® subclavian CVP attached to monitor with pressure bag
		setup of 500 ml NSS. Line zeroed per protocol. Normal
		CVP waveform on monitor shows reading of 4 cm H₂O.
		Urine output 25 ml in past hr. Mucous membranes dry,
		Skin turgor poor. P 110, BP 110/72, RR 18, oral T 99° F.
		Dr. Joe Brown notified of CVP reading and physical
		assessment findings. Fluid challenge of 500 ml NSS over
		1 hr via CVP line started. —————— Joanne Nunez, RN

Chest pain

When your patient complains of chest pain, act quickly to determine its cause. Chest pain may be caused by a disorder as benign as epigastric distress (indigestion) or as serious and life-threatening as acute myocardial infarction. (See *Responding to chest pain.*)

Responding to chest pain

Mr. A., a 69-year-old male, was admitted to the hospital after knee replacement surgery. His past medical history includes hypertension, laminectomy for a ruptured disk, two-packs-per-day smoker, and obesity. He was reluctant to participate with physical therapy because he was experiencing a lot of pain. He spent most of his time in bed and refused to use the continuous passive motion machine except at night.

At 0300 on his third postoperative day, Mr. A. called the nurse to tell her that he was having crushing substernal chest pain with radiation to his left arm. He rated the pain as a 10 on a scale of 0 to 10. He was diaphoretic and short of breath.

His vital signs were:
- temperature: 98° F (36.7° C)
- heart rate (HR): 118 beats/minute
- respiratory rate (RR): 26 breaths/minute
- blood pressure (BP): 170/88 mm Hg
- pulse oximetry: 96% on room air.

The nurse placed Mr. A. on oxygen at 4 L/minute and called the rapid response team (RRT), who arrived within 3 minutes and performed a quick assessment of Mr. A.'s diagnosis, medications, and present status. Continuous cardiac monitoring was started and showed the heart rhythm to be sinus tachycardia with ST elevation. Mr. A. was given nitroglycerin 1/150 gr sublingual. A 12-lead electrocardiogram (ECG) was obtained. Aspirin 325 mg was given by mouth.

Vital signs were:
- HR: 108 beats/minute
- RR: 22 breaths/minute
- BP: 140/80 mm Hg
- pulse oximetry: 97%.

Mr. A. continued to complain of chest pain, although he now rated it 6 out of 10. Another nitroglycerin 1/150 gr sublingual was administered. Normal saline solution was started at a "keep-vein-open" rate. A blood sample was obtained and sent to the laboratory for cardiac enzyme and troponin levels.

Mr. A.'s chest pain was nearly resolved, rating 4 out of 10. Because Mr. A. already had a medication order for morphine for postoperative pain, it was decided to administer the drug to relieve his pain. He was given morphine 2 mg I.V. and he stated that the chest pain was gone.

The attending physician was notified and Mr. A. was transferred to the cardiac care unit with orders for a stat spiral computed tomography scan to rule out pulmonary embolism, repeat laboratory work and ECG, and a nitroglycerin infusion.

Essential documentation

Record the date and time of the onset of chest pain. Question your patient about his pain, and record the responses using the patient's own words, when appropriate. Include the following:
- What was the patient doing when the pain started?
- How long did the pain last? Had it ever occurred before? Was the onset sudden or gradual?
- Did the pain radiate? If so, where did it radiate?
- What factors improve or aggravate the pain?
- Where exactly is the pain? (Ask the patient to point to the location of the pain and record the patient's response. For example, he may move his hand vaguely around his abdomen or may point with one finger to his left chest.)
- How severe is the pain? (Ask the patient to rate the pain on a scale of 0 to 10, with 0 indicating no pain and 10 indicating the worst pain imaginable.)

Record the patient's vital signs and a quick assessment of his body systems. If the patient's condition becomes critical, document the time and name of any individuals notified, such as the physician, nursing supervisor, or rapid response team. Record your actions and the patient's responses. Include any patient education and emotional support you provided.

| 4/9/08 | 0410 | Pt. c/o sudden onset of a sharp chest pain while sleeping. Points to center of chest, over sternum. States, "It feels like an elephant is sitting on my chest." Pain radiates to the neck and shoulders. Rates pain as 7 on a scale of 0 to 10. P 112, BP 90/62, RR 26. O₂ sat 94% on 2L O₂. Lungs have fine crackles in the bases on auscultation. Dr. Roger Romano notified and orders received. Morphine 2 mg I.V. given. 12-lead ECG obtained. All procedures explained to pt. and all questions answered. Reassured pt. that he's being closely monitored. — Martha Wolcott, RN |
| | 0415 | Pt. states pain is now a 5 on a scale of 0 to 10. Morphine 2 mg I.V. repeated. Pt. prepared for transport to CCU per Dr. Romano ———————————— Martha Wolcott, RN |

Chest physiotherapy

Chest physiotherapy includes postural drainage, chest percussion and vibration, and coughing and deep-breathing exercises. Together, these techniques help loosen and eliminate secretions, reexpand lung tissue, and promote efficient use of respiratory muscles. Of critical importance to the bedridden patient, chest physiotherapy helps prevent or treat atelectasis and may help prevent pneumonia. Use of an incentive spirometer is also important to pulmonary health.

Essential documentation

Whenever you perform chest physiotherapy, document the date and time of your interventions; the patient's position for secretion drainage and the length of time the patient remains in each position; the chest segments percussed or vibrated; and the characteristics of the secretion expelled, including color, amount, odor, viscosity, and the presence of blood. Document coughing and deep breathing exercises, as well as the use of the incentive spirometer and the volume the patient obtains with this device. Also, record the patient's tolerance of the treatment.

1/20/08	1415	Pt. placed on Ⓛ side with foot of bed elevated. Chest PT and
		postural drainage performed for 10 min. from lower to
		middle then upper lobes, as ordered. Pt. had productive cough
		and expelled large amt. of thick, yellow, odorless sputum. Lungs
		clear after chest PT. After chest PT, pt. stated he was tired
		and asked to lie down. ———————————— Jane Goddard, RN

Chest tube care

Inserted into the pleural space, a chest tube allows blood, fluid, pus, or air to drain and promotes lung reexpansion. Chest tube drainage may use gravity or suction to restore negative pressure and remove material or air that collects in the pleural cavity. An underwater seal in the drainage system allows air and fluid to escape from the pleural cavity but doesn't allow air to reenter.

Caring for the patient with a chest tube involves maintaining appropriate suction, monitoring for and preventing air leaks, monitoring drainage amount and characteristics, promoting pulmonary hygiene, promoting patient comfort, performing dressing changes and site care, and preventing, detecting, and treating complications. It also involves assessment of oxygenation and ventilation of the patient, as well as evaluation of lung sounds and presence of subcutaneous air.

Essential documentation

Record the date and time of your entry. Identify the chest tube location; type and amount of suction; type, amount, and consistency of drainage; and presence or absence of bubbling or fluctuation in the water-seal chamber. If site care was performed, record the appearance of the site and the type of dressing applied. Document the patient's respiratory status, including pulse oximetry readings, and any pulmonary hygiene performed. Note the patient's level of pain, any comfort measures performed, and the results. Note the presence of subcutaneous air, documenting location and extent of occurrence. Include interventions to prevent complications. If any complications occurred, record your interventions and the results. Note the name of the physician notified of problems and the time of notification. At the end of the shift, record the amount of drainage on the intake and output record, and mark the level of drainage with the date and time on the collection device.

4/30/08	1350	Received pt. from recovery room at 1325. ® midaxillary CT with 20 cm of H₂O in Pleurevac suction control chamber. Collection chamber with 100 ml of serosanguineous fluid. No clots noted. Level of drainage dated and timed. No air leak noted. All CT connections taped, and 2 rubber-tipped clamps placed at bedside. Dried blood on CT dsg. No crepitus noted. Breath sounds clear with diminished breath sounds in ® lower lobe. P 98, BP 132/82, RR 28 shallow and labored, oral T 99.1° F. Skin pale, warm, and dry, mucous membranes pink. O₂ sat. 97% on 50% face mask. Pt. c/o aching pain at CT site and refused to take deep breaths and cough due to pain. Morphine sulfate 2 mg I.V. given at 1335. ————————————————————— Mary Ann Pfister, RN
4/30/08	1415	Pt. states "Pain is gone." Incentive spirometer used x 10. —— ————————————————————— Mary Ann Pfister, RN

Chest tube insertion

Insertion of a chest tube permits drainage of air or fluid from the pleural space to allow lung reexpansion. Usually performed by a physician with a nurse assisting, this procedure requires sterile technique. Insertion sites depend on the reason for the chest tube. For pneumothorax, the second intercostal space is the usual site because air rises to the top of the intrapleural space. For hemothorax or pleural effusion, the sixth to the eighth intercostal spaces are common sites because fluid settles to the lower levels of the intrapleural space. For removal of air and fluid, a chest tube is inserted into a high site as well as a low site.

Following insertion, one or more chest tubes are connected to a thoracic drainage system that removes air, fluid, or both from the pleural space using gravity or suction, and prevents backflow into that space, thus promoting lung reexpansion. Post-insertion care requires close observation of the patient and monitoring of lung reexpansion via X-ray.

Essential documentation

Before the procedure, verify that a signed consent is on the chart. Document the date and time of chest tube insertion. Include the name of the physician performing the procedure. Identify the insertion site and the type of drainage system and amount of suction used. Record the presence of drainage and bubbling. Drainage amount should also be included on the patient's intake and output record. Record the type, amount, and consistency of drainage. Document the patient's vital signs, auscultation findings, any complications, and nursing actions taken. Record patient teaching performed and the patient's understanding of the teaching. This may also need to be recorded on a patient teaching record, depending on your facility's policy. Document X-rays obtained and the date and time of abnormal findings reported to the physician.

| 2/28/08 | 1100 | Chest tube procedure explained and informed consent signed. Preinsertion P 98, RR 32, BP 118/72, oral T 97.9° F. #22 CT inserted into pt.'s Ⓛ lower midaxillary area by Dr. Joe Brown. Tube secured with one suture. Occlusive dressing applied. CT connected to Pleur-evac with 20 cm of suction, which immediately drained 100 ml of serosanguineous drainage. No air leaks evident with the system. Postinsertion P 80, RR 24, BP 120/72. Respirations shallow, unlabored. Slightly decreased breath sounds in Ⓛ post. lower lobe, otherwise breath sounds clear bilaterally. O_2 sat. 99% after CT insertion. Equal lung expansion noted. No crepitus palpated. Pt. reports only minimal discomfort at insertion site. Upright portable CXR obtained, and Dr. Brown notified. C&DB exercises and use of incentive spirometer reviewed with pt.; pt. verbalized understanding and was able to inspire 900 ml of volume. —————————————— Carol Slane, RN |

Chest tube removal

After the patient's lung has reexpanded, you may assist the physician in removing the chest tube. In many facilities, other health care professionals such as advanced practice nurses (clinical nurse specialists or nurse practitioners) are trained to perform chest tube removal. A chest X-ray is usually obtained after removal to evaluate lung condition.

Essential documentation

Document the date and time of chest tube removal and the name of the person who performed the procedure. Record the patient's vital signs and the findings of your respiratory assessment before and after chest tube removal. Note whether an analgesic was administered before the removal and how long after administration the chest tube was removed. Describe the patient's tolerance of the procedure. Record the amount of drainage in the collection bottle and the appearance of the wound at the chest tube site. Describe the type of dressing applied. Include patient teaching performed and the patient's understanding of the teaching. Document X-rays obtained after removal with date and time of abnormal findings reported to the physician.

1/9/08	1300	Procedure regarding CT removal explained to pt. Explained how to perform Valsalva's maneuver when tube is removed. Pt. was able to give return demonstration. VS P 88, BP 120/80, RR 18, oral T 97.8° F. Respirations regular, deep, unlabored. No use of accessory muscles. Full respiratory excursion bilaterally. Breath sounds clear bilaterally. No drainage in collection chamber since 0800. Percocet 2 tablets given. ———————— Marcy Wells, RN
1/9/08	1330	#20 CT removed without difficulty by Dr. Harvey Smith. CT wound clean. No drainage or redness noted. Petroleum jelly gauze dressing placed over insertion site, covered with 4" X 4" gauze dressing, and secured with 2" tape. Breath sounds remain clear. Equal lung expansion. Breathing comfortably in semi-Fowler's position, no subcutaneous crepitus noted. P 86, BP 132/84, RR 20. Pt. without complaints of pain or shortness of breath. Used incentive spirometer x 10. CXR ordered for 1400 ———————— Marcy Wells, RN

Cold therapy application

The application of cold therapy causes constriction of blood vessels; inhibits local circulation, suppuration, and tissue metabolism; relieves vascular congestion; slows bacterial activity in infections; reduces body temperature; and may act as a temporary anesthetic during brief, painful procedures. Because use of cold therapy also relieves inflammation, prevents edema, and slows bleeding, it may provide effective initial treatment after eye injuries, strains, sprains, bruises, muscle spasms, and burns. However, cold therapy won't reduce existing edema because it inhibits reabsorption of excess fluid.

Essential documentation

Record the date, time, and duration of cold application; the site of application; and the type of device used, such as an ice bag or collar, K pad, cold compress, or chemical cold pack. Indicate the temperature or temperature setting of the device, if possible. Before and after the procedure, record the patient's vital signs and the appearance of his skin. Document any signs of complications, interventions, and the patient's response. Describe the patient's tolerance of treatment.

1/14/08	1300	Before cold application, oral T 98.6° F, BP 110/70, P 80, RR 18.
		® groin site warm and dry, without redness, edema, or
		ecchymosis. Ice bag covered with towel applied to ® groin for
		20 min. Postprocedure T 98.6° F, BP 120/70, P 82, RR 20.
		® groin site cool and dry, without redness, edema, graying,
		mottling, blisters, or ecchymosis. No c/o burning or numbness.
		Pt. is resting comfortably. ——————— Greg Pearson, RN

Confusion

An umbrella term for puzzling or inappropriate behavior or responses, *confusion* reflects the inability to think quickly and coherently. Depending on its cause, confusion may arise suddenly or gradually and may be temporary or irreversible. Aggravated by stress and sensory deprivation, confusion commonly occurs in older hospitalized patients and may be mistaken for dementia.

When severe confusion arises suddenly and the patient also has hallucinations and psychomotor hyperactivity, his condition is classified as *delirium*. Long-term progressive confusion with deterioration of all cognitive functions is classified as *dementia*.

Confusion may result from metabolic, neurologic, cardiopulmonary, cerebrovascular, or nutritional disorders or can result from infection, toxins, drugs, or alcohol.

Essential documentation

If your patient is confused, document when you became aware of his confusion. Record the results of your neurologic and cardiopulmonary assessments. Record possible contributing factors, such as abnormal laboratory values, drugs, poor nutrition, poor sleep patterns, infection, surgery, pain, sensory overload or deprivation, and the use of alcohol and nonprescription drugs. Record the time and name of the physician notified. Note any new orders such as blood work to assess laboratory values or drug changes. Describe your interventions to reduce confusion and to keep your patient safe, and include the patient's response. Document patient teaching, including patient understanding of the teaching, and emotional support given.

4/22/08	1300	Upon entering pt.'s room, noted pt. putting on his pajamas. When
		asked what he was doing pt. stated, "It's my bedtime. I'm going to
		sleep." Told pt. it was 1230, lunchtime, and I had his lunch for
		him. Pt. alert, oriented to person, but not place and time. Knows
		the year he was born but stated he was at home and that it was
		fall of 1955. Speech clear but fragmented. Unable to repeat back
		5 numbers. Moving all extremities, hand grasps firm bilaterally.
		Gait steady with walker. P 102, BP 96/62, RR 18, oral T 101.8° F.
		Lungs clear, no use of accessory muscles, skin pink. S₁ and S₂
		heart sounds, no edema noted, radial and dorsalis pedis pulses
		strong, capillary refill less than 3 sec, skin hot and dry. Pt.
		needed to urinate X2 during assessment. Urinated 100 ml each
		time, urine cloudy, foul odor. No c/o burning on urination. Dr.
		Ramon Blake notified at 1245. Urine culture sent to lab for C/S.
		Tylenol 650 mg P.O. given for fever. Blood cultures x2, CBC
		w/diff., BUN, creatinine, and electrolytes ordered. Pt. reoriented
		to time and place. Encouraged pt. to drink fluids. Will check on
		pt. q15min. Family in to visit. —————— Matilda Jennings, RN

Continuous renal replacement therapy

Continuous renal replacement therapy (CRRT) is a type of dialysis that filters fluid, solutes, and electrolytes from the patient's blood and infuses a replacement solution. CRRT is used to treat patients with fluid overload or renal failure who can't tolerate hemodialysis.

CRRT carries a much lower risk of hypotension than conventional hemodialysis because it withdraws fluid more slowly, at about 200 ml/hr. CRRT reduces the risk of other complications and makes maintaining a stable fluid volume and regulating fluid and electrolyte balance easier. CRRT methods vary in complexity and include slow continuous ultrafiltration, continuous arteriovenous hemofiltration, and continuous venovenous hemofiltration. It's performed on a continuous basis by a specially trained nurse in an intensive care unit.

Essential documentation

When performing CRRT, record the time that the treatment began and the time it ended, and record fluid balance information per facility protocol. Document baseline and hourly vital signs and weight. Record laboratory studies, such as electrolytes, coagulation factors, complete blood count, and blood urea nitrogen and creatinine levels. Weight, vital signs, intake and output, and laboratory studies may be documented on a specialized flow sheet. Describe the appearance of the ultrafiltrate. Document your inspection of the insertion sites as well as any site care and dressing changes. Make sure you mark the dressing with the date and time of the dressing change. Record your assessment of circulation in the affected leg. Document any drugs given during the procedure. Note any complications, your interventions, and the patient's response. Include the patient's tolerance of the procedure.

3/27/08	0815	CRRT started at 0800. See CRRT flow sheet for labs, and hourly
		VS and I/O. Baseline weight 132.4 lb, P 92, BP 132/74, RR 20,
		oral T 98.2° F. Ultrafiltrate clear yellow. Ⓛ femoral access site
		without hematoma, redness, swelling, or warmth. Ⓛ foot warm,
		dorsalis pedis and posterior tibial pulses strong, capillary refill
		less than 3 sec. Insertion site cleaned according to protocol
		and covered with occlusive dressing. Pt. states he's tired and
		would like to sleep. ————————— Tom Costanza, RN

Critical test values, reporting

According to The Joint Commission's 2005 National Patient Safety Goals, critical test results must be reported to a responsible licensed caregiver in a timely manner so that immediate action may be taken. Critical test results include diagnostic tests, such as imaging studies, ECGs, laboratory tests, and other diagnostic studies. These critical test results may be reported verbally (including by telephone) or by fax, e-mail, or other technologies. If the results aren't reported verbally, the person sending the results should confirm that they have been received. Critical test values may be reported to another individual (such as a nurse, unit secretary, or physician's office staff) who will then report the values to the physician or licensed caregiver.

Essential documentation

Record the date and time you received the critical test result, the person who gave the results to you, the name of the test, and the critical value. Document the name of the physician or licensed health care provider you notified, the time of the notification, the means of communication used, and any orders given. If the message wasn't relayed verbally, include confirmation that the physician received the critical test result. Note any instructions or information given to the patient. If the message was given to a nurse, unit secretary, or office staff personnel, include that individual's name.

3/4/08	1000	Nanette Lange called from lab at 0945 to report critical PT value of 52 seconds. Results reported by telephone to Dr. Cynthia Potter at 0948, orders given to hold warfarin, obtain PT level in a.m., and call Dr. Potter with results. Pt. informed about elevated PT and the need to hold warfarin until PT levels drop to therapeutic range. Pt. instructed to report any bleeding to nurse. ———————————— Karen Lane, RN

Cultural needs identification

To provide culturally competent care to your patient, you must remember that your patient's cultural behaviors and beliefs may be different than your own. For example, most people in the United States make eye contact when talking with others. However, people in a number of cultures—including Native Americans, Asians, and people from Arab-speaking countries—may find eye contact disrespectful or aggressive. Recognizing your patient's cultural needs is the first step in developing a culturally sensitive care plan.

Essential documentation

Record the date and time of your assessment. Depending on your facility's policy, cultural assessment may be part of the admission history form or there may be a separate, more in-depth cultural assessment tool.

Assess the patient's communication style. Find out if he can speak and read English, his ability to read lips, his native language, and whether an interpreter is required. Observe his nonverbal communication style for eye contact, expressiveness, and ability to understand common signs. Determine social orientation, including culture, race, ethnicity, family role function, work, and religion. Document the patient's spatial comfort level, particularly in light of his conversation, proximity to others, body movement, and space perception. Ask about food preferences, family health history, religious and cultural health practices, and definitions of health and illness.

1/20/08	1500	Pt. states that he follows Jewish tradition of a kosher diet.
		Discussed types of foods the pt. could eat. Suggested family
		bring in some food for pt. Dr. David Sacco informed during
		morning rounds. Nutritional department notified of change
		to "kosher" diet. —————————————— — Diane Reale, RN

D

Death of a patient

After a patient dies, care includes preparing him for family viewing, arranging transportation to the morgue or funeral home, and determining the disposition of the patient's belongings. In addition, postmortem care entails comforting and supporting the patient's family and friends and providing them with privacy for grieving.

Postmortem care usually begins after a physician or nurse certifies the patient's death. If the patient died violently or under suspicious circumstances, postmortem care may be postponed until the coroner completes an examination.

Follow your facility's policy for release of the patient's body to a funeral home. Some facilities take the patient's body to a morgue, whereas other facilities have the representative from the funeral home obtain the body directly from their room.

Essential documentation

Document the date and time of the patient's death and the name of the physician (or in some states, the nurse) who pronounced the death. If resuscitation was attempted, indicate the time it started and ended, and refer to the code sheet in the patient's medical record. Note whether the case is being referred to the coroner. Include all postmortem care given, noting whether medical equipment was left in place. List all belongings and valuables and the name of the family member who accepted and signed the appropriate valuables or belongings list. Record any belongings left on the patient. If the patient has dentures, note whether they were left in the patient's mouth or given to a family member. (If given to a family member, include the family member's name.) Document the disposition of the patient's body and the name, telephone number, and address of the funeral home. Note the family members who were present at the time of death. If the family wasn't present, note the name of the family member who was notified. Be sure to include any care, emotional support, and education given to the family.

Document notification of death to organ donation centers per facility or state requirements. If the patient is removed from his room by a representative from a funeral home, complete the body release form required by the facility stating which family member granted permission for release of the body and which funeral home assumed care of the body.

3/22/08	1420	Called to room by pt.'s daughter stating pt. not breathing. Pt. found unresponsive in bed at 1345, not breathing, no pulse, no heart or breath sounds auscultated. Pt. is a DNR. Case not referred to coroner. Death pronouncement made by Dr. James Holmes at 1350. Postmortem care complete. Dentures placed in mouth. Belongings given to daughter. Pt. identification placed on body. Sent to morgue at 1415. Stayed with daughter throughout her visit and provided emotional support. Declined visit by chaplain. ————————————— Jeanne Ballinger, RN

Deep vein thrombosis, risk assessment

Deep vein thrombosis (DVT) is the formation of a blood clot inside a deep vein. It affects up to 200,000 people in the United States each year. It can occur in anyone; however, certain factors increase a patient's risk for developing DVT, including surgery, immobility, and such illnesses as cancer or inflammatory disease. Many facilities are instituting a DVT risk assessment form to be completed on admission and during each shift. Completion of the assessment gives the patient a score that indicates his risk—low, moderate, or high. Interventions are then ordered (such as application of sequential compression stockings or administration of a low-dose anticoagulant) based on the risk score.

Essential documentation

Document your DVT risk assessment per facility policy. Be sure to add the date and time of each assessment. If interventions have already been instituted, be sure to document that they're being carried out. Administration of medications will be documented on the medication administration record, but documentation of use of sequential compression devices needs to be added to your nurse's notes or on the flow sheet. Document any teaching that occurs. If your patient develops a DVT, be sure to document any treatment and teaching that you do.

4/14/08	1930	Risk assessment score shows pt. to be high risk. Dr. Steven
		Kane notified and SCDs placed on patient. Pt. instructed to
		keep SCDs in place while in bed. —————— Julie Herrick, RN

Dietary restriction noncompliance

All mentally competent adults may legally refuse treatment, including following dietary restrictions. The patient or family may tell you about noncompliance, or you may suspect noncompliance based on test results, such as blood glucose levels or blood pressure readings or the patient's general presentation. The patient may be noncompliant with diet for many reasons, including lack of motivation; lack of understanding; high cost of food items; lack of support; incompatibility with lifestyle, religion, or culture; immobility or lack of transportation to stores; unfamiliarity with new food preparation and cooking techniques; and diminished sense of taste.

Assess your patient to determine his reasons for not complying with dietary restrictions. Help him develop a plan that will be compatible with his needs and cognitive ability. Explain the relationship between proper nutrition and health. Teach about the consequences of not complying with dietary restrictions. Refer the patient to the dietitian for consultation and teaching. Consult social services if finances, mobility, food preparation, or accessibility to a food store is a problem. The home care department may be able to arrange for a home delivery meal service, such as Meals On Wheels, or arrange assistance with obtaining food items. Arrange for follow-up care and provide the patient with the names and telephone numbers of people to call with questions and concerns.

Essential documentation

Document noncompliance objectively. Use the patient's own words, if appropriate, or describe the data that suggest noncompliance. Record the reasons for the noncompliance, if known. Document your teaching about the diet, its relationship to the patient's medical problem, and the consequences of noncompliance. Include the patient's response to the teaching. Record the date and time of health care referrals made and the names of agencies and persons to whom the patient was referred.

4/15/08	1500	Pt. found in room eating a large piece of chocolate cake. Pt. is on 1800-calorie ADA diet. Discussed importance of proper nutrition in the treatment of diabetes. Pointed out that his blood glucose levels by fingerstick have been elevated. Pt. states, "I understand the importance of diet, but I'm frustrated with the food I'm getting in the hospital." Dietitian Pam Walker, RD, notified and will meet with pt. in a.m. ———————— May Brown, RN

Difficult patient

Most likely you have cared for dissatisfied patients at some point and heard remarks like "I've been ringing and ringing for a nurse. I could have died before you got here!" or "I've never seen such filth in my life. What kind of a hospital is this anyway?" These are the sounds of unhappy patients. If you dismiss them, you may be increasing your risk of a lawsuit.

The first step in defusing a potentially troublesome situation is to recognize that it exists. Note the following signs of a difficult patient: constant grumpiness, endless complaints, negative or no response to friendly remarks, and journaling of situations he views as wrong or causing him unnecessary distress. Use statements such as "You seem angry. Let's talk about what's bothering you." After acknowledging the situation, continue to attempt to communicate with the patient, even if you don't get a positive response. Never argue with the patient or try to convince him that a situation didn't happen the way he thinks it did. Don't make judgments and don't become defensive. Provide reassurance that you'll try your best to improve the situation, as appropriate. As necessary, involve other members of the health care team, such as the charge nurse, manager of the unit, or nursing supervisor. This may help the patient feel that his complaints are being taken seriously.

Essential documentation

Document the patient's complaints using his own words in quotes. Record the specific care given to your patient in direct response to complaints. If the patient threatens to file suit against you or the hospital, document this and notify your nursing supervisor or your facility's legal department. Record details of your contacts with the patient. Update your care plan to include more frequent contact with the patient.

| 1/16/08 | 1500 | Pt. stated, "No one comes when I ask for pain medication or when I put on my call light to go to the bathroom. Doesn't anyone work around here?" Calmly reminded pt. that she couldn't receive pain medication any earlier because it wasn't 2 hours since last dose. Administered morphine sulfate 2 mg I.V. at 1445 for c/o incisional pain rated as 8 on a scale of 0 to 10, w/ 10 being worst pain imaginable. At 1500 pt. reported pain as 2 out of 10. Reassured pt. that nurse will assess pain and administer pain medication on time if needed. Also assisted pt. to the bathroom and told her a nurse would check on her every 30 minutes. Nursing care plan updated accordingly. ————— Sue Stiles, RN |
| | 1630 | Pt. reports pain is 4/10, states she doesn't want any pain medication at this time. Assisted pt. to more comfortable position on Ⓛ side. Pt. reports not needing assistance to the bathroom at this time. ————————— Sue Stiles, RN |

Discharge instructions

Hospitals today commonly discharge patients earlier than they did in years past. As a result, the patient and his family must learn to change dressings; assess wounds; administer medication, handle medical equipment, tube feedings, and I.V. lines; and perform other functions that a nurse traditionally performed.

To perform these functions properly, the patient and his home caregiver must receive adequate instruction. The nurse is usually responsible for these instructions. If a patient receives improper instructions and injury results, you could be held liable.

Many hospitals distribute printed instruction sheets that adequately describe treatments, home care procedures, and medications. The patient's chart should indicate which materials were given and to whom. Generally, the patient or responsible person must sign that he received and understood the discharge instructions.

Courts typically consider these teaching materials evidence that instruction took place. However, to support testimony that instructions were given, the materials should be tailored to each patient's specific needs and refer to any verbal or written instructions that were provided. If caregivers practice procedures with the patient and family in the hospital, this should be documented, too, along with the results.

Essential documentation

Many facilities combine discharge summaries and patient instructions in one form. This form contains sections for recording patient assessment, patient education, detailed special instructions, and the circumstances of discharge. (See *The discharge summary form*, page 234.)

When writing a narrative note about discharge instructions, include:
- date and time of discharge
- vital signs on discharge
- family members or caregivers present for teaching
- treatments, such as dressing changes, or use of medical equipment
- signs and symptoms to report to the physician
- patient, family, or caregiver understanding of instructions or ability to give a return demonstration of procedures
- whether a patient or caregiver requires further instruction
- prescriptions for home medications, reconciled medication list, follow-up tests, or treatments
- physician's name and telephone number
- date, time, and location of any follow-up appointments or the need to call the physician for a follow-up appointment
- details of instructions given to the patient, including medications, activity, and diet (include any written instructions given to patient).

2/1/08	1530	Pt. to be discharged to home today. Reviewed discharge
		instructions with pt. and wife. Reviewed all medications,
		including drug name, purpose, doses, administration times,
		routes, and adverse effects. Drug information sheets and a
		complete and reconciled medication list given to pt. Pt.
		able to verbalize proper use of medications. Prescriptions
		given to pt. Wife will be performing dressing change to
		pt.'s Ⓡ foot. Wife was able to change dressing properly using
		sterile technique. Pt. and wife were able to state signs and
		symptoms of infection to report to doctor. Reinforced low-
		cholesterol, low-sodium diet and progressive walking guidelines.
		Wife has many questions about diet and will meet with
		dietitian before discharge. Pt. understands he's to follow
		up with Dr. Michael Carney in his office on 2/8/08 at
		1400. Wrote doctor's phone number on written instructions.
		Written discharge instructions given to pt. — Marcy Smythe, RN

The discharge summary form

By combining the patient's discharge summary with instructions for care after discharge, you can fulfill two requirements with a single form. When using this documentation method, be sure to give one copy to the patient and keep one for the legal record.

DISCHARGE INSTRUCTIONS

Name: *Tara Nicholas*   Date *2/1/08*

1. **Summary** *Admitted with c/o of severe headache and hypertensive crisis.*
   Treatment: Nitroprusside gtt for 24 hours
   Started Lopressor for hypertension
   Recommendation: Lose 10-15 lb
   Follow low-sodium, low-cholesterol diet

2. **Allergies** *penicillin*

3. **Medications (drug, dose time)** *Lopressor 25 mg by mouth at 6 a.m. and 6 p.m.*
   temazepam 15 mg by mouth at 10 p.m.

4. **Diet** *Low-sodium, low-cholesterol*

5. **Activity** *As tolerated*

6. **Discharged to** *Home*

7. **If questions arise, contact Dr.** *James Pritchett*   **Telephone No.** *(233) 555-1448*

8. **Special instructions** *Call doctor with headaches, dizziness*

9. **Return visit Dr.** *Pritchett*   **Place** *Health Care Clinic*
   On Date *2/15/08*   **Time** *0845 a.m.*

Tara Nicholas   *Donna Morales, RN*
Signature of patient or person responsible for   **Signature of doctor or nurse**
receipt of instructions from doctors   **reviewing instructions**

Do-not-resuscitate order

When a patient is terminally ill and death is expected, his physician and family (and the patient if appropriate) may agree that a do-not-resuscitate (DNR), or no-code, order is appropriate. The physician writes the order, and the staff carries it out if the patient goes into cardiac or respiratory arrest.

Because DNR orders are recognized legally, you'll incur no liability if you don't try to resuscitate a patient and that patient later dies. You may, however, incur liability if you initiate resuscitation on a patient who has a DNR order.

Every patient with a DNR order should have a written order on file. The order should be consistent with the facility's policy, which commonly requires that such orders be reviewed every 48 to 72 hours.

Increasingly, patients are deciding in advance of a crisis whether they want to be resuscitated. Health care facilities must provide written information to patients concerning their rights under state law to make decisions regarding their care, including the right to refuse medical treatment and the right to formulate an advance directive.

This information must be provided to all patients upon admission. You must also document that the patient received this information and whether he brought a written advance directive with him. A photocopy of the directive should be in the patient's record.

Essential documentation

If a terminally ill patient without a DNR order tells you that he doesn't want to be resuscitated in a crisis, document his statement as well as his degree of awareness and orientation. Then contact the patient's physician and your nursing supervisor, and ask for assistance from administration, legal services, or social services.

As a nurse, you have a responsibility to help the patient make an informed decision about continuing treatment. If the patient's wishes differ from those of his family or physician, make sure the discrepancies are thoroughly recorded in the chart. Then document that you notified your charge nurse, nursing supervisor, or social services.

| 4/19/08 | 1700 | Pt. stated, "If my heart should stop or if I stop breathing, just let me go. I've suffered with this cancer long enough." Pt.'s wife was present for this conversation and stated, "I don't want to see him in pain anymore. If he feels he doesn't want any heroic measures, then I stand by his decision." Pt. is alert and oriented to time, place, and person. Dr. Edward Patel notified of pt.'s wishes concerning resuscitation and stated he'll be in this evening to discuss DNR status with pt. and wife and write DNR orders. Elizabeth Sawyer, charge nurse, notified of pt.'s wishes for no resuscitation. ———— Joan Byers, RN |

Doctor's orders, clarification of

Although unit secretaries may transcribe orders, the nurse is ultimately responsible for the accuracy of the transcription. You have the authority and knowledge to question the validity of orders and to spot errors.

Follow your health care facility's policy for clarifying orders that are illegible, vague, ambiguous, or possibly erroneous. If you don't have a policy to cover a particular situation, contact the prescribing physician and always document your actions.

An order may be correct when issued but improper later because of changes in the patient's status. When this occurs, delay treatment until you've contacted the physician and clarified the situation. Follow your facility's policy for clarifying an order. If you are uncomfortable about the appropriateness of an order and the physician is adamant about keeping it, contact your charge nurse or the nursing supervisor to activate the chain of command until the situation is adequately resolved. Document your efforts to clarify the order, and document whether the order was carried out.

Essential documentation

When you question a physician's order, document your assessment and other data leading you to question the order. Record your conversation with the physician and whether the order was carried out. Also note whether the order was clarified or rewritten. If you refuse to carry out an order you believe to be written in error, record your refusal, your reasons for refusing, the names of the physician and nursing supervisor you notified, the time of notification, and their responses.

1/7/08	1235	Order written by Dr. Henry Corrigan at 1155 for Darvocet N 1
		tab P.O. q4hr prn incision pain. Called Dr. Corrigan at 1210 to
		clarify Darvocet dose. Clarification written on dr.'s orders and
		faxed to pharmacy. Dose changed on MAR to Darvocet 100 mg
		po q4hr prn pain. ———————————— Penelope Green, RN

Doctor's orders, telephone

Ideally, you should accept only written orders from a physician. However, when your patient needs immediate treatment and the physician isn't available to write an order, telephone orders are acceptable. Telephone orders may also be taken to expedite care when new information, such as laboratory data, is available that doesn't require a physical examination. Keep in mind that telephone orders are for the patient's well-being and not strictly for convenience. They should be given directly to you, rather than through a third party. Carefully follow your facility's policy on accepting and documenting a telephone order. When you receive a telephone order, write it down immediately and then read it back verbatim to the person who gave you the order for verification.

Essential documentation

Record the telephone order on the physician's order sheet while the physician is still on the telephone. Note the date and time. Write the order verbatim. On the next line, write "V.T.O." for verified telephone order, which means that you read the order back and received confirmation that it was correct. Write the physician's name and sign your name. If another nurse listened to the order with you, have her sign the order, too. Draw lines through any blank spaces in the order.

Make sure the physician countersigns the order within the set time limits. Without his signature, you may be held liable for practicing medicine without a license.

2/4/08	0900	Demerol 75 mg and Vistaril 50 mg I.M. now for pain. ———
		——————— V. T.O. Dr. Michael White/*Cathy Phillips*, RN

Doctor's orders, verbal

Errors made interpreting or documenting verbal orders can lead to mistakes in patient care and liability problems for you. Clearly, verbal orders can be a necessity, especially in an emergent situation, when actions are required quickly. Another common instance for verbal orders involves assisting a physician with a procedure or treatment. When the physician can't take the time to write an order, such as for sedation during a procedure, a verbal order is an appropriate action.

In most cases, do-not-resuscitate and no-code orders shouldn't be taken verbally. Carefully follow your facility's policy for documenting a verbal order, and use a special form if one exists.

Essential documentation

If possible, write the order out while the physician is still present. Read the order back for verification and note it in the chart. Note the date and time, and record the order verbatim. On the following line, write "V.V.O." for verified verbal order, which indicates that the order was repeated back to the physician. Write the physician's full name and sign your name. The physician will need to countersign the order within the time limits set by your facility. Without this countersignature, you may be held liable for practicing medicine without a license.

3/23/08	1500	Digoxin 0.125 mg P.O. now and daily in a.m. Furosemide 40 mg
		P.O. now and daily starting in a.m.
		———————— V.V.O. Dr. Martin Blackstone/ Judith Schilling, RN

Drug administration

Your employer must include a medication administration record (MAR) in your documentation system if you administer medications to patients. Commonly included in a card file (a medication Kardex), on a separate medication administration sheet, or in a computerized system, the MAR is the central record of medication orders and their execution and is part of the patient's permanent record. (See *The medication Kardex.*)

Drug administration is also included in the nurse's notes if the medication was given in response to a particular situation or problem, such as pain or agitation.

Essential documentation

When using the MAR, follow these guidelines:
■ Know and follow your facility's policies and procedures for checking and recording drug orders and charting drug administration.
■ Make sure all drug orders include the patient's full name, the date, and the drug's name, dosage, administration route or method, and frequency. When appropriate, include the specific number of doses given or the stop date. A reason for the use of as-needed drugs must be stated.
■ Be sure to include drug allergy information.
■ Write legibly in black ink.
■ Use only standard abbreviations approved by The Joint Commission. When doubtful about an abbreviation, write out the word or phrase.

The medication Kardex

One type of Kardex is the medication Kardex. It contains a permanent record of the patient's medications. The medication Kardex may also include the patient's diagnosis and information about allergies and diet. Routine and p.r.n. drugs may be on separate forms. A sample form is shown below.

NAME: *Jack Lemmons* MEDICAL RECORD #: *1234567*

NURSE'S FULL SIGNATURE, STATUS, AND INITIALS

	INIT.		INIT.		INIT.
Roy Charles, RN	*RC*				
Theresa Hopkins, RN	*TH*				

DIAGNOSIS: *Heart failure, atrial flutter, COPD*

ALLERGIES: *ASA*   DIET: *Cardiac*

ROUTINE/DAILY ORDERS.			DATE: *1/24/08*		DATE: *1/25/08*		DATE: *1/26/08*		DATE: *1/27/08*		DATE: *1/28/08*		DATE: *1/29/08*		DATE: *1/30/08*	
ORDER DATE	MEDICATIONS DOSE, ROUTE, FREQUENCY	TIME	SITE	INT.	SITE	INT.	SITE	INT.	SITE	INT.	SITE	INT.	SITE	INT.	SITE	INT.
1/24/08	*digoxin 0.125 mg*	*0900*		*RC*		*(RC)*										
RC	*I.V. daily*	*HR*	*68*			*52*										
1/24/08	*furosemide 40 mg*	*0900*		*RC*		*RC*										
RC	*I.V. q12hr*	*2100*		*TH*												
1/24/08	*enalaprilat 1.25 mg*	*0511*		*TH*		*TH*										
RC	*I.V. q6hr*	*1100*		*RC*												
		1700		*RC*												

(continued)

The medication Kardex *(continued)*

				P.R.N. MEDICATION			
	Addressograph			ALLERGIES: ASA			
INITIAL	SIGNATURE & STATUS	INITIAL	SIGNATURE & STATUS	INITIAL	SIGNATURE & STATUS	INITIAL	SIGNATURE & STATUS
RC	Roy Charles, RN						
TH	Theresa Hopkins, RN						

YEAR 20 _08_   P.R.N. MEDICATIONS

ORDER DATE: 1/24/08	RENEWAL DATE:	DISCONTINUED DATE:	DATE	1/24/08						
MEDICATION: acetaminophen		DOSE: 650 mg	TIME GIVEN	0930						
DIRECTION: p.r.n. mild pain		ROUTE: P.O.	SITE	P.O.						
			INIT.	RC						
ORDER DATE: 1/24/08	RENEWAL DATE:	DISCONTINUED DATE:	DATE	1/24/08						
MEDICATION: Milk of Magnesia		DOSE: 30 ml	TIME GIVEN	2115						
DIRECTION: q6hr p.r.n. constipation		ROUTE: P.O.	SITE							
			INIT.	TH						
ORDER DATE: 1/25/08	RENEWAL DATE:	DISCONTINUED DATE: 1/25/08	DATE	1/25/08	1/25/08					
MEDICATION: prochlorperazine		DOSE: 5 mg	TIME GIVEN	1100	2230					
DIRECTION: q8hr p.r.n. N/V		ROUTE: P.O.	SITE							
			INIT.	RC	TH					
ORDER DATE: 1/25/08	RENEWAL DATE:	DISCONTINUED DATE: 1/25/08	DATE	1/25/08						
MEDICATION: fluzone		DOSE: 0.5 ml	TIME GIVEN	1100						
DIRECTION: x1 dose only		ROUTE: I.M.	SITE	@ delt.						
			INIT.	RC						
ORDER DATE: 1/25/08	RENEWAL DATE:	DISCONTINUED DATE: 1/25/08	DATE	1/25/08						
MEDICATION: furosemide		DOSE: 40 mg	TIME GIVEN	1300						
DIRECTION: stat now		ROUTE: I.V.	SITE							
			INIT.	RC						
ORDER DATE:	RENEWAL DATE:	DISCONTINUED DATE:	DATE							
MEDICATION:		DOSE:	TIME GIVEN							
DIRECTION:		ROUTE:	SITE							
			INIT.							
ORDER DATE:	RENEWAL DATE:	DISCONTINUED DATE:	DATE							
MEDICATION:		DOSE:	TIME GIVEN							
DIRECTION:		ROUTE:	SITE							
			INIT.							

■ Sign your name in the appropriate space on the Kardex, with your initials next to it.

■ Record drugs immediately after administration so that another nurse doesn't give the drug again.

■ If you document by computer, chart your information for each drug immediately after you administer it. If the facility uses bar codes (an electronic medication administration record) for medication administration, charting will occur at the time of administration because the scanning system requiring both the bar code on the patient's identification bracelet and the bar code on the medication to match before administration of the drug.

■ If a specific assessment parameter must be monitored during administration of a drug, such as a pulse, document this requirement on the MAR.

3/1/08	2000	Pt. given Tylenol 650 mg P.O. for temp of 102°F. Tepid bath also given. Will recheck temp in 1/2 hour. ——— ——————————————— Catherine Douglas, RN

Drug administration, adverse effects of

Also called a *side effect,* an adverse drug effect is an undesirable response that may be mild, severe, or life-threatening. Any clinically useful drug can cause an adverse effect.

As a nurse, you play a key role in reporting adverse drug effect events. Reporting adverse effects helps ensure the safety of drugs regulated by the Food and Drug Administration (FDA). The FDA's Medical Products Reporting Program supplies health care professionals with MedWatch forms on which they can report adverse events.

Complete a MedWatch form when you suspect that a drug is responsible for:

■ death
■ life-threatening illness
■ initial or prolonged hospitalization
■ disability
■ congenital anomaly
■ need for any medical or surgical intervention to prevent a permanent impairment or an injury.

Also, promptly inform the FDA of product quality problems, such as:

- defective devices
- inaccurate or unreadable product labels
- packaging or product mix-ups
- intrinsic or extrinsic contamination or stability problems
- particulates in injectable drugs
- product damage.

Essential documentation

When filing a MedWatch form, keep in mind that you aren't expected to establish a connection between the drug and the problem. You don't have to include a lot of details; you only have to report the adverse event or the problem with the drug. FDA regulations protect your identity and the identities of your patient and employer. Send completed forms to the FDA by using the fax number or mailing address on the form. For voluntary reporting, nurses can also report adverse events online using the MedWatch Voluntary Reporting Online Form (3500). The mandatory reporting MedWatch form (3500a) may be downloaded, but can't be submitted online. Many hospitals have a telephone number where anonymous reports are possible. Check with your facility's policy.

File a separate MedWatch form for each event, and attach additional pages if needed. Also, remember to comply with your health care facility's protocols for reporting adverse events associated with drugs.

Product lot numbers are used in product identification, tracking, and product recall; therefore, the lot number should be retained and your supervisor should keep a copy of the report on file.

The FDA will report back to you on the actions it takes and will continue to work to instruct health care professionals about adverse events. See *MedWatch form for reporting adverse drug reactions,* for an example of a completed form.

An adverse effect may also need to be charted in the nurse's notes if it involves a physical effect, such as a rash or nausea. Note assessment findings related to the drug on the chart and the date, time, and name of the physician notified. Also follow your facility's requirements for completing an incident report.

| 1/13/08 | 0930 | Called in by pt. to see rash developing on abdomen. Rash also noted to be covering back, scapula area. Ampicillin 1 g given at 0900. Call placed to Dr. Phillip Joshi. —— *Ronald Devine, RN* |

MedWatch form for reporting adverse drug reactions

MEDWATCH
THE FDA MEDICAL PRODUCTS REPORTING PROGRAM

For **VOLUNTARY** reporting
by health professionals of adverse
events and product problems

Form Approved: OMB No. 0910-0291 Expires: 4/30/96
See OMB statement on reverse

FDA Use Only

Triage unit
sequence #

Page _____ of _____

A. Patient information

1. Patient identifier
01234
In confidence

2. Age at time of event:
or _____
Date of birth: **3/11/58**

3. Sex
☑ female
☐ male

4. Weight
_____ lbs
or
59 kgs

B. Adverse event or product problem

1. ☐ Adverse event and/or ☑ Product problem (e.g., defects/malfunctions)

2. Outcomes attributed to adverse event (check all that apply)
☐ death _____ (mo/day/yr)
☐ life-threatening
☐ hospitalization – initial or prolonged
☐ disability
☐ congenital anomaly
☐ required intervention to prevent permanent impairment/damage
☐ other: _____

3. Date of event (mo/day/yr) **3/8/08**

4. Date of this report (mo/day/yr) **3/8/08**

5. Describe event or problem

After reconstituting 100-mg vial with 10 ml of bacteriostatic water, the drug crystallized and turned yellow.

Drug wasn't given.

6. Relevant tests/laboratory data, including dates

7. Other relevant history, including preexisting medical conditions (e.g., allergies, race, pregnancy, smoking and alcohol use, hepatic/renal dysfunction, etc.)

PLEASE TYPE OR USE BLACK INK

C. Suspect medication(s)

1. Name (give labeled strength & mfr/labeler, if known)
#1 *Leucovorin calcium for*
#2 *Injection — 100-mg vial*

2. Dose, frequency & route used
#1 *100 mg IV X1*
#2

3. Therapy dates (if unknown, give duration) from/to (or best estimate)
#1 *3/8/08*
#2

4. Diagnosis for use (indication)
#1 *Megaloblastic anemia*
#2

5. Event abated after use stopped or dose reduced
#1 ☐ yes ☐ no ☐ doesn't apply
#2 ☐ yes ☐ no ☐ doesn't apply

6. Lot # (if known)
#1 *#891*
#2

7. Exp. date (if known)
#1
#2

8. Event reappeared after reintroduction
#1 ☐ yes ☐ no ☐ doesn't apply
#2 ☐ yes ☐ no ☐ doesn't apply

9. NDC # (for product problems only)

10. Concomitant medical products and therapy dates (exclude treatment of event)

D. Suspect medical device

1. Brand name

2. Type of device

3. Manufacturer name & address

4. Operator of device
☐ health professional
☐ lay user/patient
☐ other:

5. Expiration date (mo/day/yr)

6.
model # _____
catalog # _____
serial # _____
lot # _____
other # _____

7. If implanted, give date (mo/day/yr)

8. If explanted, give date (mo/day/yr)

9. Device available for evaluation? (Do not send to FDA)
☑ yes ☐ no ☐ returned to manufacturer on _____ (mo/day/yr)

10. Concomitant medical products and therapy dates (exclude treatment of event)

E. Reporter (see confidentiality section on back)

1. Name & address
Patricia Cohen
987 Elm Ave.
Cincinnati, Ohio

phone # **(123) 456-7890**

2. Health professional? ☑ yes ☐ no

3. Occupation *RN*

4. Also reported to
☐ manufacturer
☐ user facility
☑ distributor

5. If you do NOT want your identity disclosed to the manufacturer, place an "X" in this box. ☐

Mail to: MEDWATCH
5600 Fishers Lane
Rockville, MD 20852-9787

or FAX to:
1-800-FDA-0178

FDA

FDA Form 3500 (1/96)   Submission of a report does not constitute an admission that medical personnel or the product caused or contributed to the event.

Drug administration, withholding ordered drug

Under certain circumstances, a prescribed drug can't or shouldn't be given as scheduled. For example, you may decide to withhold a stool softener for a patient with diarrhea. A patient may be scheduled for a test that requires him to not take a certain drug or a change in the patient's condition may make the drug inappropriate to give. For example, an antihypertensive drug may have been prescribed for a patient who now has low blood pressure. In some circumstances, a patient may refuse a drug. For example, a patient may refuse to take his cholestyramine because he believes it's causing abdominal upset. If a drug is withheld, notify the physician.

Essential documentation

In your nurse's note, document the date and time the drug was withheld, the reason for withholding the drug, the name of the physician notified, and the physician's response. If the physician changed a drug order, record and document the new order and the time it was carried out. Document any actions taken to safeguard your patient.

On the medication administration record (MAR) or medication Kardex, initial the appropriate box as usual but circle your initials to indicate the drug wasn't given. (See *Withholding an ordered medication.*) Record the correct code indicating why the drug wasn't given, or fill in the appropriate section on the MAR with the date, time, name, and dose of the drug withheld, as well as the reason for withholding the drug. For a computerized record, follow your program's guidelines for recording a held medication.

3/3/08	1800	Digoxin 0.125 mg P.O. not given due to pulse less than 60. Dr. Miller notified that medication was withheld. ——————————————————— Betty Griffin, RN

Withholding an ordered medication

When withholding an ordered medication, it's necessary to document it on the medication administration record as indicated below. This is usually indicated by circling your initials.

NAME: *Jack Lemmons*   MEDICAL RECORD #: *987654*

NURSE'S FULL SIGNATURE, STATUS, AND INITIALS

NAME	INIT.		INIT.		INIT.
Roy Charles, RN	*RC*				
Theresa Hopkins, RN	*TH*				

DIAGNOSIS: *Heart failure, atrial flutter, COPD*

ALLERGIES: ASA   DIET: *Cardiac*

ORDER DATE	MEDICATIONS DOSE, ROUTE, FREQUENCY	TIME	DATE: 1/24/08 SITE	INT.	DATE: 1/25/08 SITE	INT.	DATE: 1/26/08 SITE	INT.	DATE: 1/27/08 SITE	INT.	DATE: 1/28/08 SITE	INT.	DATE: 1/29/08 SITE	INT.	DATE: 1/30/08 SITE	INT.
1/24/08	digoxin 0.125 mg	0900		RC		(RC)										
RC	I.V. daily	HR	68		52											
1/24/08	furosemide 40 mg	0900		RC		RC										
RC	I.V. q12hr	2100		TH												
1/24/08	enalaprilat 1.25 mg	0511		TH		TH										
RC	I.V. q6hr	1100		RC												
		1700		RC												
		2300	.	TH												

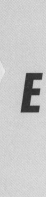

E

Endotracheal extubation

When your patient no longer requires mechanical ventilation or airway protection, the endotracheal (ET) tube can be removed. The ET tube is also removed when a tracheostomy is performed. When done at the bedside, the ET tube is often removed by the respiratory therapist. Explain the procedure to your patient and provide assistance to prevent traumatic manipulation of the tube when it's untaped or unfastened. Teach the patient to cough and deep breathe after the ET tube is removed, and assess him frequently for signs of respiratory distress.

Essential documentation

Record the date and time of extubation, presence or absence of stridor or other signs of upper airway edema, breath sounds, type of supplemental oxygen administered, any complications and required subsequent therapy, and the patient's tolerance of the procedure. Document patient teaching and support given.

4/26/08	1700	Explained extubation procedure to pt. Pt. acknowledged
		understanding by nodding his head "yes." Placed pt. in
		high Fowler's position and suctioned for scant amount of
		thin white secretions. ET tube removed at 1630 by respiratory
		therapist. No stridor or respiratory distress noted, breath
		sounds clear. RR 22, P 92, BP 128/82, oral T 98.4° F.
		Pulse oximetry 97% on O_2 2 L by NC. Instructed pt. on
		importance of coughing and deep breathing every hr. Pt.
		was able to give proper return demonstration. Cough
		nonproductive. ———————————————— Margie Egan, RN

Endotracheal intubation

Endotracheal (ET) intubation involves the oral or nasal insertion of an ET tube through the larynx into the trachea, providing a controlled airway and mechanical ventilation and oxygenation. Performed by a doctor, anesthetist, respiratory therapist, or nurse educated in the procedure, ET intubation may occur in emergencies such as cardiopulmonary arrest, to manage illnesses such as epiglottiditis, or under more controlled circumstances such as surgery. (See *Responding to breathing problems,* pages 248 and 249.)

ET intubation establishes and maintains a patent airway, protects against aspiration by sealing off the trachea from the digestive tract, permits removal of tracheobronchial secretions in patients who can't cough effectively, and provides a route for mechanical ventilation. Teaching about ET intubation should be provided when appropriate.

Essential documentation

Document whether the doctor explained the procedure, risks, complications, and alternatives to the patient or person responsible for making decisions concerning the patient's health care. Record the date and time of intubation and the name of the person performing the procedure. Include indications for the procedure and success or failure. Chart the type and size of tube, cuff size, amount of inflation, and the ET tube marking at the lip. Indicate whether drugs were administered before or after the procedure. Document the initiation of supplemental oxygen or ventilation therapy. Record the results of carbon dioxide detection, chest auscultation, and chest X-ray study. Note the occurrence of any complications or necessary interventions, and the patient's response. Describe the patient's reaction to the procedure. Also, document any teaching done before and after the procedure.

3/16/08	1015	Pt. informed by Dr. Tina Eagan of the need for intubation, the risks, potential complications, and alternatives. Pt. consented to the procedure. Pt. given etomidate 10 mg I.V. and intubated by Dr. Eagan at 0945 with size 8 oral cuffed ET tube. Tube taped at #23 at the lip, in right corner of mouth. Pt. on ventilator set at TV 750, FIO_2 45%, 5 cm PEEP, AC of 12. RR 20, nonlabored. Portable CXR confirms proper placement. ® lung with basilar crackles and expiratory wheezes. Ⓛ lung clear. Pt. opening eyes when name is called. When asked if he's comfortable and in no pain, pt. nods head yes. ———— ———————————————————————— Jim Haner, RN

CASE CLIP

Responding to breathing problems

Mr. J. is a 52-year-old male patient admitted to the hospital with pneumonia. He has no other past medical history. He smokes two packs of cigarettes per day and drinks two to three beers each evening. He's a police officer and he's currently going through a divorce. He's angry that he's in the hospital and questions all of his care. Vital signs on admission were:

- temperature: 100.1° F (37.8° C)
- heart rate (HR): 108 beats/minute
- respiratory rate (RR): 22 breaths/minute
- pulse oximetry: 95% on room air.

Mr. J. was on the medical-surgical unit. He was permitted to be out of bed and ambulating. He requested to walk outside but was told he had to wait until his I.V. antibiotic was complete. At change of shift, 1810, Mr. J. called the nurse to tell her that he was having trouble breathing. He had audible gurgling respirations and a moist cough. His vital signs at this time were:

- temperature: 98.8° F (37.1° C)
- HR: 120 beats/minute
- RR: 28 breaths/minute
- pulse oximetry: 91% on room air.

The nurse placed him on oxygen at 4 L/minute via nasal cannula. Her assessment revealed bibasilar crackles and wheezing. She noticed that the I.V. antibiotic that she had just started at 1800 was empty. When questioned, Mr. J. admitted that he "opened up" the I.V. because he wanted to go outside to smoke. Mr. J. was becoming increasingly anxious and restless. His pulse oximetry reading decreased to 86% and he began coughing up pink-tinged sputum.

The rapid response team (RRT) was notified and arrived within 3 minutes. Mr. J.'s vital signs at this time were:

- HR: 120 beats/minute
- RR: 30 breaths/minute
- pulse oximetry: 83% on 100% non-rebreather mask.

Mr. J. was becoming more lethargic. His respirations were more labored. The RRT quickly reviewed Mr. J.'s history and medications. Results of arterial blood gas (ABG) analysis were:

- pH: 7.15
- Po_2: 60
- Pco_2: 55
- HCO_3^-: 28
- O_2 sat: 79%.

Responding to breathing problems *(continued)*

Mr. J. was given 40 mg Lasix I.V. but because of his poor ABG results and decreasing level of consciousness, the RRT decided to call the emergency department (ED) physician to insert an endotracheal tube to assist with ventilation and oxygenation. The ED physician responded to the call and intubated Mr. J. He was placed on mechanical ventilation and transferred to the intensive care unit (ICU). The attending physician was notified about the occurrence and additional orders for care were obtained. The family was notified of the change in Mr. J.'s condition and his transfer to ICU.

Enema administration

An enema is a solution introduced into the rectum and colon for the administration of medication, to clean the lower bowel in preparation for diagnostic or surgical procedures, or to relieve distention and promote expulsion of flatus. An enema may also lubricate the rectum and colon and soften hardened stool for removal. Enema solutions and methods vary to suit your patient's condition or treatment requirements.

Essential documentation

Record the date, time, type, and amount of enema administration. Describe the color, consistency, amount of the return, and any abnormalities with the return. Record complications that occurred, actions taken, and the patient's response. Document the patient's tolerance of the procedure.

Depending on your facility's policy, you may also need to document the enema on the medication Kardex or treatment record.

2/28/08	0900	Pt. c/o constipation. States she hasn't had a BM for 2 days. Dr.
		Mary Martin notified and ordered Fleet enema 1 daily p.r.n.
		constipation. Received Fleet enema, 100 ml, at 0830 and held
		for 20 minutes. Pt. had large amount of brown, solid stool.
		No c/o abd. pain; no abd. distention noted. —— Sue Smith, RN

Epidural analgesia

Epidural analgesia is medication administered to the epidural space to provide pain relief. It causes less sedation and allows patients to perform coughing and deep-breathing exercises and to ambulate earlier after surgery. It's also useful in patients with chronic pain that isn't relieved by less invasive methods of pain therapies. An epidural catheter is placed by an anesthesiologist in the epidural space outside the spinal cord between the vertebrae. Pain relief with minimal adverse effects is the result of drug delivery so close to the opiate receptors.

Opioids, such as preservative-free morphine (Duramorph) and fentanyl, are administered through the catheter and move slowly into the cerebrospinal fluid to opiate receptors in the dorsal horn of the spinal cord. The opioids may be administered by bolus dose, continuous infusion by pump, or patient-controlled analgesia. They may be administered alone or in combination with bupivacaine (a local anesthetic).

Adverse effects of epidural analgesia include sedation, nausea, urinary retention, orthostatic hypotension, itching, respiratory depression, headache, back soreness, leg weakness and numbness, and respiratory depression. The nurse must monitor the patient for these adverse reactions and notify the doctor or anesthesiologist if they occur. Most facilities have policies or standards of care that address interventions for adverse effects and monitoring parameters.

Essential documentation

Record the date and time of your entry. Document the type and dose of the drug administered. Include the patient's level of consciousness, pain level (using a 0 to 10 scale, with 0 being no pain and 10 being the worst pain imaginable), and respiratory rate and quality. Also record the amount of drug received per hour and the number of dose attempts by the patient if the analgesia is patient-controlled. Be sure to include site assessment, dressing changes, infusion bag changes, tubing changes, and patient education. Document complications, such as numbness, leg weakness, and respiratory depression, your interventions, and the patient's response.

Most facilities use a flow sheet to document drug dosage, rate, route, vital signs, respiratory rate, pulse oximetry, pain scale, and sedation scale. Follow your facility's policy; however, these parameters should be monitored frequently for the first 12 hours and then every 4 hours after that. If you don't have a specific flow sheet for epidural documentation, use your regular flow sheet and document in the progress notes other assessments, as needed, or unusual circumstances.

5/22/08	1500	Pt. received from PACU with epidural catheter in place.
		Dressing covering site clean, dry, and intact. Pt. receiving
		bupivacaine 0.125% and fentanyl 5 mcg/ml in 250 ml NSS at
		rate of 2 ml/hr. Respiratory rate 20 and deep, level of
		sedation 0 (alert), O₂ sat. by pulse oximetry on O₂ 2L by NC
		99%, BP 120/80, P 72. Pt. reports pain as 2 on a scale of 0
		to 10. No c/o nausea, itching, H/A, leg weakness, back soreness.
		Pt. voided 300 ml yellow urine. Told pt. to report any pain
		greater than 3 out of 10, inability to void, and numbness in
		legs. See flow sheet for frequent monitoring of drug dose,
		rate, VS, resp. rate, pulse ox., level of pain, and sedation level.
		—————————————————— — Mary Holmes, RN

Evidence collection, suspected criminal case

If you're asked to care for an injured suspect who's accompanied by the police, you may be asked to give the police the patient's belongings and a sample of his blood. If you fail to follow proper protocol, the evidence you turn over to the police may not be admissible in court. The patient may later be able to sue you for invasion of privacy. However, if an accused person consents to a search, any evidence found is considered admissible in court. (See *To search or not to search.*)

 LEGAL LOOKOUT

To search or not to search

The Fourth Amendment to the U.S. Constitution provides that "the right of the people to be secure in their persons, houses, papers, and effects, against unreasonable searches and seizures shall not be violated, and no warrants shall be issued, but upon probable cause." This means that every individual, even a suspected criminal, has a right to privacy, including a right to be free from intrusions that are made without search warrants. However, the Fourth Amendment doesn't absolutely prohibit all searches and seizures, only the unreasonable ones.

In general, searches that occur as part of medical care don't violate a suspect's rights. However, searches made for the sole purpose of gathering evidence—especially if done at police request—very well may. Several courts have said that a suspect subjected to an illegal private search has a right to seek remedy against the unlawful searcher in a civil lawsuit.

LEGAL LOOKOUT

Collecting blood as evidence

Opinions differ as to whether a blood test, such as a blood alcohol test, is admissible in court if the person refused consent for the test. In *Schmerber v. California (1966),* the U.S. Supreme Court said that a blood extraction obtained without a warrant, incidental to a lawful arrest, isn't an unconstitutional search and seizure and is admissible evidence. Many courts have held this to mean that a blood sample must be drawn after the arrest to be admissible.

Further, the blood sample must be drawn in a medically reasonable manner. In *People v. Kraft (1970),* a suspect was pinned to the floor by two police officers while a doctor drew a blood sample. In *State v. Riggins (1977),* a suspect's fractured arm was twisted while a police officer sat on him to force consent to a blood test. In both cases, the courts ruled the test results inadmissible. The courts have also ruled as inadmissible — and as a violation of due process rights—evidence gained by the forcible and unconsented insertion of a nasogastric tube into a suspect to remove stomach contents (*Rochin v. California [1952]*).

Courts have admitted blood tests as evidence when the tests weren't for medically necessary purposes such as blood typing (*Commonwealth v. Gordon [1968]*). Some courts have also allowed blood work to be admitted as evidence when it was drawn for nontherapeutic reasons and voluntarily turned over to the police.

Be careful, though. A doctor or nurse who does blood work without the patient's consent may be liable for committing battery, even if the patient is a suspected criminal and the blood work is medically necessary.

Opinions differ as to whether a blood test, such as an alcohol blood test, is admissible in court if the person refused consent for the test. A doctor or nurse who does blood work without the patient's consent may be liable for committing battery, even if the patient is a suspected criminal and the blood work is medically necessary. (See *Collecting blood as evidence.*)

Because the laws of search and seizure are complex and subject to change by new legal decisions, consult an administrator or hospital attorney before complying with a police request to turn over a patient's personal property.

Essential documentation

Be precise in documenting all medical and nursing procedures related to collecting evidence or dealing with a patient in police custody. Note any blood work done. List all treatments and the patient's response to them. Record anything you turn over to the police or administration and the name of the person you gave it to. Statements made by the patient should be recorded only if they're directly related to his care. If your patient keeps a journal during his stay, document this in your note. Document the presence of a police officer and your interactions with the officer. Document the name of the administrator or hospital attorney with whom you consulted before turning anything over to the police.

If you discover evidence, use your facility's chain of custody form to document the identity of each person handling the evidence as well as the dates and times it was in that person's possession. If your facility doesn't have a chain of custody form, keep careful notes of exactly what was taken, by whom, and when. Give this information to the administrator when you deliver the evidence. Until such time as the evidence can be turned over, it should be kept in a locked area.

3/7/08	2300	Pt. escorted by a police officer to the ED with four
		lacerations on Ⓛ leg. Pt. calm but easily agitated. While
		removing his pants, a ziplock bag with a white powder
		fell to the floor. In addition, a pocketknife, $6.87, and a
		pen were collected. Officer J. Smitts requested the knife
		and bag of white powder. After discussing the request
		with Arnold Beckwith, Chief Administrator, the knife and
		bag of powder were turned over to Officer J. Smitts.
		The remaining items and clothing, which consisted of
		pen, brown belt, and lightweight blue jacket, were bagged
		and left with pt. Pt. states he had tetanus shot last
		year. Lacerations of Ⓛ leg were irrigated with sterile
		NSS, sutured by Dr. Will Rogers after administering local
		anesthetic injections, antibiotic ointment applied, and
		covered with dry sterile dressings. Pt. reports only
		minimal discomfort at laceration site. Explained care of
		lacerations and signs and symptoms of infection to
		report. Pt. verbalized understanding. Written ED guide-
		lines for care of sutures given to pt. —— L. Salamon RN

F

Falls, patient

Falls are a major cause of injury and death among older adults. For this reason, many facilities have a fall risk identification system in place to help identify those at risk for a fall. Once identified, additional measures are taken to heighten patient safety and decrease the incidence of falls.

If your patient falls despite your preventive measures, call for help, perform a quick head to toe assessment, and check his vital signs before you move him, if possible. Provide any emergency measures necessary, such as securing an airway, controlling bleeding, or stabilizing a deformed limb. Ask the patient or a witness what happened. If you don't detect any problems, return the patient to bed. Notify the physician of the event, and obtain orders for additional care or evaluation, such as X-ray examination.

Essential documentation

After a patient falls, chart the event and file an incident report. Record how and where the patient was found and the time he was discovered. Keep notes objective, avoiding any judgments or opinions. Assess the patient and record any bruises, lacerations, or abrasions. Describe any pain or deformity in the extremities, particularly the hip, arm, leg, or lumbar spine. Record vital signs. Document your patient's neurologic assessment. Include confusion, slurred speech, weakness in the extremities, or a change in mental status. Record the date, time, and name of the doctor and other persons notified, such as family members. Include instructions or orders given. Also document any patient education.

1/6/08	1500	Pt. found on floor between bed and chair on left side of bed
		at 1330. Pt. c/o pain in her ® hip area and difficulty moving
		® leg. No abrasions or lacerations noted. BP elevated at
		158/94. P 94, RR 22, oral T 98.2° F. Pt states, "I was trying
		to get into the chair when I fell." Pt. alert and oriented to
		time, place, and person. Speech clear and coherent. Hand
		grasps strong bilaterally. ® leg externally rotated and shorter
		than Ⓛ leg. Dr. Ali Dayoub notified at 1338. Pt. assisted back to
		bed with assist of 3, maintaining ® hip and leg in alignment.
		Hip X-ray ordered and showed ® hip fracture. Dr. Dayoub
		aware and family notified. Pt. to be evaluated by orthopedic
		surgeon. Pt. medicated for pain with Demerol 50 mg I.M.
		Maintaining bed rest at present time. Siderails up, bed in low
		position. Explained all procedures to pt. Call bell in hand and
		verbalizes she understands to call for help with moving. ———
		——————————— Beverly Kotsur, R.N

Falls, precautions against

Patient falls resulting from slips, slides, weakness, fainting, or tripping over equipment can lead to prolonged hospitalization, increased hospital costs, and liability problems. Because falls can cause so many problems, your facility may require you to assess each patient for his risk of falling and to take measures to prevent falls. (See *Reducing the risk of falls,* page 256.) If your facility requires a risk assessment form for patients, complete it and keep it in the patient's chart. (See *Risk assessment for falls,* page 257.) Those at risk require documentation of interventions performed to prevent falls. (See *Reducing your liability in patient falls,* page 258.)

Essential documentation

Record the date and time of your entry. Describe the reasons for implementing fall precautions for your patient, such as a high score on a risk for falls assessment tool. Document your interventions, such as frequent toileting, reorienting the patient to his environment, and placing needed objects within his reach. Include the patient's response to these interventions. If the patient is confined to bed, document safety measures, such as the bed in low position and call light within reach. Note measures taken to alert other health care workers of the risk of

(Text continues on page 258.)

Reducing the risk of falls

There are no foolproof ways to prevent a patient from falling, but The Joint Commission recommends the following steps to reduce the risks of falls and injuries. Be sure to document your safety interventions in the appropriate place in the medical record.

Physical measures
- Provide adequate exercise and ambulation.
- Offer frequent food and liquids.
- Provide regular toileting.
- Evaluate medications (hypnotics, sedatives, analgesics, psychotropics, antihypertensives, laxatives, diuretics, and polypharmacy increase the risk of falling).
- Assess and manage pain.
- Promote normal sleep patterns.

Psychological measures
- Reorient the patient to his environment.
- Communicate with the patient and his family about the risk of falls and the need to call for help before getting up on his own.
- Teach relaxation techniques.
- Provide companionship, such as sitters or volunteers.
- Provide diversionary activities.

Environmental measures
- Orient the patient to his environment.
- Use appropriate lighting and noise control.
- Consider a bed alarm.
- Provide a safe space layout (long-term care), such as a low-lying bed or mattress or pads on the floor.
- Place assistive devices within the patient's reach at all times.
- Provide bed adaptations (long-term care).
- Provide accessibility to needed objects at all times.
- Ensure frequent observation of any patient at risk, such as moving the patient closer to the nurses' station and involving family.
- Provide side rail adaptations and alternatives.
- Use appropriate seating and equipment.
- Provide identifiers of high-risk status, such as an arm band or an identifier on the patient's bed or door.

Education
- Provide staff, patient, and family education on identifying and reducing the risk of falls.

Risk assessment for falls

Because falls create so many problems, your facility may require documented risk assessment and prevention actions. For example, if your facility requires a risk assessment form for patients, complete it and keep it in the patient's chart.

Certain patients have a greater risk of falling than others. Using a list such as the one below, which was developed for use with older patients, can help you determine the extent of the risk. To use the chart, check each applicable item and total the number of points. A score of 10 or more indicates a risk of falling.

DETERMINING A PATIENT'S RISK OF FALLING

Points	Patient category	Points	Patient category
	Age		**Gait and balance**
1	80 or older		Assess gait by having the patient stand in one spot with both feet on the ground for 30 seconds without holding onto something. Then have him walk straight ahead and through a doorway. Next, have him turn while walking.
2 ✓	70 to 79 years old		
	Mental state		
0	Oriented at all times or comatose	1	Wide base of support
2	Confused at all times	1	Loss of balance while standing
4 ✓	Confused periodically	1 ✓	Balance problems when walking
	Duration of hospitalization	1	Diminished muscle coordination
0 ✓	Over 3 days	1	Lurching or swaying
2	0 to 3 days	1	Holds on or changes gait when walking through a doorway
	Falls within the past 6 months	1	Jerking or instability when turning
0	None	1	Needs an assistive device such as a walker
2 ✓	1 or 2		
5	3 or more		**Medications** How many different drugs is the patient taking?
	Elimination	0	None
0 ✓	Independent and continent	1	1
1	Uses catheter, ostomy, or both	2 ✓	2 or more
3	Needs help with elimination		___ Alcohol ___ Cathartics
5	Independent and incontinent		___ Anesthetics ___ Diuretics
			___ Antihistamines ___ Opioids
1 ✓	**Visual impairment**		✓ Antihyperten- ___ Psychotropics
			sives Sedative-
3	**Confinement to chair**		___ Antiseizure drugs hypnotics
			___ Antidiabetics ___ Other drugs
2	**Blood pressure** Drop in systolic pressure of 20 mm Hg or more between lying and standing positions		✓ Benzodiazepines (specify)
		1 ✓	Check if the patient has changed drugs, dosage, or both in the past 5 days.
		/3	**TOTAL**

LEGAL LOOKOUT

Reducing your liability in patient falls

Patient falls are a very common area of nursing liability. Patients who are debilitated, infirm, sedated, or mentally incapacitated are the most likely to fall. The case of *Stevenson v. Alta Bates* (1937) involved a patient who had a stroke and was learning to walk again. As two nurses, each holding one of the patient's arms, assisted her into the hospital's sun room, one of the nurses let go of the patient and stepped forward to get a chair for her. The patient fell and sustained a fracture. The nurse was found negligent: The court said she should have anticipated the patient's need for a chair and made the appropriate arrangements before bringing the patient into the sun room.

falls, such as placing a band on the patient's wrist and communicating this risk on the patient's Kardex. Record any patient and family teaching and their level of understanding. In some facilities, patient and family education may be documented on an education flow sheet.

| 1/26/08 | 1000 | Score of 13 on admission Risk Assessment for Falls form. High risk for falls communicated to pt. and family. Risk for falls ID placed on pt.'s Ⓛ wrist, high-risk for falls checked off on care plan and Kardex. Pt. alert and oriented to time, place, and person. Oriented pt. and family to room and call bell system. Instructed pt. to call for help before getting out of bed or up from chair on his own. Pt. demonstrated proper use of call bell and verbalized when to use it. Personal items and call bell placed within reach. ———————— Betty Floyd, RN |

G

Gastric lavage

After poisoning or a drug overdose, especially in patients who have central nervous system depression or an inadequate gag reflex, gastric lavage is used to flush the stomach and remove ingested substances through a gastric lavage tube. For patients with gastric or esophageal bleeding, a lavage with normal saline solution may be used to stop bleeding. Gastric lavage is contraindicated after ingestion of a corrosive substance, such as lye, ammonia, or mineral acids, because the lavage tube may perforate the already compromised esophagus.

Typically, a doctor, gastroenterologist, or nurse performs this procedure in the emergency department or intensive care unit. Correct lavage tube placement is essential for patient safety because accidental misplacement (in the lungs, for example) followed by lavage can be fatal.

Essential documentation

If possible, note the type of substance ingested, when the ingestion occurred, and how much substance was ingested. Obtain and record preprocedure vital signs and level of consciousness (LOC). Record the date and time of lavage, the size and type of nasogastric tube used, the volume and type of irrigant, and the amount, color, and consistency of aspirated gastric contents. Document the amount of irrigant solution instilled and gastric contents drained on the intake and output record sheet. Note whether drainage was sent to the laboratory for analysis.

Also record any drugs instilled through the tube. Assess and record vital signs every 15 minutes on a frequent vital signs assessment sheet and LOC on a Glasgow Coma Scale sheet until the patient is stable. Indicate the time that the tube was removed, how the patient tolerated the procedure, and comfort measures provided.

| 4/22/08 | 2300 | Single lumen #30 Fr. Ewald tube placed by Dr. Brian Jones at 2230, without difficulty, for gastric lavage following ingestion of unknown quantity of diazepam. Prelavage P 56, BP 90/52, RR 14 and shallow, rectal T 97° F. Pt. lethargic, unresponsive to verbal stimuli, but responsive to painful stimuli, gag reflex present but hypoactive, PEARL. Lavage performed with 250 ml NSS, returned contents liquid green with small blue flecks and some undigested food. Sample collected and sent to lab for analysis. Postprocedure P 58, BP 90/54, RR 15, LOC unchanged. ———————————————— Lisa Greenwald, RN |
| | 2315 | Lavage repeated x2 with 500 ml NSS each. Gastric return clear after third lavage. Total return 1375 ml. P 60, BP 94/52, RR 15. Lethargic but responsive to verbal stimuli, reflexes still sluggish. q15min VS and LOC documented on frequent vital signs and Glasgow Coma Scale sheets. Gastric tube will be left in place until pt. alert. ———————————— Lisa Greenwald, RN |

H

Health Insurance Portability and Accountability Act

The Health Insurance Portability and Accountability Act (HIPAA) of 1996 went into effect in spring 2003 to strengthen and protect patient privacy. Health care providers (such as physicians, nurses, pharmacies, hospitals, clinics, and nursing homes), health insurance plans, and government programs (such as Medicare and Medicaid) must notify patients about their right to privacy and how their health information will be used and shared. This includes information in the patient's medical record, conversations about the patient's care between health care providers, billing information, health insurers' computerized records, and other health information. Employees must also be taught about privacy procedures.

Under HIPAA, the patient has the right to access his medical information, know when health information is shared, and make changes or corrections to his medical record. Patients also have the right to decide whether they want to allow their information to be used for certain purposes, such as marketing or research. Patient records with identifiable health information must be secured so that the records aren't accessible to those who don't have a need for them. Identifiable health information may include the patient's name, Social Security number, identification number, birth date, admission and discharge dates, and health history.

Documenting patient authorization to use personal health information

Your agency probably has an authorization form similar to the one below to be used for release of a patient's personal health information for reasons other than routine treatment or billing. Make sure all the required information is completed before having the patient or legal guardian sign the form.

AUTHORIZATION FORM

By signing, I authorize Community Hospital to use and/or disclose certain protected health information (PHI) about me to *Dr. Geoffrey Bedarnz*. This authorization permits Community Hospital to use and/or disclose the following individually identifiable health information about me (specifically describe the information to be used or disclosed, such as dates(s) of services, type of services, level of detail to be released, origin of information, etc.):

X-ray films and report, notes on care from 2/6/08 Emergency Department visit

The information will be used or disclosed for the following purpose:

f/u care with Dr. Geoffrey Bedarnz

(If disclosure is requested by the patient, purpose may be listed as "at the request of the individual.")

The purpose(s) is/are provided so that I can make an informed decision whether to allow release of the information. This authorization will expire on *2/7/08*.

The practice _____ will *X* will not receive payment or other remuneration from a third party in exchange for using or disclosing the PHI.

I do not have to sign this authorization in order to receive treatment from Community Hospital. In fact, I have the right to refuse to sign this authorization. When my information is used or disclosed pursuant to this authorization, it may be subject to redisclosure by the recipient and may no longer be protected by the federal HIPAA Privacy Rule. I have the right to revoke this authorization in writing except to the extent that the practice has acted in reliance upon this authorization. My written revocation must be submitted to the Privacy Office at:

Community Hospital
123 Main Street
Oakwood, PA

Marcy Thayer	*2/6/08*	*self*
Signed by:	Date:	Relationship to patient:

Marcy Thayer	
Print patient's name	Print name of Legal Guardian, if applicable

---

When a patient receives health care, he will need to sign an authorization form before protected health information can be used for purposes other than routine treatment or billing. The form should be placed in the patient's medical record. (See *Documenting patient authorization to use personal health information.*)

For patients who can't read or understand English, be sure to explain it to them or provide an interpreter. Document this procedure in your notes.

Essential documentation

Use your agency's HIPAA authorization form to document your patient's consent for the use and disclosure of protected health information. An authorization form must include a description of the health information that will be used and disclosed, the person authorized to use or disclose the information, the person to whom the disclosure will be made, an expiration date, and the purpose for sharing or using the information. The form is to be signed by the patient or legal guardian and placed in the patient's medical record.

1/7/08	1130	Pt. unable to understand HIPAA notice due to poor English
		skills. Speaks mostly Spanish. Privacy rights explained with the
		assistance of AT&T interpreter, Judy Rivera. Pt. acknowledges
		understanding of these per J. Rivera, and form signed by pt.
		Copy given to the pt. ———————————— Jennifer Good, RN

Heat application

Heat applied directly to the patient's body raises tissue temperature and enhances the inflammatory process by causing vasodilation and increasing local circulation. This promotes leukocytosis, suppuration, drainage, and healing. Heat also increases tissue metabolism, reduces pain caused by muscle spasm, and decreases congestion in deep visceral organs. Moist heat softens crusts and exudates and penetrates deeper than dry heat.

Essential documentation

Record the date and time of the heat application. Document the reason for the use of heat, the site of application, and the type of heat used, such as dry or moist. Describe the type of heating device used, such as hyperthermia blanket, K pad, chemical hot pack, or warm compresses; the temperature or heat setting; measures taken to protect the patient's skin; and the duration of time the heat was applied. Include the condition of the skin before and after the application of heat, signs of complications, and the patient's response to the treatment. Record any patient education provided.

1/4/08	0900	Warm moist compress (128° F by bath thermometer) applied to
		lumbar region of the back for 20 min. for c/o stiffness and
		discomfort. Skin pink, warm, dry, and intact before application.
		Told pt. to lay compress over back and not to lie directly on
		compress. Instructed pt. to call for nurse if he experienced
		any pain. Skin pink, warm, dry, and intact after the procedure.
		Pt. reports decrease in stiffness and discomfort. ————————
		———————————————————————— Brian Petry, RN

Hemodynamic monitoring

Continuous pulmonary artery pressure (PAP) and intermittent pulmonary artery wedge pressure (PAWP) measurements provide important information about left ventricular function and preload. This information is useful not only for monitoring, but also for aiding diagnosis, refining your assessment, guiding interventions, and projecting patient outcomes.

Many acutely ill patients are candidates for PAP monitoring—especially those who are hemodynamically unstable, who need fluid management or continuous cardiopulmonary assessment, or who are receiving multiple or frequently administered cardioactive drugs. PAP monitoring is also crucial for patients with shock, trauma, pulmonary or cardiac disease, or multiorgan disease. It's also used before some major surgeries to obtain baseline measurements.

Current pulmonary artery (PA) catheters can have up to six lumens. In addition to distal and proximal lumens used to measure pressures, a balloon inflation lumen inflates a balloon for PAWP measurement and a thermistor connector lumen allows cardiac output measurement. Some catheters also have a pacemaker wire lumen that provides a port for pacemaker electrodes and measures continuous mixed venous oxygen saturation.

The PA catheter is inserted into the heart's right side with the distal tip lying in the pulmonary artery. Fluoroscopy may not be required during catheter insertion because the catheter is flow directed, following venous blood flow from the right heart chambers into the pulmonary artery.

Essential documentation

Document the date and time of catheter insertion and the name of the physician who performed the procedure. Identify the number of catheter lumens, catheter insertion site, the pressure waveforms and the pressure readings of the right atrium, right ventricle, PAP, and PAWP. Include the balloon inflation volume required to obtain a wedge tracing. Note whether any arrhythmias occurred during or after the procedure. Document any solution infusing through the catheter ports. Record the type of flush solution used and its heparin concentration (if any). Describe the type of dressing applied and the patient's tolerance of the procedure. Document that a chest X-ray study was obtained after insertions, and document the results. Chart all site care, dressing changes, tubing, and solution changes.

3/19/08	1300	PA catheter insertion procedure and need for hemodynamic
		monitoring explained to pt. and informed consent obtained
		by Dr. Jill Monroe. Four-lumen thermodilution catheter
		inserted via the ℝ subclavian vein. Pressures on insertion:
		RA 6 mm Hg. RV 30/5 mm Hg. PAP 24/10 mm Hg. PAWP
		10 mm Hg. Wedge tracing obtained with 1.5 ml of air for
		balloon inflation. Portable CXR completed to confirm place-
		ment. Standard flush solution infusing into distal port. NS
		infusing at 30 ml/hr into proximal port. Cardiac monitor
		shows sinus tachycardia with rate of 102; no arrhythmias
		noted during insertion. Site covered with sterile occlusive
		dressing. Pt. resting comfortably in bed with HOB at 30°, no
		c/o pain; breathing unlabored. ———— Kathy Osborne RN

Home care referral

Before you begin caring for a patient in his home, your agency will receive information about that patient on a referral, or intake, form. Before taking the new case, either you or someone in your agency will use this form to make sure the patient is eligible for home care and that the agency can provide the services he needs.

To meet Medicare's criteria for home care reimbursement, the patient will need to meet the following conditions:

■ Patient must be confined to his home.

■ Patient must need skilled services on an intermittent basis.

■ The care must be reasonable and medically necessary.

■ Patient must be under the care of a physician.

Essential documentation

Document your patient's demographic information, including the name and telephone number of the physician and primary caregiver, and insurance information. Record orders and services required, specifying

Home care referral

Also called the *intake form,* this form is used to document a new patient's needs when you begin your evaluation. Use the form below as a guide.

ELECTION BENEFIT PERIOD ① 2 3 4

Date of Referral: _3/2/08_ Branch _____ Chart#: _0001234_ H _____
Info Taken By: _Jane Smith, RN_ Admit Date: _3/2/08_
Patient's Name: _Terry Elliot_
Address: _11 Second St._
City: _Hometown_ State: _PA_ Zip: _10981_
Phone: _881-555-2937_ Date of Birth: _07/08/26_
Primary Caregiver Name & #: _Susan Elliot_ _881-555-2937_
Insurance Name: _Medicare_ Ins.#: _123-45-6789A_
Is this a managed care policy (HMO): _No_
Primary Dx: (Code _891.00_) _Open wound Foot/Complications (Onset)_ Date: _3/2/08_
　　　　　(Code _250.72_) _Type 2 DM Uncontrolled_ _(Exac.)_ Date: _3/2/08_
　　　　　(Code _443.89_) _Periph Vascular Disease_ _(Exac.)_ Date: _3/2/08_
Procedures: (Code _86.28_) _Debridement Wound_ _(Onset)_ Date: _3/2/08_
Referral Source: _Doctor's office_ Phone: _881-555-6900_
Physician Name & Phone #: (UPIN _22222_) _Dr. Kyle Stevens_
Phone: _881-555-6900_
Physician Address: _Dr's Medical Center, Hometown, PA 10981_
Hospital _N/A_ Admit _N/A_ Discharge _N/A_
Functional Limitations: Pain Management, _Pain, ambulation dysfunction_

ORDERS/SERVICES (specify amount, frequency, and duration):
SN: _5-7 visits/wk X 9 wks for assessment and wound care ① foot: Saline wet to dry drsg_
AI: _3-5 visits/wk X 9 wks for assistance with ADLs and personal care_
PT, OT, ST: _PT 1-3 visits/wk X 9 wks to assess mobility and safety and develop home exercise program._
MSW: _1-2 visits X 1 mo. for financial assessment and long-term planning_
Spiritual Coordinator: _N/A_ Counselor: _N/A_
Volunteer: _N/A_
Other Services Provided: _N/A_
Goals: _Wound healing without complications._
Equipment: _walker and dressing supplies_
Company & Phone #: _Best Med Equip. Co 881-260-1026_
Safety Measures: _Correct use of supportive devices_ Nutritional Req: _20% protein 30% fat_

FUNCTIONAL LIMITATIONS: (Circle Applicable)

①Amputation	5 Paralysis	9 Legally Blind
2 Bowel/Bladder	⑥Endurance	A Dyspnea With
3 Contracture	⑦Ambulation	Minimal Exer
4 Hearing	8 Speech	B Other

ACTIVITIES PERMITTED: (Circle Applicable)

1. Complete Bedrest	5. Partial Wgt Bearing	A. Wheelchair
2. Bedrest BRP	6. Independent at Home	⑧Walker
3. Up as Tolerated	7. Crutches	C. No Restriction
④Transfer Bed/Chair	8. Cane	D. Other— specify

Home care referral *(continued)*

Accessibility to Bath Y (N)   Shower Y (N)   Bathroom (Y) N   Exit Y (N)
Mental Status: (Circle) (Oriented) Comatose (Forgetful) Depressed Disoriented Lethargic Agitated Other
Allergies: _NKA_
• Hospice Appropriate Meds   • Med company: _N/A_
MEDICATIONS: _Humulin N 24 units subQ every am_ _____ _changed_
Tylenol 325-1000 mg q4hr prn pain P.O. _____ _unchanged_
Darvocet N 100 one tab q4hr prn pain P.O. _____ _new_
MOM 30 ml at bedtime prn P.O. _____ _unchanged_
Living Will   Yes _____ No _X_ Obtained _____ Family to mail to office _____
Guardian, POA, or Responsible Person: _wife_
Address & Phone Number: _same_
Other Family Members: _N/A_
ETOH: _O_ _____ Drug Use: _X_ _____ Smoker _1-2 ppd X 25 yrs_
HISTORY: _Chronic peripheral vascular disease with periodic open wounds of feet and legs._
Seen by doctor in office 3/2/08 and new wound of Ⓛ foot debrided.
Social History (place of birth, education, jobs, retirement, etc.): _Korean War veteran retired (X 18 yrs)_
construction worker

ADMISSION NOTES: VS: T _99°F orally_ ____ AP _88_ _____ RR _22_ _____ BP _150/82_
Lungs: _diminished bilat. at bases_ _____ Extremities: Ⓡ BKA, Ⓛ foot pale, DP and PT pulses +._
Wgt: _155 lb_ _____ Recent wgt loss/gain of _denies_
Admission Narrative: _Pt. independent in Insulin administration and instructed in Insulin_
dosage change with good understanding. Wound of Ⓛ ankle-outer malleolar area = 4 cm
X 5 cm X 1 cm deep; open with beefy red appearance, wound edges pink, moderate
amount serosanguineous drainage present. Wound care performed by RN per care plan.
Pain controlled with Darvocet prn.
Psychosocial Issues _N/A_
Environmental Concerns _None_
Are there any cultural or spiritual customs or beliefs of which we should be aware before providing Hospice services? _____
_N/A_
Funeral Home: _N/A_ _____ Contact made YES _____ NO _____
DIRECTIONS: _1 block before intersection of Main St, on Second St._

Agency Representative
Signature: _Jane Smith, RN_ _____ Date: _3/2/08_

the amount, frequency, and duration. Note the patient's functional limitations and activities permitted. List drug orders and allergy information. Record advance directive information. Include your patient's medical and psychosocial histories, cultural and religious considerations, environmental assessment, vital signs, and physical assessment findings. Date and sign your entry.

See *Home care referral,* for sample documentation.

Hyperthermia-hypothermia blanket

A blanket-sized aquathermia pad—the hyperthermia-hypothermia blanket—raises, lowers, or maintains body temperature through conductive heat or cold transfer between the blanket and the patient. It can be operated manually or automatically.

The blanket is used most commonly to reduce high temperatures when more conservative measures, such as baths, ice packs, and antipyretics, are unsuccessful. Its other uses include maintaining normal temperature during or after surgery or shock; inducing hypothermia during surgery to decrease metabolic activity and thereby reducing oxygen requirements; reducing intracranial pressure; controlling bleeding and intractable pain in patients with amputations, burns, or cancer; and providing warmth in cases of severe hypothermia.

Essential documentation

Record the date and time of your entry. Document that the procedure was explained to the patient and the family and a signed informed consent form is in the chart if required by your facility. Record the patient's vital signs, neurologic signs, fluid intake and output, skin condition, and position change. Record vital signs every 15 minutes until the temperature is stable or as ordered. Document the type of hyperthermia-hypothermia unit used and control settings (manual or automatic, and temperature settings). Note the duration of the procedure and the patient's tolerance of treatment. Describe any measures taken to prevent skin injury. Record signs of complications, such as shivering, marked changes in vital signs, increased intracranial pressure, respiratory distress or arrest, cardiac arrest, oliguria, and anuria; the name of the physician notified; the time of notification; the orders given; your actions; and the patient's response.

1/19/08	1000	Need for hypothermia blanket explained to pt.'s wife by Dr.
		Thomas Albright. Wife signed consent form. Preprocedure VS:
		Rectal T 104.3° F, P 112 and regular, RR 28, BP 138/88. Automatic
		hypothermia blanket, set at 99° F, placed under pt. at 0945.
		Sheet placed between pt. and hypothermia blanket. Lanolin
		applied to back, buttocks, and undersides of legs, arms, and feet.
		Skin intact, flushed, warm to the touch. Rectal probe in place
		and secured with tape. Pt. drowsy, but easily arousable and
		oriented to place and person but not time, able to feel light
		touch in all extremities, moving all extremities on own, no c/o
		numbness or tingling, PEARL. See I/O and frequent vital signs
		flow sheets for hourly intake and output, and q5min. VS and
		neuro. assessments. No shivering noted, Foley catheter intact
		draining clear amber urine, no dyspnea. ——— Jane Walters, RN

IJK

Infection control

Meticulous record keeping is an important contributor to effective infection control. Various federal agencies require documentation of infections so that the data can be assessed and used to help prevent and control future infections. In addition, the data you record help your health care facility meet national and local accreditation standards.

Typically, you must report to your facility's infection control department any culture result that shows a positive infection and any surgery, drug, elevated temperature, X-ray finding, or specific treatment related to infection.

Essential documentation

Record the date, time, and to whom you reported the signs and symptoms of suspected infection, instructions received, and treatments initiated. Record that you have followed standard precautions against direct contact with blood and body fluids, and any additional precautions required, based on the type of infection. Record that you have taught the patient and his family about these precautions. Record the dates and times of your interventions in the patient's chart and on the Kardex.

Note the name of the doctor whom you notified of the results of any culture and sensitivity studies, and record the time of notification. Note any new orders given regarding the culture results. Also, inform the infection control practitioner.

1/28/08	1300	Standard precautions maintained. P 96, BP 132/82, rectal T
		102.3° F. Large amount of purulent yellow-green, foul-smelling
		drainage from incision soaked through 6 4" X 4" gauze pads in
		2 hr. Dr. Samuel Levin notified. Ordered Tylenol 650 mg P.O. q
		4hr prn for temp greater than 101° F, given at 1250. Repeat
		C&S obtained and sent to lab. Wound cleaned w/NSS and covered
		with 4 sterile 4" X 4" pads using sterile technique. Reinforced
		standard precautions to pt. and wife. ———— Lynne Kasoff, RN

Intake and output

Many patients require 24-hour intake and output monitoring. They include surgical patients, patients in intensive care, patients with fluid and electrolyte imbalances, and patients with burns, hemorrhage, or on dialysis.

See *Intake and output record* for an example of proper documentation.

For easy reference, list the volumes of specific containers. Infusion devices make documenting enteral and I.V. intake more accurate. However, keeping track of intake that isn't premeasured—for example, food such as gelatin that's normally fluid at room temperature—requires the cooperation of the patient, family members (who may bring the patient snacks and soft drinks or help him eat at the health care facility), and other caregivers. Therefore, you must make sure that everyone understands how to record or report all foods and fluids that the patient consumes orally.

Don't forget to count I.V. piggyback infusions, drugs given by I.V. push, patient-controlled analgesics, and any irrigation solutions that aren't withdrawn. You'll also need to know whether the patient receives any fluids orally or intravenously while he's off your unit, for example, at physical therapy.

Recording fluid output accurately requires the cooperation of the patient and staff members in any other departments where your patient goes.

The amount of fluid lost through the GI tract is normally 100 ml or less daily. However, if the patient's stools become excessive or watery, they must be counted as output. Vomiting, drainage from suction devices and wound drains, and bleeding are other measurable sources of fluid loss. If the patient is incontinent, document this as well as tube drainage and irrigation volumes.

Intake and output record

As the sample shows, you can monitor your patient's fluid balance by using an intake and output record.

Name: _Josephine Klein_
Medical record #: _49731_
Admission date: _2/13/08_

INTAKE AND OUTPUT RECORD

	INTAKE						OUTPUT				
	Oral	Tube feeding	Instilled	I.V. and IVPB	TPN	Total	Urine	Emesis	NG Tube	Other	Total
Date *2/15/08*											
0700–1500	250	320	H_2O 50	1100		1720	1355				1355
1500–2300	200	320	H_2O 50	1100		1670	1200				1200
2300–0700		320	H_2O 50	1100		1470	1500				1500
24-hr total	450	960	H_2O 150	3300		4860	4055				4055
Date											
24-hr total											
Date											
24-hr total											
Date											
24-hr total											

Key: IVPB = I.V. piggyback   TPN = total parenteral nutrition   NG = nasogastric

Standard measures

Styrofoam cup	240 ml	Water (large)	600 ml	Milk (large)	600 ml	Ice cream,	120 ml
Juice	120 ml	Water pitcher	750 ml	Coffee	240 ml	sherbet, or gelatin	
Water (small)	120 ml	Milk (small)	120 ml	Soup	180 ml		

Essential documentation

Make sure your patient's name is on the intake and output record. Record the date and time of your shift on the appropriate line. Record the total intake and output for each category of fluid for your shift, then total these categories and provide a shift total for intake and output. At the end of 24 hours, a daily total is calculated, usually by the night nurse. Make sure all nurses use the same units of measurement. In most cases, this is in milliliters.

Intracranial pressure monitoring

Intracranial pressure (ICP) monitoring measures pressure exerted by the brain, blood, and cerebrospinal fluid (CSF). Indications for monitoring ICP include head trauma with bleeding or edema, overproduction or insufficient absorption of CSF, cerebral hemorrhage, cerebral aneurysm, and space-occupying brain lesions. ICP monitoring can detect elevated ICP early, before clinical danger signs develop. Your prompt interventions can then help avert or diminish neurologic damage caused by cerebral hypoxia and shifts of brain mass. The procedure is always performed by a neurosurgeon in the operating room, emergency department, or critical care unit.

Essential documentation

Document that the procedure has been explained to the patient or his family and that the patient or a responsible family member has signed the consent form. If done at the bedside, before the insertion, take a "time out" and identify the patient using two identifiers and review the procedure to be done with the health care team present and with the patient, if appropriate. Record the date and time of the insertion procedure, the name of the doctor performing the procedure, and the patient's response. Note the insertion site and the type of monitoring system used. Record ICP digital readings and waveforms and cerebral perfusion pressure hourly in your notes, on a flow sheet, or directly on readout strips, depending on your facility's policy. Document any factors that may affect ICP (for example, drug administration, stressful procedures, or sleep).

Record routine and neurologic vital signs hourly (including temperature, pulse, respirations, blood pressure, level of consciousness, pupillary activity, and orientation to time, place, person, and date), and describe the patient's clinical status. Note the amount, character, and frequency of any CSF drainage (for example, "between 1800 and 1900, 15 ml of blood-tinged CSF"). Also, record the ICP reading in response to drainage. Describe the insertion site and any site care and dressing changes performed. Describe any patient and family education and support given.

4/29/08	1100	ICP insertion and monitoring procedures explained to pt.'s
		wife by Dr. Bruce Norton. Wife verbalized understanding of
		procedure and signed consent form. Subarachnoid bolt placed
		by Dr. Norton on ① side of skull behind hairline. Initial ICP
		16 mm Hg, MAP 110 mm Hg, monitor strip mounted below. Site
		clean, no drainage or redness, covered with sterile dressing.
		See flow sheets for hourly ICP readings, VS, neuro. checks. BP
		154/88, P 98 and regular, RR 24 and regular, rectal T 99.4° F.
		Opens eyes and moves ® extremities to painful stimuli, makes
		incomprehensible sounds. PERRLA. No purposeful movement on
		① side. Breath sounds clear, normal heart sounds, peripheral
		pulses palpable. Skin pale, cool. Foley catheter drained 100 ml
		of clear amber urine last hr. ———————— Mary Steward, RN
		Mr. Paul Smith 1100
		4/29/08 ID#: 563421

I.V. catheter insertion

Peripheral I.V. line insertion involves the selection of a venipuncture device and an insertion site, application of a tourniquet, preparation of the site, and venipuncture. Selection of a venipuncture device and site depends on the type of solution to be used; frequency and duration of infusion; patency and location of accessible veins; the patient's age, size, and condition; and, when possible, the patient's preference.

I.V. catheters are inserted to administer medications, blood, or blood products or to correct fluid and electrolyte imbalances.

Essential documentation

In your note or on the appropriate I.V. sheets, record the date and time of the venipuncture; the type, gauge, and length of the needle or catheter; and the anatomic location of the insertion site. Also document the number of attempts at venipuncture (if you made more than one), the type and flow rate of the I.V. solution, the name and amount of medication in the solution (if any), and any adverse reactions and actions taken to correct them. If the I.V. site was changed, document the reason for the change. Document patient teaching and evidence of patient understanding. Document appearance of the insertion site every 4 hours and any site care given.

1/3/08	1100	20G 1½" catheter inserted in Ⓡ forearm without difficulty on the first attempt. Site dressed with transparent dressing. I.V. infusion of 1000 ml D₅W started at 100 ml/hr. I.V. infusing without difficulty. Pt. instructed to notify nurse if the site becomes swollen or painful or catheter becomes dislodged or leaks. No c/o pain after insertion. ———— David Stevens, RN

I.V. catheter removal

A peripheral I.V. line is removed on completion of therapy, for cannula site changes, and for suspected infection or infiltration. A peripheral I.V. may also be removed by the patient, either accidentally during activity or purposely.

Essential documentation

After removing an I.V. line, document the date and time of removal. Document whether the catheter was intact when it was removed. Describe the condition of the site. If drainage was present at the puncture site, document that you sent the tip of the device and a sample of the drainage to the laboratory for culture, according to your facility's policy. Record any site care given and the type of dressing applied. Include any patient instructions. Document the date, time, and circumstances if the catheter is accidentally removed or if the patient deliberately removes it.

1/15/08	1000	I.V. catheter removed from Ⓡ forearm vein. Catheter intact. Pressure held for 2 min. until bleeding stopped. Site clean and dry, no redness, drainage, warmth, or pain noted. Dry sterile dressing applied to site. Pt. instructed to call nurse if bleeding, swelling, redness, or pain occurs at the removal site. ———— *Jane Newport, RN*

I.V. site care

Proper I.V. site care is an important intervention for prevention of infection and other complications. Typically, I.V. dressings are changed every 48 hours or whenever the dressing becomes wet, soiled, or nonocclusive. The site should be assessed every 2 hours if a transparent semipermeable dressing is used or with every dressing change otherwise. Check your facility's policy for frequency of I.V. dressing changes and the type of site care to be performed.

Essential documentation

In your notes or on the appropriate I.V. sheets, record the date and time of the dressing change. Chart the condition of the insertion site, noting whether there are signs of infection (redness and pain), infiltration (coolness, blanching, and edema), or thrombophlebitis (redness, firmness, pain along the path of the vein, and edema). If complications are present, note the name of the doctor notified, the time of notification, the orders given, your interventions, and the patient's response. Record site care given and the type of dressing applied. Document patient education.

2/3/08	0910	Transparent I.V. dressing wet and curling at edges.
		Dressing removed. Skin cleaned with alcohol, air dried.
		No redness, blanching, warmth, coolness, edema, drainage,
		or induration noted. No c/o pain at site. New trans-
		parent dressing applied. Pt. told to report any pain at
		site. ———————————— Gina Antenucci, R.N.

I.V. site infiltration

Infiltration of an I.V. site occurs when an I.V. solution enters the surrounding tissue as a result of a punctured vein or leakage around a venipuncture site. If vesicant drugs or fluids infiltrate, severe local tissue damage may result. Because infiltration can occur without pain or in unresponsive patients, the I.V. site must be monitored every 4 hours or more frequently, depending on the type of solution infusing through it.

Document your assessments of the I.V. site and the site care you provide. Such documentation is important in the prevention and early detection of infiltration and other complications. Many malpractice cases are brought annually because of the severe nerve and tissue damage resulting from infiltrated I.V. sites that nurses failed to monitor. In some cases, amputations have been necessary because of the nerve and tissue damage.

Essential documentation

Record the date and time of your entry. Record signs and symptoms of infiltration at the I.V. site, such as swelling, burning, discomfort, or pain; tight feeling; decreased skin temperature; and blanching. Chart your assessment of circulation to the affected and unaffected limbs, such as skin color, capillary refill, pulses, and circumference. Document your actions, such as stopping the infusion. Estimate the amount of fluid infiltrated. Record the name of the doctor notified, the time of notification, the orders given (such as vesicant antidotes, limb elevation, and ice or warm soaks), your actions, and the patient's response. Restart the infusion and note the new location above the infiltration or in the unaffected limb. Record any emotional support and patient education.

1/31/08	1900	I.V. site in ® forearm edematous and cool at 1820. Pt.
		c/o of some discomfort at the site. Hands warm with
		capillary refill less than 3 seconds, strong radial pulses
		bilaterally. ® forearm circumference 9½", Ⓛ forearm
		circumference 9". I.V. catheter removed intact and
		sterile gauze dressing applied. ® arm elevated on 2
		pillows and ice applied in wrapped towel for 20 min.
		After ice application, skin cool, intact. No c/o burning or
		numbness. Explained importance of keeping arm elevated
		and to call nurse immediately for any pain, burning,
		numbness in ® forearm. New I.V. catheter #18G inserted
		in Ⓛ forearm without difficulty on first attempt. ———
		——————————————————— Betsy Rothman, RN

L

Last will and testament, patient request for witness of

A patient, especially one who believes he's dying, may ask you to witness a last will and testament. In many states, a nurse can witness a patient's signature on a will. However, you don't have a legal or ethical responsibility to act as a witness. Check your facility's policy or ask your facility's legal consultant before you witness a will. (See *Witnessing a will,* page 278.)

If a patient asks you to be a witness when he draws his will, notify the doctor and your supervisor before you act as a witness. Don't give any legal advice or offer assistance in wording the document. Don't comment on the nature of the patient's choices. Document your actions in your nurse's note.

Essential documentation

When you witness a written will, document that it was signed and witnessed, who signed and witnessed it, who was present, what was done with it after signing, and what the patient's condition was at the time. Document the name of the doctor, facility attorney, or any other person (such as the nursing supervisor) who was notified, and note the time of notification. Record instructions that were given and your actions. Record that you heard the maker of the will declare it to be his will and that all witnesses and the maker of the will were actually present during the signing.

LEGAL LOOKOUT

Witnessing a will

In many states, your signature on a will certifies that:
■ you witnessed the signing of the will
■ you heard the maker of the will declare it to be his will
■ all witnesses and the maker of the will were actually present during the signing.

By attesting to the last two facts, you help ensure the authenticity of the will and the signatures. However, your signature doesn't certify that the maker of the will is competent.

Before you sign any document, read at least enough of it to make sure it's the type of document the maker represents it to be. Usually you won't have to read all the text and, legally, that isn't necessary for your signature to be valid. You should, however, always examine the document's title and first page and give careful attention to what's written immediately above the place for your signature.

| 1/17/08 | 1300 | Asked to witness pt's will. Dr. William Pershing; Edward Ewing, hospital attorney; and Nancy Strom, RN, nursing supervisor, were contacted at 1245. Mr. Ewing; Ms. Strom; pt.'s daughter, Mrs. Pope; pt.; and I were present at the signing. The document was entitled "My last will and testament." Pt. signed the will. It was witnessed by the above people and myself. Will was placed with pt.'s personal belongings in his closet after signing. At pt.'s request, a copy was given to Mrs. Pope. At the signing, pt. was alert and oriented to time, place, and person. ———————— Sally Ball, RN |

Late documentation entry

Late documentation entries are appropriate in several situations:
■ if the chart was unavailable when it was needed—for example, when the patient was away from the unit (for X-rays or physical therapy)
■ if you need to add important information after completing your notes
■ if you forgot to write notes on a particular chart.

LEGAL LOOKOUT

Avoiding late entries

If the court uncovers alterations in a patient's chart during the course of a trial, suspicions may be aroused. The court may logically infer that additional alterations were made. In such situations, the value of the entire medical record may be brought into question.

That's what happened to the nurse involved in one case. She failed to chart her observations of a patient for 7 hours after a surgery, during which time the patient died. The patient's family later sued the hospital, charging the nurse with malpractice. The nurse insisted that she had observed the patient but, because her particular unit was understaffed and overpopulated, she wasn't able to record her observations. She explained that the assistant director of nursing later instructed her about the hospital's policy on charting late additions. The nurse subsequently added her observations to the patient's medical record.

However, the court wasn't convinced that the nurse had indeed observed the patient during the postoperative period. Suspicious of the altered record, it ruled that the nurse's failure to chart her observations at the proper time supported the plaintiff's claim that she had made no such observations.

Keep in mind, however, that a late or altered chart entry can arouse suspicions and can be a significant problem in the event of a malpractice lawsuit. (See *Avoiding late entries*.)

Essential documentation

If you must make a late entry or alter an entry, find out if your facility has a protocol for doing so (many do). If not, the best approach is to add the entry to the first available line and to label it "late entry" to indicate that it's out of sequence. Then record the date and time of the entry and, in the body of the entry, record the date and time it should have been made.

2/14/08	0900	(Chart not available 2/13/08 at 1500; pt. was in radiology) On
	Late entry	2/13/08 at 1300, pt. stated she felt faint when getting OOB on
		2/13/08 at 1200 and she fell to the floor. Pt. states she didn't
		hurt herself at the time and didn't think she had to tell anyone
		about this until her husband encouraged her to report it. Ⓡ
		wrist bruised and slightly swollen. Pt. c/o some tenderness. Dr.
		Andrew Muir notified at 1310 and came to see pt. at 1320 on
		2/13/08. X-ray of wrist ordered. ———— *Elaine Kasmer, R.N.*

Learning needs

Every patient will have learning needs when they are admitted to a facility. Even something as simple as room orientation is a learning need. After your admission assessment, basic learning needs should be identified. Basic learning needs may be room orientation, equipment orientation, or teaching about tests or medications. Along with identifying learning needs is the identification of learning barriers, that is, anything that may hinder the patient's learning. Learning barriers may include language barrier, reading difficulty, cultural differences, or disease process.

Essential documentation

Some facilities have a section on their admission form for the identification of learning needs and learning barriers. If so, complete this while completing the admission assessment. If your facility has a separate patient teaching form, be sure to initiate it when the patient is admitted to the facility and to update it during the patient's stay, as needed. Enter the date and time of the teaching and what information was taught or reviewed. If your facility doesn't have a separate teaching form, enter any learning needs that are identified in your nurse's notes, as well as any teaching that was done and the patient's response.

| 2/13/08 | 1300 | Pt. learning needs identified regarding medication use, diet restrictions, and blood sugar testing. Pt. demonstrated noncompliance with these topics in the past. Will consult nutritional dept. for assistance with diet. Will consult diabetic educator for assistance with medication teaching and blood sugar testing. ———————— Tiffany Noree, RN |

Level of consciousness, changes in

A patient's level of consciousness (LOC) provides information about his respiratory and cardiovascular status and is the most sensitive indicator of neurologic status. The Glasgow Coma Scale provides a standard reference for assessing or monitoring the LOC of a patient with a suspected or confirmed brain injury. This scale measures three responses to stimuli—eye opening response, motor response, and verbal response—and assigns a number to each of the possible responses within these categories. The lowest possible score is 3; the highest is

---

CASE CLIP

Responding to a change in level of consciousness

Mr. D. is a 60-year-old black male admitted to the hospital for new-onset atrial fibrillation. He has a past medical history of hypertension, he's a two-pack-per-day smoker, and he's overweight with a body mass index of 32. His blood pressure (BP) wasn't under good control because Mr. D. often forgot to take his medication. His admission vital signs were:

- temperature: 97.2° F (36.2° C)
- heart rate (HR): 143 beats/minute
- respiratory rate (RR): 20 breaths/minute
- BP: 156/94 mm Hg
- pulse oximetry: 97% on room air.

Mr. D. was admitted to the telemetry floor and was started on a Cardizem drip at 10 mg/hour after a 10-mg bolus. One hour after the start of the infusion, neither his HR nor heart rhythm had changed. While bringing in his lunch tray, the nurse found Mr. D. difficult to arouse. His speech was also garbled when he attempted to talk. She called the rapid response team (RRT), who arrived within 3 minutes.

The RRT quickly reviewed Mr. D.'s history and medications. At this time, his vital signs were:

- HR: 138 beats/minute
- RR: 16 breaths/minute
- BP: 160/88 mm Hg
- pulse oximetry: 97%.

It was determined that Mr. D. had a stable airway. A capillary blood sugar reading was done and results were 100. Further assessment findings identified a flaccid left arm and left facial droop. Mr. D. was taken for a stat computed tomography (CT) scan of the head. The attending physician was notified and the patient was taken to the intensive care unit. A neurosurgeon was consulted to review the CT scan results and to direct care.

---

15. A score of 7 or lower indicates a coma. (See *Responding to a change in level of consciousness.*)

Essential documentation

Record the date and time of your assessment. Depending on your facility's Glasgow Coma Scale flow sheet, you'll either circle the number that describes your patient's response to stimuli or you'll write in the

Using the Glasgow Coma Scale

The Glasgow Coma Scale is a standard reference that's used to assess or monitor level of consciousness in a patient with a suspected or confirmed brain injury. This scale measures three responses to stimuli—eye opening response, motor response, and verbal response—and assigns a number to each of the possible responses within these categories.

The lowest possible score is 3; the highest is 15. A score of 7 or lower indicates coma. This scale is commonly used in the emergency department, at the scene of an accident, and for the evaluation of a hospitalized patient.

GLASGOW COMA SCALE

Characteristic	Response	Score
Eye opening response	▪ Spontaneous	4
	▪ To verbal command	③
	▪ To pain	2
	▪ No response	1
Best motor response	▪ Obeys commands	⑥
	▪ To painful stimulus:	
	– Localizes pain; pushes stimulus away	5
	– Flexes and withdraws	4
	– Abnormal flexion	3
	– Extension	2
	– No response	1
Best verbal response (arouse patient with painful stimulus, if necessary)	▪ Oriented and converses	5
	▪ Disoriented and converses	④
	▪ Uses inappropriate words	3
	▪ Makes incomprehensible sounds	2
	▪ No response	1
	Total:	*13*

number of the corresponding response. Then record the total of these three responses.

See *Using the Glasgow Coma Scale,* for an example of how to document your patient's LOC.

M

Mechanical ventilation

A mechanical ventilator moves air in and out of a patient's lungs. Although the equipment ventilates a patient, it doesn't ensure adequate gas exchange. Mechanical ventilation may use either positive or negative pressure to ventilate a patient.

Positive-pressure ventilators exert a positive pressure on the airway, which causes inspiration while increasing tidal volume. The inspiratory cycles of these ventilators may vary in volume, pressure, or time. A high-frequency ventilator uses high respiratory rates and low tidal volume to maintain alveolar ventilation.

Negative-pressure ventilators create negative pressure, which pulls the thorax outward and allows air to flow into the lungs. Examples of such ventilators are the iron lung, the cuirass (chest shell), and the body wrap. Negative-pressure ventilators are used mainly to treat neuromuscular disorders, such as Guillain-Barré syndrome, myasthenia gravis, and poliomyelitis. They aren't used for the treatment of acutely ill patients.

Other indications for ventilator use include central nervous system disorders, such as cerebral hemorrhage and spinal cord transsection, acute respiratory distress syndrome, pulmonary edema, chronic obstructive pulmonary disease, flail chest, and acute hypoventilation.

Essential documentation

Document the date and time that mechanical ventilation began. Note the type of ventilator used as well as its settings, such as ventilatory mode, tidal volume, rate, fraction of inspired oxygen, positive end-expiratory pressure, and peak inspiratory flow. Record the size of the endotracheal (ET) tube, centimeter mark of the ET tube at the lip, and cuff pressure. Describe the patient's response to mechanical ventilation, including vital signs, breath sounds, use of accessory muscles, comfort level, and physical appearance.

Throughout use of mechanical ventilation, list any complications and subsequent interventions. Record pertinent laboratory data, including arterial blood gas (ABG) analyses and oxygen saturation findings. Also record tracheal suctioning and the amount and characteristics of secretions.

If the patient is receiving pressure-support ventilation or is using a T-piece or tracheostomy collar, note the duration of spontaneous breathing and the patient's ability to maintain the weaning schedule. If the patient is receiving intermittent mandatory ventilation, with or without pressure-support ventilation, record the control breath rate, time of each breath reduction, and rate of spontaneous respirations.

Record adjustments made in ventilator settings as a result of ABG levels, and document changing, cleaning, or discarding of the tubing, although this action and documentation is done by a respiratory therapist in many facilities. Also, record teaching efforts and emotional support given.

| 3/16/08 | 1015 | Pt. on Servo ventilator set at TV 750, F IO₂ 45%, 5 cm PEEP, Assist-control mode of 12, RR 20 and nonlabored; #8 ET tube in Ⓡ corner of mouth taped securely at 22-cm mark. Suctioned via ET tube for large amt. of thick white secretions. Pulse oximetry reading 98%. Ⓛ lung clear. Ⓡ lung with basilar crackles and expiratory wheezes. Dr. Robert Short notified at 1000; no treatment at this time. Explained all procedures including suctioning to pt. Pt. nodded head "yes" when asked if he understood explanations. ————— Janice Del Vecchio, RN |
| | | |

Medication error

Medication errors are the most common, and potentially the most dangerous, nursing errors. Mistakes in dosage, patient identification, drug selection, drug preparation, or drug administration by the incorrect

LEGAL LOOKOUT

Lawsuits and medication errors

Unfortunately, lawsuits involving nurses' drug errors are common. The court determines liability based on the standards of care required of nurses who administer drugs. In many instances, if the nurse had known more about the proper dosage, administration route, or procedure connected with a drug's use, she might have avoided the mistake.

In *Norton v. Argonaut Insurance Co. (1962)*, an infant died after a nurse administered injectable digoxin at a dosage level appropriate for elixir of Lanoxin, an oral drug. The nurse was unaware that digoxin was available in an oral form. The nurse questioned two doctors who weren't treating the infant about the order but failed to mention to them that the order was written for elixir of Lanoxin. She also failed to clarify the order with the doctor who wrote it.

The nurse, the doctor who ordered the drug, and the hospital were found liable.

route by nurses have led to vision loss, brain damage, cardiac arrest, and death. (See *Lawsuits and medication errors.*)

A medication event report or incident report should be completed when a medication error is discovered. The nurse who discovers the medication error is responsible for completing the medication event report or incident report and for communicating the error to the patient's doctor and to the charge nurse, unit manager, and nursing supervisor. If the medication error may potentially result in, or actually does result in, serious injury or death, it's considered a sentinel event and must reported as such by the facility. Appropriate follow-up investigation into how the event occurred and an action plan to prevent it from occurring again are usually initiated by the unit manager.

Essential documentation

In your nurse's notes, describe the situation objectively and include the name of the physician notified, the time of notification, and the physician's response. Avoid the use of such terms as "by mistake," "somehow," "unintentionally," "miscalculated," and "confusing," which can be interpreted as admissions of wrongdoing.

Medication event quality review form

When a medication error occurs, most facilities require the nurse to complete a medication event report. The information is used to investigate the incident and develop an action plan to avoid future incidents.

QUALITY REVIEW FORM

Confidential— This is a peer review document and may be protected by applicable law. ***Not for distribution.***

Patient information

Event data

Date and time of event: _1/8/08_ _1300_   Date and time reported: _1/8/08_ _1315_

Primary event type (check one only):
- ☐ Wrong drug   ☐ Wrong dose
- ☐ Omitted dose   ☐ Wrong route
- ☑ Wrong time   ☐ Wrong patient
- ☐ Other _____

For wrong dose or omitted doses,
doses involved: _____

Event severity (check only one):
- ☐ 0 - potential error only
- ☐ 1 - error occurred, no harm to the patient
- ☑ 2 - error occurred, increased monitoring only
- ☐ 3 - error occurred, change in VS, additional labs, no permanent harm
- ☐ 4 - error occurred, required additional treatment, increased LOS
- ☐ 5 - error occurred, permanent harm to patient
- ☐ 6 - error resulted in patient's death

Contributing causes of event

Order related (check all that apply):
Type of order: ☐ Written   ☐ Oral   ☐ Telephone
- ☐ Order incomplete:
  - ☐ Not dated   ☐ No frequency
  - ☐ Not timed   ☐ No route
  - ☐ No dose   ☐ No drug parameters indicated
  - ☐ No signature   ☐ Signature illegible
- ☐ Order illegible
- ☐ Unacceptable abbreviation used: _____
- ☐ Decimal misplaced
- ☐ Inappropriate use of leading or trailing zeros
- ☐ Order not flagged correctly
- ☐ Order written on wrong patient's chart
- ☐ Inappropriate drug selection
- ☐ Inappropriate route selection
- ☐ Patient drug allergies not identified or documented
- ☐ Drug not renewed
- ☐ Drug not discontinued
- ☐ Drug not reordered postop
- ☐ Nonformulary request

Transcription related (check all that apply):
- ☐ Order not faxed
- ☐ Order not transcribed
- ☐ Pharmacy clarification of order not transcribed
- ☐ Incomplete order not clarified
- ☐ Order not completely signed off
- ☐ Incorrect transcription onto:
  - ☐ MAR   ☐ Recopied MAR

- ☐ Transcription illegible on:
  - ☐ MAR   ☐ Recopied MAR
- ☐ Incomplete allergy documentation
- ☐ Allergies not transcribed onto:
  - ☐ Order sheets ☐ MAR   ☐ Recopied MAR
- ☐ Unacceptable abbreviations

Patient related (check all that apply):
- ☐ Took own meds
- ☐ Altered infusion rate
- ☐ Loss of venous access
- ☐ Medication refused

Dispensing related (check all that apply):
- ☐ Drug incompatibility
- ☐ Outdated product dispensed
- ☐ Patient allergies not identified
- ☐ Incorrect product chosen
- ☐ Product incorrectly labeled
- ☐ Product not delivered to nursing unit
- ☐ Delay in delivery due to:
  - ☐ Nonformulary request   ☐ Illegible order
  - ☐ Out of stock   ☐ Illegible fax
  - ☐ Further investigation required
  - ☐ Pneumatic tube problem ☐ Other: _____
- ☐ Product incorrectly prepared in:
  - ☐ Pharmacy ☐ Nursing unit ☐ Other: _____
- ☐ Miscalculation
- ☐ No physician order

Medication event quality review form *(continued)*

☐ Incomplete physician order not clarified
☐ Unacceptable abbreviation used: _____
☐ Computer entry errors (pharmacy only):
   ☐ Duplicate   ☐ Wrong patient   ☐ Wrong drug
   ☐ Missed order   ☐ Other _____
☐ Pharmacy clarification of order not documented

Administration related (check all that apply):
☐ Incorrect drug storage method
☐ Patient allergies not correctly checked against:
   ☐ Allergy band   ☐ MAR
☐ Patient allergy band not intact
☐ Patient not correctly identified
☐ No physician order
☐ Drug incompatibility
☐ Available product incorrectly prepared
☐ Miscalculation

☐ Incorrectly labeled
☐ Medication or I.V. not checked with MAR, order, I.V. record
☑ Time of last p.r.n. medication administration not checked
☐ Patient not observed taking medication
☐ Med. or I.V. not charted at time of administration
☐ Med. or I.V. not charted correctly
☐ Incorrect I.V. line used
☐ Incorrect setting on infusion pump
☐ Lock-out on infusion pump not used
☐ Outdated product given
☐ Forgotten or overlooked
☐ Product not available
☐ Extra or duplicated dose
☐ Monitoring, insufficient or not done

Event analysis

(Include additional information, such as staffing patterns, activity level, patient outcome, action plan, and conclusion) _____

   Susan Jones, RN, had administered and documented giving p.r.n. Demerol 100 mg I.M. to the pt. at 1215. I did not review the p.r.n. MAR and administered the dose again at 1300. Pt. monitored q 15 min. for 2 hours. No adverse effects. Pt. alert and oriented to time, place, and person. Dr. George Miller notified at 1305 and came to see pt. ————————————————

Completed by: *Aleisha Adams, RN* _____   Date completed: *1/8/08*

Document the medication error on an incident report or medication event report. (See *Medication event quality review form*.)

| 1/8/08 | 1315 | Pt. was given Demerol 100 mg I.M. 1215 and again at 1300 for abdominal pain. Dr. George Miller was notified at 1305 and is on his way to see pt. P 80, BP 120/82, RR 20, oral T 98.4° F. Alert and oriented to time, place, and person. ———————— ————————————————— *Aleisha Adams, RN* |

N

Nasogastric tube insertion

Usually inserted to decompress the stomach, a nasogastric (NG) tube is also used for preventing vomiting after major surgery, helping with assessing and treating upper GI bleeding, allowing collection of gastric contents for analysis, performing gastric lavage, aspirating gastric secretions, and administering drugs and nutrients.

An NG tube is typically in place for 48 to 72 hours after surgery, by which time peristalsis usually resumes. However, the NG tube may remain in place for shorter or longer periods, depending on its use. Insertion of an NG tube demands close observation of the patient and verification of proper tube placement.

Essential documentation

Record the type and size of the NG tube inserted; the date, time, and route of insertion; and confirmation of proper placement. Note if placement was confirmed by X-ray study. Describe the type and amount of suction, if applicable; the drainage characteristics, such as amount, color (for example, green, brown, or brown-flecked), character, consistency, and odor; and the patient's tolerance of the insertion procedure. Document any tube feedings or medications instilled, with confirmation of proper tube placement, and the amount of any residual fluid aspirated from the stomach.

Include in your note signs and symptoms signaling complications, such as nausea, vomiting, and abdominal distention. Document subsequent irrigation procedures and continuing problems after irrigations.

Document oral and nasal care given while the NG tube was in place.

4/22/08	1700	Procedure explained to pt. #12 Fr. NG tube inserted via ℚ
		nostril without difficulty. Placement verified by aspiration of
		green stomach contents and pH test strip result of 5. Tube
		attached to low intermittent suction as ordered. Tube taped
		to nose. Drainage pale green, Hematest negative. Irrigated
		with 30 ml NSS per order. Hypoactive bowel sounds in all 4
		quadrants. ———————————— Carol Allen, RN

Nasogastric tube removal

A nasogastric (NG) tube typically remains in place for 48 to 72 hours after surgery and is removed when peristalsis resumes. If it was used for other purposes, such as feeding, it may be removed when the patient can resume oral feedings on his own or has a gastric tube inserted. Depending on its use, it may remain in place for shorter or longer periods.

Essential documentation

Record the date and time that the NG tube is removed. Chart that you have explained the procedure to the patient. Describe the color, consistency, and amount of gastric drainage, if connected to suction. Note the patient's tolerance of the procedure. Note when oral and nasal care were performed.

4/24/08	0900	Explained the procedure of NG tube removal to pt. Active
		bowel sounds heard in all 4 quadrants. Drained 25 ml of pale
		green odorless drainage over last 2 hr. Tolerating ice chips
		without nausea, vomiting, discomfort, or abdominal distention.
		NG tube removed without difficulty. Pt. taking small sips of
		water without c/o nausea. ——————— Carol Allen, RN

O

Organ donation

A federal requirement enacted in 1998 requires facilities to report deaths to the regional organ procurement organization (OPO). This regulation was enacted so that no potential donor would be missed. The regulation ensures that the family of every potential donor will understand the option to donate. It's important to be familiar with the legal aspects of organ donation, because legislation varies in every state.

Collection of most organs, including the heart, liver, kidney, and pancreas, requires that the patient be pronounced brain dead and be kept physically alive until the organs are harvested. Tissue, such as eyes, skin, bone, and heart valves, may be taken after death.

Follow your facility's policy for identifying and reporting a potential organ donor. Contact your local or regional OPO when a potential donor is identified. Typically, a specially trained person from your facility along with someone from your regional OPO will speak with the family about organ donation. The OPO coordinates the donation process after a family consents to donation.

Essential documentation

Your documentation will vary depending on the stage of, and your role in, the organ donation process. You'll need to write a separate note for each stage. Make sure that you record the date and time of each note. Record the date and time that the patient is pronounced brain dead and the physician's discussions with the family about the prognosis. (See "Brain death," page 202.) If the patient's driver's license or other documents indicate his wish to donate organs, place copies in the medical record and document that you have done so. The individual who contacts the regional OPO must document the conversation, including the date and time, the name of the person he spoke with, and instructions given. If you were part of the discussion about organ donation with the family, document who was present, what the family was told and by whom, and their response. Record your nursing care of the donor until the time he's taken to the operating room for organ procurement. Chart teaching, explanations, and emotional support given to the family.

1/12/08	0900	Dr. Regina Silverstone explained to pt's family (wife and son)
		at 0815 that pt. was brain dead and the prognosis. Family
		asked about organ donation. Driver's license located with pt.'s
		belongings confirmed pt.'s request for organ donation. Copy
		of license placed in medical record. Dr. Silverstone explained
		the criteria for organ donation and the process to the
		family. Mrs. Hubbard stated she would like more information
		from the regional OPO. OPO was contacted at 0830. Intake
		information was taken by Rhonda Tierney. Appointment made
		for today at 1100 for OPO coordinator to meet with family
		in conference room on nursing unit. Family also requested
		to speak with a chaplain. Chaplain was paged, and Fr. Stone
		will be here at 0915 to meet with family. Checking with family
		every hour to see if there is anything they need, to answer
		questions, and to provide support. ———— Patty Fisher, RN

Ostomy care

An ostomy is a surgically created opening used to replace a normal physiologic function. Ostomies are used to facilitate the elimination of solid or liquid waste or to support respirations if placed in the trachea. The type and amount of care an ostomy requires depend on the output and location of the stoma. The nurse is responsible for providing ostomy care, protecting the skin surrounding the stoma, and assessing the condition of the skin and stoma. The nurse may also need to help the patient adapt to the care and wearing of an appliance while helping him accept the body change.

Essential documentation

Record the date and time of ostomy care. Describe the location of the ostomy and the condition of the stoma, including size, shape, and color. Chart the condition of the peristomal skin, noting any redness, irritation, breakdown, bleeding, or other unusual conditions. Note the character of drainage, including color, amount, type, and consistency. Record the type of appliance used, appliance size, and type of adhesive used. Document patient teaching, describing the teaching content. Record the patient's response to self-care, and evaluate his learning progress. Some facilities use a patient-teaching record to document patient teaching.

4/11/08	1000	Ostomy located in ⊕ upper abdomen. Appliance removed, minimal amount of dark brown fecal material in bag. Stoma 4 cm in diameter, round, beefy red in color; no drainage or bleeding. Skin surrounding stoma is pink and intact. Karaya ring applied to skin surrounding stoma after applying skin adhesive. New appliance snapped onto ring. Pt. helped measure stoma and applied skin adhesive. Pt. currently reading material on ostomy care. Discussed proper measurement of stoma and cutting hole in skin barrier to proper size. Pt. understands and agrees to cut skin barrier with next change. ——— Dawn March, RN

Oxygen administration

Oxygen therapy is initiated in circumstances in which the body has a higher metabolic demand or increased oxygen consumption. Arterial blood gas (ABG) analysis, oximetry monitoring, and clinical assessments determine the adequacy and amount of oxygen therapy. The patient's disease, physical condition, and age help determine the most appropriate method of administration. The physician prescribes the oxygen concentration and method of delivery.

Essential documentation

Record the date and time of oxygen administration. Document the oxygen delivery device and the concentration of oxygen used or the oxygen flow rate. Record your assessment findings, including vital signs, skin color and temperature, respiratory effort, use of accessory muscles, breath sounds, and level of consciousness (LOC). Signs of hypoxia may include a decreased LOC, increased heart rate, arrhythmias, restlessness, dyspnea, use of accessory muscles, flared nostrils, cyanosis, and cool, clammy skin. Record ABG or oximetry values. If a physician was notified, include the name of the physician, time of notification, and any orders given. Record the patient's response to oxygen therapy and include any patient and family teaching and emotional support given.

2/16/08	1200	When walking in room at 1130 to bring pt. his lunch tray, noted
		pt. sitting upright, pale, diaphoretic, taking deep labored respira-
		tions using accessory muscles with nasal flaring. O_2 currently at
		2 L by nasal cannula. Pt. only able to speak 1-2 words at a time,
		stated his breathing has been "getting short" over the last hour.
		P 124 regular, BP 134/88, RR 32 and labored, tymp temp 97.2° F.
		Skin cool and pale, cyanosis noted around lips. Normal heart
		sounds, wheezes heard posteriorly on expiration. Pt. alert and
		oriented to time, place, and person, but appears anxious and
		restless. Pulse oximetry 87%. Dr. David Desmond notified. Orders
		given. O_2 increased to 4 L by nasal cannula. Albuterol 2 puffs
		administered by inhaler. 1145 pt. stated he's "breathing easier."
		P 92 and regular, BP 128/82, RR 24 and unlabored. Pulse oxime-
		try 96%. No use of accessory muscles noted, skin warm and pink.
		Lungs clear. Pt. resting comfortably in bed. Explained to pt the
		importance of immediately reporting SOB to the nurse. Pt. ver-
		balized understanding. Per orders, O_2 to be titrated to keep O_2
		sat greater than 92%. 1150 O_2 sat by pulse oximetry 96%, O_2
		reduced back to 2 L. Will recheck O_2 sat in 10 min. ————————
		————————————————— Mindy Pressler, RN

P

Pacemaker, initiation of transcutaneous

A temporary pacemaker is usually used in an emergency. In a life-threatening situation, when time is critical, a transcutaneous pacemaker is the quickest treatment. (See *Responding to cardiac arrhythmia*.) This device sends an electrical impulse from the pulse generator to the patient's heart by way of two electrodes, which are placed on the front and back of the patient's chest. Transcutaneous pacing is quick and effective, but it's used only until a transvenous or permanent pacemaker is inserted.

Essential documentation

Chart the date and time of the procedure. Record the reason for transcutaneous pacing and pacemaker settings. Note the patient's response to the procedure along with complications and interventions. If possible, obtain rhythm strips before, during, and after pacemaker use; whenever settings are changed; and when the patient is treated for a complication caused by the pacemaker. As you monitor the patient, record his response to pacing and note changes in his condition. Record patient teaching and patient under-

CASE CLIP

Responding to cardiac arrhythmia

Mr. R. is a 65-year-old male admitted to the emergency department with complaint of crushing chest pain. He reported his pain level to be at 10/10. Cardiac enzymes and troponin levels were elevated and electrocardiogram (ECG) showed acute inferior wall myocardial infarction.

Vital signs on admission were:
- temperature: 99.1° F (37.3° C)
- heart rate (HR): 110 beats/minute
- respiratory rate (RR): 22 breaths/minute
- blood pressure (BP): 130/78 mm Hg
- pulse oximetry: 95% on 2 L/minute.

Mr. R. was given aspirin, sublingual nitroglycerin, and morphine 2 mg I.V., and was started on oxygen at 4 L/minute and nitroglycerin drip. Pain level decreased to 1/10. Mr. R. was taken to the intensive care unit. While waiting to go to the cardiac catheter laboratory, his cardiac rhythm changed from normal sinus rhythm (rate 97) to third-degree heart block (rate 40). Vital signs at this time were:
- temperature: 100.1° F (37.8° C)
- HR: 40 beats/minute
- RR: 25 breaths/minute
- BP: 80/50 mm Hg
- pulse oximetry: 93%.

Mr. R. started to complain of chest pain that he rated at 5/10. Skin was diaphoretic. Dr. George Gonzales was paged but didn't respond within 5 minutes. The patient was less alert. The rapid response team (RRT) was notified and arrived within 3 minutes.

The RRT quickly reviewed Mr. R.'s history, medications, and cardiac rhythm. An ECG confirmed that Mr. R. had third-degree heart block. A transcutaneous pacemaker was applied with the following settings: rate 70, mA 80. Cardiac monitor showed pacemaker rhythm with 100% fire and capture. Vital signs after initiation of pacemaker were:
- HR: 70 beats/minute
- RR: 20 breaths/minute
- BP: 114/68 mm Hg
- pulse oximetry: 97%.

Mr. R. was more alert. Chest pain resolved to a rating of 2/10. Mr. R. was given morphine 1 mg and Ativan 1 mg to completely resolve his chest pain and to help him tolerate the pacemaker function. Dr. Gonzalez saw the patient. Mr. R. was transported to the catheter laboratory for cardiac catheterization and transve-

standing of the procedure. Document emotional support and comfort measures provided.

2/15/08	1420	Pt. with VS: Apical HR 48, BP 84/50, RR 16, arousable with verbal and physical stimulation, speech incomprehensible. Skin pale and clammy, peripheral pulses weak. Monitor shows sinus bradycardia. Transcutaneous pacing initiated. Output set at 40 mA, rate at 60. Apical HR 60, BP 94/60, RR 18. Cardiac monitor shows PMR with 100% fire and capture. Medicated with Ativan 1 mg I.V. Pt. alert and oriented; no c/o chest pain, dyspnea, or dizziness. Peripheral pulses strong; skin warm and dry. Explained to pt. that he may feel a thumping or twitching sensation during pacing. ———————————————————————— Sally Hanes, RN

Pacemaker, insertion of permanent

A permanent pacemaker is a self-contained unit designed to operate for 3 to 20 years. In an operating room or cardiac catheterization laboratory, a surgeon places pacing wires into the heart chambers to be paced and then implants the generator device in a pocket under the patient's skin.

A permanent pacemaker allows the patient's heart to beat on its own but begins pacing when the patient's heart rate reaches a preset rate. Pacemakers may pace at a rate that varies in response to intrinsic conditions such as skeletal muscle activity, and pacemakers may have antitachycardia and shock functions.

Candidates for permanent pacemakers include patients with symptomatic bradyarrhythmia, complete heart block, or slow ventricular rates stemming from congenital or degenerative heart disease or cardiac surgery. Patients who suffer Stokes-Adams attacks and those with Wolff-Parkinson-White syndrome may also benefit from a permanent pacemaker.

Essential documentation

Record the date and time of your entry. Record the time that your patient returned to the unit. Document the type of pacemaker used, pacing rate, where the generator is located, and practitioner's name. Verify that the chart contains information on the pacemaker's serial number and its manufacturer's name. Note cardiac rhythm and obtain rhythm strips to place in the chart. If the pacemaker is functioning, record firing and capturing ability. Document the condition of the incision site dressing. Chart the patient's vital signs and level of consciousness every 15 minutes for the first hour, every hour for the next 4 hours, every 4 hours for the next 24 hours, and then once every shift, or according to facility policy or practitioner's order. You may record these frequent assessments on a critical care or frequent vital signs flow sheet. Assess for and record signs and symptoms of complications, such as infection, perforated ventricle, cardiac tamponade, or pacemaker malfunction. Record the name of the practitioner notified, the time of notification, interventions, and the patient's response. Document your patient teaching and the patient's understanding of the procedure. This may be recorded on a patient-teaching flow sheet.

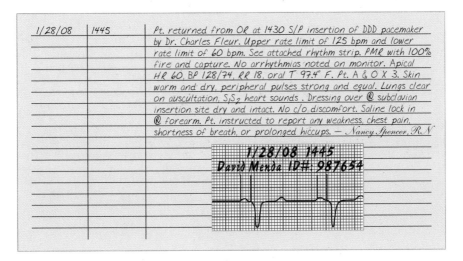

1/28/08	1445	Pt. returned from OR at 1430 S/P insertion of DDD pacemaker
		by Dr. Charles Fleur. Upper rate limit of 125 bpm and lower
		rate limit of 60 bpm. See attached rhythm strip. PMR with 100%
		fire and capture. No arrhythmias noted on monitor. Apical
		HR 60, BP 128/74, RR 18, oral T 97.4° F. Pt. A & O X 3. Skin
		warm and dry, peripheral pulses strong and equal. Lungs clear
		on auscultation, S₁S₂ heart sounds . Dressing over Ⓡ subclavian
		insertion site dry and intact. No c/o discomfort. Saline lock in
		Ⓡ forearm. Pt. instructed to report any weakness, chest pain,
		shortness of breath, or prolonged hiccups. — Nancy Spencer, R.N

Pacemaker, insertion of transvenous

A transvenous pacemaker is usually inserted in an emergency by threading an electrode catheter through the brachial, femoral, subclavian, or jugular vein, into the patient's right atrium, right ventricle, or both. The electrodes are then attached to an external battery-powered pulse generator. Some pulmonary artery catheters have transvenous pacing electrodes.

Essential documentation

Record the date and time that the pacemaker was inserted, the reason for pacing, and the location of the insertion site. Chart the pacemaker settings and the patient's cardiac rhythm, and place a rhythm strip in the chart. Document the patient's level of consciousness and cardiopulmonary assessment, including vital signs and pain assessment. Note the patient's response to the procedure, complications, and interventions. Document your assessment of the insertion site and your neurovascular assessment of the involved limb, if appropriate. Record your patient teaching and the patient's understanding of the procedure. Document emotional support and comfort measures provided.

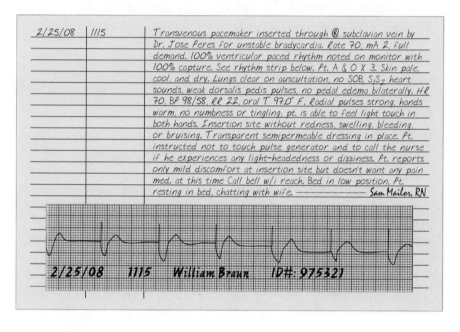

2/25/08	1115	Transvenous pacemaker inserted through ® subclavian vein by
		Dr. Jose Peres for unstable bradycardia. Rate 70, mA 2, full
		demand. 100% ventricular paced rhythm noted on monitor with
		100% capture. See rhythm strip below. Pt. A & O X 3. Skin pale,
		cool, and dry. Lungs clear on auscultation, no SOB, S₁S₂ heart
		sounds, weak dorsalis pedis pulses, no pedal edema bilaterally. HR
		70, BP 98/58, RR 22, oral T 97.0° F. Radial pulses strong, hands
		warm, no numbness or tingling; pt. is able to feel light touch in
		both hands. Insertion site without redness, swelling, bleeding,
		or bruising. Transparent semipermeable dressing in place. Pt.
		instructed not to touch pulse generator and to call the nurse
		if he experiences any light-headedness or dizziness. Pt. reports
		only mild discomfort at insertion site but doesn't want any pain
		med. at this time Call bell w/i reach. Bed in low position. Pt.
		resting in bed, chatting with wife. ————— Sam Mailor, RN

2/25/08   1115   William Braun   ID#: 975321

Pain management

Pain is a subjective complaint. It's whatever the patient says it is. The perception of pain produces anxiety, which in turn can increase the patient's pain. Your primary goal is to eliminate or minimize your patient's pain through appropriate actions. You can use a number of tools to assess pain. Always document the results of your assessments. (See *Assessing and documenting pain*.)

Interventions to manage pain include administering analgesics, providing emotional support and comfort measures, and using cognitive techniques to distract the patient. Patients with severe pain usually require an opioid analgesic. Invasive measures, such as epidural or patient-controlled analgesia, may also be required.

Assessing and documenting pain

Used appropriately, standard assessment tools, such as the McGill-Melzack Pain Questionnaire and the Initial Pain Assessment Tool (developed by McCaffery and Beebe), provide a solid foundation for your nursing diagnoses and care plans. If your health care facility doesn't use standardized pain questionnaires, you can devise other pain measurement tools, such as the pain flow sheet or the visual and graphic rating scales that appear below. Whichever pain assessment tool you choose, remember to document its use and include the graphic record in your patient's chart.

Pain flow sheet

Possibly the most convenient tool for pain assessment, a flow sheet provides a standard for reevaluating a patient's pain at regular intervals. It's also beneficial for patients and families who may feel too overwhelmed by the pain experience to answer a long, detailed questionnaire.

If possible, incorporate the pain assessment into the flow sheet that you're already using. Generally, the easier the flow sheet is to use, the more likely you and your patient will be to use it.

PAIN FLOW SHEET					
Date and time	Pain rating (0 to 10)	Patient behaviors	Vital signs	Pain rating after intervention	Comments
1/16/08 0800	7	Wincing, holding head	186/88 98–22	5 @ 0830	Dilaudid 2 mg I.M. given
1/16/08 1200	3	Relaxing, reading	160/80 84–18	2 @ 1300	Tylox † P.O. given

Visual analog pain scale

With a visual analog pain scale, the patient marks a linear scale containing words or numbers that correspond to his perceived degree of pain. Draw a scale to represent a continuum of pain intensity. Verbal anchors describe the pain's intensity; for example, "no pain" begins the scale and "pain as bad as it could be" ends it. Ask the patient to mark the point on the continuum that best describes his pain.

VISUAL ANALOG SCALE

No pain   **X**   Pain as bad as it could be

(continued)

Assessing and documenting pain *(continued)*

Graphic rating scale
Other rating scales have words that represent pain intensity. Use one of these scales as you would the visual analog scale. Have the patient mark the spot on the continuum.

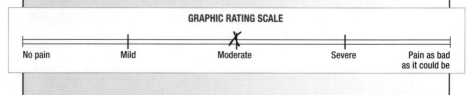

GRAPHIC RATING SCALE

No pain — Mild — Moderate — Severe — Pain as bad as it could be

Essential documentation

When charting pain levels and characteristics, describe the location of the pain and note if it's internal, external, localized, or diffuse. Record whether the pain interferes with the patient's sleep or activities of daily living. In the chart, describe the pain in the patient's own words, using quotation marks. Chart when the pain started, whether the patient has had this pain in the past, and what the patient says relieves or worsens it. Record the patient's ranking of his pain using a pain rating scale.

Describe the patient's body language and behaviors associated with pain, such as wincing, grimacing, or body position in bed. Note sympathetic responses commonly associated with mild to moderate pain, such as pallor, elevated blood pressure, dilated pupils, skeletal muscle tension, dyspnea, tachycardia, and diaphoresis. Record parasympathetic responses commonly associated with severe, deep pain, including pallor, decreased blood pressure, bradycardia, nausea and vomiting, dizziness, and loss of consciousness.

Document interventions taken to alleviate your patient's pain and the patient's responses to these interventions. Also note patient teaching and the patient's understanding of any treatment and medication. Document emotional support and comfort measures provided.

3/19/08	1630	Pt. c/o severe pain in LLQ. Pt. states, "It feels like my insides
		are on fire." Pt. rates pain as 6/10. States pain keeps him
		from sleeping and eating. States he's been taking Percocet 2
		tabs q4hr at home, but it's no longer providing relief. Pt. A &
		O X 3. Curled in bed on Ⓛ side, with arms wrapped around
		abdomen and softly moaning. Skin pale and diaphoretic, pupils
		dilated. Dr. Joyce Martin notified at 1550. Dilaudid 2 mg
		ordered and given I.V. HR 92, BP 110/64, RR 22, oral T 99° F.
		Pt. resting at present, no longer moaning or curled in a ball.
		States pain is now 2/10. Explained possible side effects of
		medication and ordered schedule. Instructed pt. to call if
		pain worsens. —————————— Kaylee Compton, RN

Paracentesis

Paracentesis is a bedside procedure in which fluid from the peritoneal space is aspirated through a needle, trocar, or cannula inserted in the abdominal wall. Paracentesis is used to diagnose and treat massive ascites when other therapies have failed. Additionally, it's used as a prelude to other procedures, including radiography, peritoneal dialysis, and surgery. It's also used to detect intra-abdominal bleeding after traumatic injury and to obtain a peritoneal fluid specimen for laboratory analysis.

Essential documentation

Document that the procedure and its risks have been explained to the patient, that a consent form has been signed, and that the patient is identified using two patient identifiers. Chart what you taught the patient about the procedure and his understanding of it. Your facility may require you to document patient education on a patient-teaching flow sheet. Record baseline vital signs, weight, and abdominal girth.

Record the date and time of the procedure. Describe the puncture site and record the amount, color, viscosity, and odor of the aspirated fluid. Also record the amount of fluid aspirated in the fluid intake and output record. Record the number of specimens sent to the laboratory. Note whether the wound was sutured and the type of dressing that was applied.

Record the patient's tolerance of the procedure, vital signs, and signs and symptoms of complications (such as shock and perforation of abdominal organs) that occur during or after the procedure. If peritoneal fluid leakage occurs, document that you notified the practitioner, any orders given, your actions, and the patient's response.

Document vital signs, drainage checks and the patient's response to the procedure every 15 minutes for the first hour, every 30 minutes for the next hour, every hour for the next 4 hours, and then every 4 hours for the next 24 hours (or according to your facility's policy). Continue to document drainage characteristics, including color, amount, odor, and viscosity. Document daily patient weight and abdominal girth measurements after the procedure.

2/12/08	0920	*Procedure explained to pt. Pt. states understanding. All*
		questions answered. Signed consent on chart. Dr. Richard
		Novello performed paracentesis in RLQ, as per protocol.
		1500 ml of cloudy pale-yellow fluid drained and sent to
		lab as ordered. Site sutured with one 3-0 silk suture.
		Sterile 4" X 4" gauze pad applied. No leakage noted at
		site. Abdomen marked at level of umbilicus with black
		felt-tipped pen for measurements. Abdominal girth 44"
		preprocedure and 42¾" postprocedure. VS and weight
		before and after procedure as per flow sheet. Before
		procedure pt. stated, "I am afraid of this procedure."
		Reinforced teaching related to the procedure and pt.
		verbalized understanding. Offered reassurances during
		the procedure. Pt. now resting comfortably in bed. ——
		—————————————————————— Carol Barsky, RN

Parenteral nutrition administration, total

Total parenteral nutrition (TPN) is the administration of a solution of high-concentrate dextrose, proteins, electrolytes, vitamins, and trace elements in amounts that exceed the patient's energy expenditure, thereby achieving anabolism. Because this solution has about six times the solute concentration of blood, it requires dilution by delivery into a high-flow central vein to avoid injury to the peripheral vasculature. The solution is delivered to the superior vena cava through a central venous (CV) catheter or a peripherally inserted central catheter. Generally, TPN is prescribed for any patient who can't absorb nutrients through the GI tract for more than 10 days.

Because TPN solution promotes bacterial growth and the CV catheter allows systemic access, contamination and sepsis are always a risk. Strict surgical asepsis is required during solution, dressing, tubing, and filter changes. Site care and dressing changes should be performed according to your facility's policy, usually at least three times per week (once per week for transparent dressings) and whenever the dressing becomes wet, soiled, or nonocclusive. Tubing and filter changes should be performed every 24 hours, according to your facility's policy.

Because of the concentration of TPN, careful cross-check of practitioner's orders should occur before administration of each bag of solution, usually by two nurses.

Essential documentation

Record the date and time of your entry. Document the type and location of the CV line and the volume and rate of the solution infused. Document cross-check of practitioner orders (two nurses). Record the amount of TPN infused on the intake and output record. Document site care, describing the condition of the insertion site, cleaning of the site, and the type of dressing applied. Many facilities document all this information on an I.V. flow sheet. Document any adverse reactions, such as air embolism, extravasation, phlebitis, pneumothorax, hydrothorax, septicemia, or thrombosis, and document your observations, interventions, and the patient's response to them. Record what you teach the patient about TPN and his understanding of the teaching.

3/31/08	2020	2-L bag of TPN hung at 2000 at 65 ml/hr via infusion
		pump through Ⓡ subclavian CV line. Transparent dressing
		intact, and site is without redness, drainage, swelling, or
		tenderness. See I/O flow sheet for intake and output.
		Reviewed reasons for TPN and answered pt.'s questions
		about its purpose. Pt. verbalized understanding.
		———————————————— Meg Callahan, RN

Patient activity level

Patient activity level is determined by the patient's present illness and patient mobility level. On admission, the practitioner orders an activity level for the patient, such as complete bed rest or bathroom privileges. This order may advance to increased activity—or decrease to bed rest, based on the patient's course of illness. A physical therapy consultation may assist the patient in advancing activity before being discharged to home or another facility.

Essential documentation

Document the patient's activity level as ordered on admission. Record whether the patient needs assistance with activity and the patient's level of mobility. When a patient's activity level changes, document the patient's compliance with that activity level. Record any physical therapy sessions and the patient's response. Upon discharge or transfer to another facility, record the patient's ability to participate at the ordered activity level. Document patient teaching and the patient's understanding of the ordered activity.

1/01/08	1030	Pt. activity increased to OOB in chair. Pt. OOB to chair with assistance, unsteady on feet. Pt. instructed to remain in chair. Call bell within reach. ———————— G. Smith, RN

Patient-controlled analgesia

Some patients receive opioids by way of a patient-controlled analgesia (PCA) infusion pump that allows patients to self-administer boluses of an opioid analgesic I.V., subcutaneously, or epidurally within limits prescribed by the practitioner. To avoid overmedication, an adjustable lockout interval inhibits premature delivery of additional boluses. PCA increases the patient's sense of control, reduces anxiety, reduces drug use over the postoperative course, and gives enhanced pain control. Indicated for patients who need parenteral analgesia, PCA therapy is typically given to trauma patients postoperatively, terminal cancer patients, and others with chronic diseases.

Essential documentation

Follow facility policy for documentation of the opioid used, lockout interval, maintenance dose, ordered dose, attempts to receive the drug, and actual amount of opioid used during your shift. Many facilities require dual verification of PCA orders, settings, and remaining amount of drug between nursing shifts. Record the patient's verbalization of pain level, any patient teaching you perform, and the patient's understanding of PCA use. Document your patient's vital signs and level of consciousness according to your facility's policy. Document adverse effects and interventions. (See *Responding to misuse of PCA pump.*)

CASE CLIP

Responding to misuse of PCA pump

Mrs. J. is a 60-year-old female admitted for an abdominal hysterectomy. Vital signs on admission were:

- temperature: 98.1° F (36.7° C)
- heart rate (HR): 70 beats/minute
- respiratory rate (RR): 16 breaths/minute
- blood pressure (BP): 110/70 mm Hg
- pulse oximetry: 98% on room air.

The procedure was performed without incident and Mrs. J. was taken to her room on the gynecology floor. She was awake and oriented three times. A Dilaudid PCA pump was initiated in the postanesthesia care unit. Teaching was reinforced on use of the pump when the patient was admitted to her room. Upon entering the patient's room after dinner, the nurse couldn't arouse Mrs. J. Vital signs at this time were:

- HR: 68 beats/minute
- RR: 8 breaths/minute
- BP: 78/50 mm Hg
- pulse oximetry: 91% on room air.

The rapid response team (RRT) was called and arrived within 3 minutes. The RRT quickly reviewed Mrs. J.'s history and medications. A 100% nonrebreather mask was applied and pulse oximetry increased to 97%. Narcan 0.4 mg was given and the patient immediately became arousable. Vital signs at this time were:

- HR: 85 beats/minute
- RR: 16 breaths/minute
- BP: 110/82 mm Hg
- pulse oximetry: 98%.

Dr. John Seaboard was notified. The patient was transported to the intensive care unit for observation. The PCA pump was discontinued and the patient placed on Percocet every 4 hours as needed for pain.

Record your observations of the insertion site. See *PCA flow sheet,* page 304, for an example of documentation using this method.

| 1/10/08 | 1300 | Pt. c/o pain 6/10 @ 1230. Pt. on PCA morphine. Teaching reinforced on use of PCA pump, benefits and possible adverse effects of morphine. Pt. encouraged to use PCA when pain starts. Pt. states understanding and administered PCA dose. Pain level reevaluated #2/10. ———— J. Devine, RN |

PCA flow sheet

The form shown below is used to document the use of patient-controlled analgesia (PCA). PCA allows the patient to self-administer an opioid analgesic as needed within limits prescribed by the practitioner.

Patient name: Martin Smith   **Medical record #:** 1234567   **Date:** 3/22/08

Medication (Circle one)   Meperidine 100 mg in 50 ml (10 mg/1 ml)
(Morphine 50 mg in 50 ml (1 mg/ml))

	7–3 Shift				3–11 Shift				11–7 Shift			
Time (enter in box)	1300	1400			1530							
New cartridge inserted	OR											
PCA settings Lockout interval 10 (minutes)	10	10			10							
Dose volume 1 (mg)	1	1			1							
One-hour limit 6 (mg)	6	6			6							
Basal rate 0 (mg/hr)	0	0			0							
Respiratory rate	18	20			20							
Blood pressure	150/70	130/62			128/10							
Sedation rating 1. Wide awake 2. Drowsy 3. Dozing, intermittent 4. Mostly sleeping 5. Only awakens when stimulated	1	2			3							
Analgesia rts (1–10) Minimal pain – 1 Maximum pain – 10	2	2			2							
Additional doses given (optional doses)	3ml/OR											
Total ml delivered (total from ampule)	3	6			9							
ml remaining	47	44			41							
RN check	JG	JG/AR			AR/KS							

RN SIGNATURE (7–3 SHIFT) _Janet Green, RN (OR)_ / _Anne Rice, RN_   Date 3/22/08

RN SIGNATURE (3–11 SHIFT) _Karen Singleton, RN_   Date 3/22/08

RN SIGNATURE (11–7 SHIFT) _____   Date _____

Patient requesting access to medical records

According to the Health Insurance Portability and Accountability Act of 1996, the patient has the right to view and obtain copies of his medical records. Many states have since enacted laws allowing patients access to such records, and health care providers are required to honor such requests. Psychologists, however, may deny a patient access to his psychotherapy records.

When a patient requests to see his medical record, assess why he wants to see it. He may simply be curious, or his request may reflect hidden fears about his treatment that you or another member of the health care team may be able to address. Be sure to follow your facility's policy when a patient requests to view his own medical record. These policies may dictate that you notify your nursing supervisor or medical records manager of the request and that you notify the risk manager to alert administrative staff and legal counsel, if necessary.

Explain the procedure for accessing medical records, and provide the patient with the appropriate forms to use. Advise him when you expect the records to be available (typically, copies are available within 30 days of the request). Also let him know whether the facility charges a fee for copying the records.

When the medical record is available, be sure to properly identify the patient and remain with him while he reads the record. Explain to the patient that he has the right to request that incorrect information be changed or that missing information be added, with verification of that information, such as a social security number. If the practitioner or health care facility believes that the medical record is correct, the patient can note his disagreement in the medical record. Observe how the patient responds while he reads. Offer to answer any questions he may have; assure him that the practitioner will also answer questions. While the patient reads, help him interpret the abbreviations and terminology used in medical charting, as well as decipher difficult handwriting.

Essential documentation

If your patient asks to see his medical record, use your facility's form or have the patient draft a written request to see his medical record, according to your facility's policy. Chart the parts of the medical record that the patient requested and whether copies were given to the patient. Record the names of the nursing supervisor, medical records personnel, risk manager, legal counsel, and practitioner who were notified of the patient's request. Record the date and time the patient reviewed his record and the name of the person who stayed with the patient while he read it. Document the patient's response to reading his record and whether he had questions or concerns.

3/3/08	1400	Pt. stated, "I want to look at my chart." Appropriate
		forms completed by pt. and request sent to medical
		records. Notified Bruce Wallins, RN, nursing supervisor;
		Loretta Reilly, RN, nurse manager; and Dr. Mary Felbin
		of pt.'s request. Identity confirmed by checking ID band
		and DOB. Dr. Felbin and I were in attendance while pt.
		read record. All questions answered. —— Monica Lutz, RN

Patient teaching

Patient and caregiver teaching is essential for maintaining the patient's health, preventing or detecting early signs of complications, and promoting self-care and independence. Patient teaching is every patient's right in any setting. Teaching is most effective when it's specific to the patient's and family's physical, financial, emotional, intellectual, cultural, and social circumstances and when the patient and family are ready to learn, are mentally alert, and are free from discomfort and distraction.

Keep teaching sessions brief, and reinforce all instructions using verbal explanations, demonstrations, videos, and written materials. Evaluate the patient's understanding by asking him to restate material, answer your questions, or give a return demonstration.

Documentation of your teaching is important and lets other health care team members know what the patient has been taught, how he responded, and what materials need to be reinforced. It also serves as a record to confirm teaching and level of understanding. (See *Documenting what you teach.*)

Essential documentation

Check your facility's policies and procedures regarding when, where, and how to document your teaching. Despite their similar content, patient-teaching forms vary according to the health care facility. The forms may ask you to document information by filling in blanks, checking boxes, or writing brief narrative notes. Typically, you'll need

LEGAL LOOKOUT

Documenting what you teach

Always document what you teach the patient and his family and their understanding of what you taught. The Court in *Kyslinger v. United States* (1975) addressed the nurse's liability for patient teaching. In this case, a Veterans Administration (VA) hospital patient with an artificial kidney was discharged to home where he would use a home hemodialysis unit. The patient eventually died (apparently while on the hemodialysis machine) and his wife sued, alleging that the hospital and its staff failed to teach either her or her late husband how to properly use and maintain a home hemodialysis unit.

After examining the evidence, the Court ruled against the patient's wife, as follows: "During those 10 months that plaintiff's decedent underwent biweekly hemodialysis treatment on the unit (at the VA hospital), both plaintiff and decedent were instructed as to the operation, maintenance, and supervision of said treatment. The Court can find no basis to conclude that the plaintiff or plaintiff's decedent were not properly informed on the use of the hemodialysis unit."

to document information about the patient's learning needs, learning abilities, barriers to learning, goals to be met, equipment or supplies used, specific content taught, response to teaching, and skills to be acquired by the time of discharge. You'll also need to chart how you evaluated the patient's learning, such as by return demonstration or verbalization of understanding. Before discharge, document the patient's remaining learning needs, and note whether you provided him with printed material or other patient-teaching aids. If there's an opportunity or need to teach caregivers when teaching the patient, document the teaching that occurred and the caregiver's response and understanding of the teaching.

See *Patient-teaching forms* in chapter 5 for an example of how to document patient education.

Patient threat of self-harm

A threat of self-harm may come as a refusal of care, a threat to injure oneself, or a threat to commit suicide. The best way to prevent self-harm is by early recognition and treatment of depression and other mental illnesses, including substance abuse.

When a patient threatens or tries to harm himself, you have a duty to protect him from harm. Use your communication skills to try to calm the patient. Let him know you care about him. Remove potentially harmful objects from the immediate area. If the patient is holding a dangerous object and is threatening to harm himself, send a coworker to call security, the nursing supervisor, and the patient's practitioner, and stay with him until assistance arrives. If constant observation is ordered, someone must stay with the patient at all times. Administer medications as ordered. Restraints should be used as a last resort, according to your facility's policy.

Essential documentation

Record the date and time of your entry. Record, in the patient's own words, his threat to harm himself. If known, document the situation that led up to this event. Objectively describe any behaviors that indicate a desire for self-harm. Note all steps taken immediately to protect the patient from harm, such as one-to-one observation and removal of any harmful objects from the immediate environment. Chart the names of the practitioner, nursing supervisor, and security officer notified and the time of notification. Document their responses, your interventions, and the patient's response. Record any explanations given to the patient and efforts to reduce anxiety. If restraints were needed, be sure to follow proper policy for restraint use and documentation.

1/1/08	1655	Heard thumping noise in room at 1625 and found pt.
		beating his Ⓡ fist against wall. Pt. stated, "I'm better,
		and my wife doesn't visit. If I was hurt, maybe she
		would visit." Asked pt. to sit on his bed and he complied.
		Listened as pt. spoke of family problems. Pt. agreed to
		talk with social worker. Pt. able to move fingers of Ⓡ
		hand, no bruising noted, no c/o pain. Called Meg Watkins,
		CNA, to sit with pt. Spoke with Dr. George Sterling at 1635
		who agreed to referral to social worker. Dr. Sterling will
		be by to see pt. at 1800. Andrew O'Toole, social worker,
		called at 1640 and will be by to see pt. Will have CNA
		stay with pt. until social worker and doctor arrive. CNA
		instructed to call immediately if pt. resumes harmful
		behaviors. ———————————————— Maria Perez, RN

Patient threat to harm another

When a patient threatens to harm someone else—whether verbally or by making threatening gestures—quick action is needed to prevent a violent act from occurring. Follow your facility's policy for dealing with a patient who threatens to harm someone else. Remove the person being threatened from the immediate area. Use your communication skills to calm the patient and reduce agitation. Call the practitioner, nursing supervisor, and security to inform them of the situation. Some facilities have a special code, such as "Mr. Atlas," that alerts other hospital personnel that assistance is needed in a certain area. Activate this code if necessary. If the situation escalates, call local police for appropriate assistance.

Essential documentation

Record the date and time of your entry in your nurse's note. Chart the location and time of the incident and any predisposing factors to the incident, if known. Describe the threat, quote exactly what the patient said, and record threatening behaviors or gestures, or use of threatening objects. Record your immediate interventions and the patient's response. Document how the situation was resolved.

Chart the names of the people you notified, such as the practitioner, nursing supervisor, security, or local police; the time of notification; and their responses. Record any changes in the care plan. Don't name another patient in your patient's chart; this violates confidentiality. Use the word "roommate" or "visitor," or give a room and bed number to describe the person threatened.

Complete an incident report, repeating the exact information that's in your nurse's note. Include names, addresses, and telephone numbers of witnesses, including the name of the threatened person.

3/29/08	0315	*Pt. pacing back and forth in room at 0300, stating "I'll take*
		care of it my way. I'll take care of him real good," while
		punching one hand into the other. Pt.'s roommate moved to
		another room. At 0310 Dr. Ma Chi, nursing supervisor Ron
		Hardy, RN, and security officer Tom Gulden were notified
		of pt.'s threats toward his roommate. Pt. alert, disoriented
		to time and date, states when asked his name, "I'm going to
		get him." c/o "bad smell in here." No foul odor noted. Face
		red, diaphoretic, draws away from touch. Trying to open
		sealed window to "let the bad smell out." Breathing easily,
		skin color other than face is pink. MAE X 4. — Carla Aiken, RN
	0345	*Dr. Chi, Mr. Hardy, and Mr. Gulden arrived on unit at 0320.*
		Assessment findings reported. Pt. less agitated. No longer
		punching his palm. Assisted back to bed. HR 88 and regular,
		BP 136/94, RR 32. I.V. line started in Ⓛ forearm with #20
		angiocath on first attempt. 1000 ml NSS running at 30 ml/hr.
		Dilantin 100 mg given as slow I.V. bolus by Dr. Chi. Dilantin
		level ordered for a.m. Will check pt. q15min. — Carla Aiken, RN

Patient transfer to assisted living facility

Many care and service options are available to older adults to help them function at their highest level of independence. Assisted living provides the older adult with meals, assistance with activities of daily living (ADLs), health care, 24-hour supervision, and other supportive systems.

Transfer to an assisted living facility requires preparation and careful documentation. Preparation includes explaining the transfer to the patient and his family, discussing the patient's condition and care plan with the assisted living staff, and arranging for transportation, if necessary. Documentation of the patient's condition before transfer and adequate communication between nursing staffs ensure continuity of nursing care and provide legal protection for the transferring facility and its staff.

Essential documentation

Record the date and time of the transfer in your nurse's note. Include the practitioner's name, and indicate that transfer orders have been written. Record the name of the assisted living facility to which the patient will be discharged and the name of the nurse who received your verbal report. Indicate that discharge instructions were written and that a copy was given to and discussed with the patient. Have the patient sign a personal belongings form acknowledging that he has all his belongings. In your note, record that the form was completed and placed in the medical record. Describe the condition of your patient at discharge. Be sure to include vital signs and descriptions of wounds as well as tubes and other equipment still in place. Chart the time of discharge, who accompanied the patient, the mode of transportation, and the name of the person at the assisted living facility who will be receiving the patient. Indicate that the medical record was copied and sent with the patient.

Document that transfer forms have been completed and that a copy is being sent to the receiving facility. (See *Transfer form.*) Although details may vary, the transfer form may contain:

■ demographic patient information
■ financial information
■ receiving facility information
■ medical information, including diagnoses, surgeries, allergies, laboratory test values, and advance directives

(Text continues on page 316.)

Transfer form

Documentation of the patient's condition before transfer and adequate communication between nursing staffs ensure continuity of nursing care and provide legal protection for the transferring facility and its staff. Transfer forms such as the one below contain basic information about the patient and his care.

TRANSFER FORM Date: _3/4/08_

PATIENT INFORMATION

Last Name: _Tomlin_   MR#: _1234_
First Name: _Vera_   MR#:
Address: _123 Main St._
City: _Newtown_   State: _VA_ Zip: _22222_
County: Marital Status: _W_
Telephone: _(123) 456-7890_ S.S. #: _111-22-3333_
Age: _90_ Sex: _F_ Height: _5'3"_ Weight: _126#_ DOB: _2/8/16_
Adm. date: _2/26/08_   Discharge date: _3/4/08_

FINANCIAL INFORMATION

Primary: Medicare #:
Medicaid: County:
Policy #:   Group #:
Secondary:
Precert #:

Level of Care: ☐ CORF   ☐ ICF   ☐ SNF   ☐ Rehab Hospital
☑ Assisted   ☐ Home Health   ☐ ICF-MR

MEDICAL INFORMATION

Primary Dx: (date) _Fx @ arm_   _2/26/08_
Secondary Dx: _Type 2 DM_

Surgery: (date) _2/27/08 open reduction_

Allergies: _none_
Prior functional status: _independent_

Advance Directives: ☑ Living Will   ☑ Power of Attorney
☑ DNR   ☐ Legal Guardian
☐ PASSAR   ☐ Level of Care

FAMILY or GUARDIAN

Last Name: _Tomlin_
First Name: _Evelyn_
Relationship: _daughter_
(H)#: _(123) 456-7890_   (W)#:

SERVICES REQUIRED

☑ PT   ☐ OT   ☐ ST   ☐ I.V. Therapy ☐ Hook Up
☐ Skilled Nursing ☐ Social Services ☐ Pain Management
☐ Home Health Aid ☐ RT   ☐ Wound Management
☐ Enteral Fdgs. ☐ TPN ☐ Nut. Tx.   ☐ Palliative Care ☐ Hospice
☐ Dialysis: ☐ Peritoneal ☐ Hemo   ☐ Ventilator Weaning/
Day/week: Maintenance
Location:
Established Post Hospital LOS: ☐ Other
☑ < 30 days   ☐ > 30 days

AGENCY ACCEPTING REFERRAL

Name: _The Oaks Assisted Living Facility_
Contact: _Cathy O'Rourke, RN_
Phone: _(123) 987-6543_   FAX:
Name:
Contact:
Phone: FAX:

PHYSICIAN

MD ordering: _Dr. Vera Chang_   Phone:
MD to follow: _Dr. John Meadows_   Phone:
Other   Phone:
Prognosis _good_

To the best of my knowledge, all information provided about the individual is a true and accurate reflection of the patient's needs. I certify that inpatient care is required at: Level: ☐ Skilled ☑ Intermediate

Physician Signature: _Dr. Vera Chang, MD_
Date signed: _3/5/08_

(continued)

Transfer form *(continued)*

Patient Name: _Vera Tomlin_

LAB ORDERS

Labs:	Labs:

Call or FAX results to: _____

Phone: _____ FAX: _____

Call or Fax results to: _____

Phone: _____ FAX: _____

GENERAL PHYSICIAN ORDERS

PT to Ⓛ arm
NAS 1800-cal ADA diet
Ambulate with walker as tolerated.

Home Medications	Last Dose Given	Dosage	Route	Frequency	Dosing Times	Start Date	End Date
Glucotrol	0730	5 mg	PO	daily	0730		
Lasix	0730	20 mg	PO	daily	0730		

☐ HIVAT (see Final HIVAT Script)

Comments/Delivery: _____

PHYSICAL THERAPY NOTES/PLAN

Assist for transfers supine to sit: ☐ Max ☐ Mod ☐ Min ☐ Contact Guard ☐ Superv ☐ Verbal Cue ☐ Tactile Cue ☑ Independ

Assist for transfers sit to stand: ☐ Max ☐ Mod ☐ Min ☐ Contact Guard ☐ Superv ☐ Verbal Cue ☐ Tactile Cue ☑ Independ

Ambulated _40_ feet with: ☑ Walker ☐ Crutches ☐ Quad cane ☐ Straight cane ☐ W/o device ☐ Nonambulatory
☐ W/wheels ☐ W/platform attachments

With assistance needed: ☐ Max ☐ Mod ☐ Min ☐ Contact Guard ☐ Superv ☐ Verbal Cue ☐ Tactile Cue ☑ Independ

Weight Bearing Status: ☐ NWB ☐ TDNWB ☐ TDWB ☐ PWB ☐ WBAT ☐ FWB ☐ On which leg: ☐ Right ☐ Left ☐ Both

Plan: _strengthen Ⓛ arm_ ☐ Therapy EX ☐ Bed Mobility Plan ☐ Transfer Training ☐ Gait Training

Goal: _regain function Ⓛ arm_ Demonstrates understanding of home safety precautions ☑ Yes ☐ No

PT Additional Comments:

Signature: _Mary Jones_   Title: _PT_   Phone: _(123) 234-8290_   Date: _3/4/08_

Transfer form *(continued)*

Patient Name: _Vera Tomlin_

	ASSESSMENT			

Cardio-pulmonary
BP _148/84_
Pulse _88_
Temp _97.0° F_
Resp _22_

☐ Oxygen
   Rate _____ Method _____
☐ Secretions (describe): _____
☐ Tracheostomy Size: _____ Type: _____

☐ Chest Tube(s)
☐ Vent Settings
☐ CXR (date): _____
☐ TB (date): _____

Nutrition and Hydration
Diet _NAS 1800 cal ADA_
Consistency _regular_
☐ Teeth ☐ No teeth
☑ Dentures type
upper/lower
☐ Dentures with patient

☑ Feeds self
☐ Assist feed ☐ Total feed
☐ Hyperalimentation
☐ Feeding tube type _____
Date inserted _____

☐ Dehydration
☐ Edema
☐ Nausea
☐ Vomiting
☐ Dysphagia
☐ Poor appetite

Access device: _____
Insertion date: _____
Last flushed: _____

Sensory-Comfort	VISION	HEARING	SPEECH	COMFORT	COMMENTS
	☑ Adequate ☐ Poor ☐ Blind ☑ Glasses ☐ Contacts	☑ Adequate ☐ Poor ☐ Deaf ☐ Aid in _R/L_ ear	☑ Good ☐ Difficult ☐ Unable Language: _____	Pain? ☐ Yes ☑ No Where? When?	

Pyscho-social	MENTAL STATUS	BEHAVIOR	SUPPORTS	
	☑ Alert ☐ Lethargic ☐ Comatose ☐ Oriented ☐ Disoriented ☐ Confused ☐ Anxious	☐ Wanders ☑ Cooperative ☐ Combative ☐ Forgetful ☐ Sleep Problems ☐ Other (specify)	Supports: _daughter – Evelyn Tomlin_ Safety:	

Elimination	BLADDER	BOWEL	TOILETING	
	☑ Continent ☐ Incontinent ☐ Retention ☐ Frequency ☐ Dribbling	☑ Continent ☐ Incontinent ☐ Constipation ☐ Diarrhea ☐ Last BM: _3/4/08_	☑ Independent ☐ Dependent ☐ Toilet ☐ Ostomy Type _____ Appliance _____	☐ Bedpan ☐ Catheter Type _____ Size _____ Date inserted: _____

Skin
Skin intact? ☑ Yes ☐ No
Describe any impairments: _Incision @ upper arm intact, healing well_

		INDEPENDENT	ASSIST	TOTAL DEPENDENT	EQUIPMENT/# PERSONS USED
Hygiene	Oral Care	✓			
	Bathing		✓		_needs help of 1 until arm heals_
	Dressing		✓		
Mobility	Wheelchair				
	Transfer	✓			
	Ambulation	✓			_uses walker_

☐ Amputation   ☐ Contractures   ☐ Paralysis   ☐ Paresis   ☐ Other

Labs	Test	Date	Result	Test	Date	Result	Test	Date	Result	
										Isolation Precautions? Last culture date: Results:

- family contacts
- services needed, such as physical, occupational, or speech therapy; dialysis; or wound management
- practitioner's information and orders
- medication information, including last dose given
- assessment of body systems
- ability to perform ADLs
- method of transportation and the company used to perform the transfer.

3/4/08	1100	Pt. transferred to The Oaks Assisted Living Facility at 1030.
		Pt. transported to front door in w/c, accompanied by pt.'s
		daughter, Evelyn Tomin, and me. Pt. assisted into car and
		transported by her daughter. Personal belongings sheet
		completed and signed by pt. Personal belongings packed by
		daughter and placed in suitcase to be transported with pt.
		Transfer orders written by Dr. Vera Chang. Verbal report
		given to Cathy O'Rourke, RN, who will be receiving pt. Transfer
		forms completed and copy sent with pt. to The Oaks with copy
		of medical record. Discharge instruction sheet completed and
		reviewed with daughter and pt. Copy given to pt. Pt. and
		daughter verbalized understanding of med schedule, times,
		doses, and adverse effects to report to Dr. Chang. On discharge,
		pt. is alert and oriented to time, place, and person. HR 88,
		BP 148/84, RR 22, oral T 97.0° F. Lungs clear on auscultation,
		S_1S_2 heart sounds, normal bowel sounds in all 4 quadrants,
		urinating without problems, skin warm, dry, and intact. On
		no-added-salt diet, ambulating on own with walker. Wears
		glasses and bilateral hearing aids, which pt. had on transfer.
		———————————————————————— Thomas Corrigan, RN

Patient transfer to long-term care facility

Many older adults are cared for at home, either by themselves or by their families. However, many will need long-term care (LTC) assistance in their later years.

Several types of LTC facilities are available. An assisted living facility provides meals, sheltered living, and some medical monitoring. This type of facility is appropriate for someone who doesn't need continuous medical attention.

An intermediate care facility provides custodial care for individuals who can't care for themselves due to mental or physical infirmities. Intermediate care facilities provide room, board, and regular nursing care. Physical, social, and recreational activities are provided, and some facilities have rehabilitation programs.

A skilled nursing facility provides medical supervision, rehabilitation services, and 24-hour nursing care by registered nurses, licensed practical nurses, and nurses' aides for patients who have the potential to regain function.

Essential documentation

In your note, record the date and time of the transfer, the practitioner's name, and that transfer orders were written. Note the LTC facility's name and the name of the nurse who received your verbal report. Note that discharge instructions were written and that a copy was discussed with the patient and given to him. You'll need to have the patient sign a personal belongings form acknowledging that he has all his belongings. Remember to record that the form was completed and placed in the medical record. In your note, describe the condition of your patient at discharge, including vital signs, descriptions of wounds, and tubes or other equipment that's still in place. Record the time of discharge, who accompanied the patient, the mode of transportation, and the name of the person at the LTC facility who will be receiving him. Indicate that the medical record was copied and sent with the patient.

Document that transfer forms have been completed and that a copy is being sent to the receiving facility.

The transfer form may contain:
- demographic patient information
- financial information
- receiving facility information
- medical information, including diagnoses, surgeries, allergies, laboratory test values, and advance directives
- family contacts
- services needed, such as physical, occupational, or speech therapy; dialysis; or wound management
- practitioner's information and orders
- medication information, including last dose given
- assessment of body systems
- ability to perform activities of daily living
- mode of transportation and company performing the transfer.

3/11/08	1300	Pt. transferred to Aristocrat Skilled Nursing Facility at
		1230. Pt. transported by stretcher via Metro ambulance.
		Personal belongings list completed and placed in chart.
		Copy placed with belongings sent with pt. Transfer
		orders written by Dr. James Desai. Verbal report given
		to Rachel Peters, RN, who will be receiving pt. Transfer
		forms completed, copy sent with pt. with copy of medical
		records. At the time of discharge, pt. alert and oriented
		to person but not to place, date, and time. HR 72, BP 128/70,
		RR 18, oral T 98.2° F. Lungs clear on auscultation with
		diminished breath sounds at bases, S_1S_2 heart sounds,
		normal bowel sounds in all 4 quadrants, incontinent of
		bladder and bowels. Skin warm, dry, pedal pulses palpable,
		no edema. Has stage 2 pressure ulcer on coccyx, 2 cm
		X 2 cm and approximately 2 mm deep, red granulation
		tissue at base, transparent dressing covering wound. See
		referral form for treatments. ————— Kristen Rice, RN

Patient transfer to specialty unit

Specialty units provide continuous and intensive monitoring of patients and constant and spontaneous care to persons who have limited tolerance for delay. Specialty units include perioperative units, labor and delivery units, burn units, and intensive care units.

Specialty units rely on close and continuous assessment by registered nurses as well as use of specialized equipment. Medication administration may be more complex and frequent, with medication infusions being titrated every couple of minutes, based on patient response. Vital signs may be measured frequently and certain procedures may be performed at the bedside.

Essential documentation

Record the date and time of the transfer, the name of the practitioner who ordered the transfer, and the name of the unit receiving the patient. Describe the patient's condition at the time of the transfer, including vital signs, condition of wounds, and locations of tubes or medical devices still in place. Record significant events that led to the need for the transfer. Chart that you gave the report to the receiving unit and include the name of the nurse who received the report. Note how the patient was transported to the specialty unit and who accompanied him. Document notification of family regarding the transfer. Document any patient teaching regarding the need for transfer to a specialty unit and the patient's understanding.

3/24/08	1430	Pt. being transferred from medical unit to MICU by
		stretcher accompanied by her daughter and medical
		resident. Report given to Sue Riff, RN. Advance
		directives in chart. Pt. unresponsive to verbal stimuli,
		opens eyes to painful stimuli. Prior to this episode,
		daughter reports pt. was alert and oriented to person
		but not always to place and time. Pt. is severely dehydrated
		despite 2000 ml over last 24 hr. Currently NPO. I.V.
		infusion with 18G catheter in ® antecubital vein with 0.45% NSS
		at 75 ml/hr. AP 124 irregular, BP 84/palp, RR 28, rectal T
		100.0° F, weight 78 lb., height 64". Allergies to molds, pollen,
		and mildew. Lungs clear on auscultation. S₁, S₂ heart sounds.
		Skin intact, pale, cool, poor skin turgor. Radial pulses weak,
		pedal pulses not palpable. Foley catheter in place draining
		approx. 30 ml/hr. Dr.'s orders written. ——— Diana Starr, RN

Patient's belongings, at admission

When a patient is admitted to a facility, encourage him to send home his money, jewelry, and other valuable belongings. If a patient refuses to do so, make a list of his possessions and store them according to your facility's policy.

Place valuable items in an envelope and other personal belongings in approved containers; then label them with the patient's identification number. Never use garbage containers, laundry bags, or other unauthorized receptacles for valuables because they could be discarded accidentally.

If the patient brings his medications to the facility and can't send them home, label them and send them to the pharmacy until the patient is discharged.

Essential documentation

Make a list of the patient's valuables and include a description of each one. Most facilities provide an area on the nursing admission form to list the belongings. To protect yourself and your employer, ask the patient (or a responsible family member) to sign or witness the list that you compile so that you both understand the items for which you're responsible.

Use objective language to describe each item, noting its color, approximate size, style, type, and serial number or other distinguishing features. Don't assess the item's value or authenticity. For example, you might describe a diamond ring as a "clear, round stone set in a yellow metal band."

Besides jewelry and money, include dentures, eyeglasses or contact lenses, hearing aids, prostheses, electronic devices, and clothing on the list. If the patient insists on keeping any valuable belongings at the bedside, be sure to chart this information. Also chart whether the patient decides to send home belongings with the family at a later time.

Document any valuables given to security and medications sent to the pharmacy.

3/9/08	1500	Pt. admitted to room 318 with one pair of brown glasses, upper and lower dentures, a yellow metal ring with a red stone on 4th ⓛ finger, a pink bathrobe, and a black radio.
		—————————————————————— Paul Cullen, RN

Patient's condition, change in

One of your major responsibilities is to document any change in a patient's condition. You'll also need to record the date, time, name of the practitioner you notified, and the practitioner's response. If a patient's care subsequently comes into question, unless you properly documented your conversation, the practitioner could claim that he wasn't notified.

Nurses commonly write, "Notified practitioner of patient's condition." This statement is too vague. In the event of a malpractice suit, it allows the plaintiff's lawyer (and the practitioner) to imply that you didn't communicate the essential data. The chart should include exactly what you told the practitioner. (See *Documenting a change in the patient's condition.*)

If the practitioner doesn't respond appropriately to the change in condition, notify the charge nurse and nursing supervisor to activate the chain of command, per facility policy.

Essential documentation

Your note should include the date and time that you notified the practitioner, the practitioner's name, and what you reported. Record the practitioner's response and orders given. If no orders are given, document that also. If the practitioner doesn't respond to the situation in an appropriate manner, initiate the chain of command and document who

Documenting a change in the patient's condition

To ensure clear documentation regarding a patient's care communicated to practitioner on the phone, remember to keep the following points in mind:

- Document the practitioner's full name.
- Include the exact time you contacted the practitioner. If you don't note the time you called, allegations may be made later that you failed to obtain timely medical treatment for the patient.
- Always note in the chart the specific change, problem, or result you reported to the practitioner, along with any orders or response. Use his own words, if possible.
- If you're reporting a critical laboratory test result (for example, a serum potassium level of 3.2 mEq/L) but don't receive an order for intervention (such as potassium replacement therapy), be sure to verify with the practitioner that he doesn't want to give an order. Then document this fact in the progress notes. For example, you would write "Dr. Raymond Jones informed of potassium level of 3.2 mEq/L. No orders received."
- If you think a practitioner's failure to order an intervention puts your patient's health at risk, follow the chain of command and notify your supervisor. Then be sure to document your actions and their outcomes.

was notified, such as the charge nurse, nursing supervisor, and appropriate chief practitioner, and the response. Complete an incident report per facility policy.

3/29/08	0900	Pt. had moderate-sized, soft, dark brown stools with red streaks, positive for blood by guaiac test. Abdomen soft, nontender, positive bowel sounds heard in all 4 quadrants. Skin warm, pink, capillary refill less than 3 sec. HR 92, BP 128/68, RR 28, oral T 97.2° F. Dr. Paul Rodriguez notified at 0915. Hemoglobin and hematocrit ordered stat. ———————————————————— Jackie Paterno, RN

Peripherally inserted central catheter site care

After inserting a peripherally inserted central catheter, proper site care and dressing changes are vital to preventing infection. Follow your facility's policy for the procedure and frequency of site care. Keep in mind, though, that a dressing should be changed any time it becomes wet or soiled or loses its integrity.

After the initial insertion, apply a new, sterile, transparent semipermeable dressing without using gauze because gauze may hold moisture, promoting bacterial growth and skin maceration. Thereafter, change the dressing every 3 to 7 days, according to your facility's policy, or as needed.

Assess the catheter insertion site through the transparent semipermeable dressing every shift or per your facility's policy. Look at the catheter and cannula pathway, and check for bleeding, redness, drainage, and swelling. Question the patient about pain at the site.

Essential documentation

Record the date and time of site care in your nurse's notes as well as on the dressing. Describe the condition of the site, noting any bleeding, redness, drainage, or swelling. Document pain or discomfort reported by the patient. Note the name of the practitioner notified of complications, the time of notification, orders given, your interventions, and the patient's response. Record how the site was cleaned and the type of dressing applied. Chart the patient's tolerance of the procedure, any patient teaching, and the patient's understanding of the procedure.

1/31/08	1100	Explained dressing change and site care for PICC to
		pt. Pt. verbalized understanding. Old dressing removed,
		no redness, bleeding, drainage, or swelling. No c/o pain at
		site. Using sterile technique, site cleaned with chlorhexidine.
		Sterile, transparent, semipermeable dressing applied and
		tubing secured to edge of dressing with tape. Instructed
		pt. to report pain or discomfort at insertion site or in Ⓛ
		arm to nurse. ———————————— Lillian Mott, RN

Peritoneal dialysis

Peritoneal dialysis is indicated for patients with chronic renal failure who have cardiovascular instability, vascular access problems that prevent hemodialysis, fluid overload, or electrolyte imbalances. In this procedure, dialysate—the solution instilled into the peritoneal cavity by a catheter—draws waste products, excess fluid, and electrolytes from the blood across the semipermeable peritoneal membrane. After a prescribed period, the dialysate is drained from the peritoneal cavity, removing impurities with it. The dialysis procedure is then repeated, using a new dialysate each time until waste removal is complete and fluid, electrolyte, and acid-base balances have been restored. Peritoneal dialysis may be performed manually or by using an automatic or semi-automatic cycle machine.

Essential documentation

Record the date and time of dialysis. During and after dialysis, monitor and document the patient's response to treatment. Record his baseline vital signs and weight. Document vital signs every 10 to 15 minutes for the first 1 to 2 hours of exchanges and then every 2 to 4 hours or as often as necessary, or per facility policy. If you detect any abrupt changes in the patient's condition, document them, notify the practitioner, and document your notification.

Record the amount of dialysate infused and drained, and record any medications added. Be sure to complete a peritoneal dialysis flowchart every shift. Keep a record of the effluent's characteristics, such as color, clarity, and odor, and the assessed negative or positive fluid balance at the end of each infusion-dwell-drain cycle. Also, record each time you notify the practitioner of an abnormality.

Chart the patient's weight (immediately after the drain phase) and abdominal girth when the treatment ends. Note the time of day and variations in the weighing-measuring technique. In addition, document physical assessment findings and fluid status daily.

Keep a record of equipment problems, such as mechanical malfunction, and your interventions. Also, note the condition of the patient's skin at the dialysis catheter site, the patient's reports of unusual discomfort or pain, and your interventions.

1/15/08	0700	Pt. receiving peritoneal exchanges q2hr of 1500 ml 4.25
		dialysate with 500 units heparin and 2 mEq KCL. Dialysate
		infused over 15 min. Dwell time 75 min. Drain time 30 min.
		Drainage clear, pale-yellow fluid. Weight 135 lb, abdominal
		girth 40" after drain phase. Lungs clear on auscultation,
		normal heart sounds, mucous membranes moist, no skin
		tenting when pinched. VSS (See flow sheets for fluid
		balance and frequent VS assessments.) No c/o abdominal
		cramping or discomfort. Skin warm, dry at RLQ catheter
		site, no redness or drainage. Dry split 4" X 4" dressing
		applied after site cleaned per protocol. — Liz Schaeffer, RN

Photographing or videotaping patient

Each patient is entitled to privacy and may not be photographed or videotaped without his informed consent. Using a photograph or videotape of a patient without his written consent violates his right to privacy and may lead to legal action against the health care facility. Before you allow anyone to photograph or videotape your patient, make sure the person has your facility's authorization as well as the patient's. Follow your facility's policy for photographing or videotaping a patient. If your facility doesn't have a policy or if you have questions, contact your nursing supervisor or risk manager. Commonly, the public affairs office handles consent for photographing or videotaping a patient.

Photographs and videotapes are frequently used in publications and for the purpose of educating health care workers. Before signing the consent form, the patient must be fully informed as to why the photograph or videotape is being taken as well as how, when, and where the photograph or videotape will be used. Patients should be advised against signing consents that speak to disguising their identity because there's always the possibility that recognition may occur.

Essential documentation

Most health care facilities use a consent form that includes the patient's name, address, and telephone number; the name of the person requesting permission for the photographs or videotapes; and the manner in which the photographs or videotapes will be used. The person signing must be of legal age, competent, and not taking any mind-altering drugs. One copy of the signed consent form should be given to the patient, and a second copy should be placed in the patient's medical record. The person requesting permission to photograph or videotape should also receive a copy of the consent.

A notation should be made in the patient's record regarding the date and time that the request was signed, the person's name who made the request, and the patient's response.

See *Consent to photograph or videotape* for documenting a request to photograph or videotape your patient.

Consent to photograph or videotape

A form such as the sample below can be used to obtain consent to videotape or photograph a patient.

CONSENT TO PHOTOGRAPH OR VIDEOTAPE

I, _____ *Barry Arnold* _____ , consent to have my surgical procedure
        (patient's name)
*coronary artery bypass* videotaped and photographed by _____
  (name of the procedure)   (Person/facility requesting permission)
for the purpose of educating nursing or medical students. I understand that the photographs or videotape will be used in nursing and medical publications.

Barry Arnold _____   _____   *3/21/08*
Patient signature   Patient address   Patient phone number   Date

Angela Steiner   *3/21/08*
Witness signature   Date

02/10/08	*1800*	*Pt.'s wife requested to photograph pt. for legal purposes*
		after a motor vehicle crash. Consent form completed. Dr.
		Larry Judson notified @ 1900. M. Riley, nurse-manager
		also aware. Photos taken by wife @ 1930. —— L. Lawson, RN

Physician notification

Reports you need to communicate to the practitioner include changes in the patient's condition, laboratory and other test results, and patient concerns. If a patient's care comes into question, the practitioner could claim that he wasn't notified; that's why proper documentation of your conversation is essential.

Nurses commonly write, "Notified practitioner of lab results." This statement is too vague. In the event of a malpractice suit, it allows the plaintiff's lawyer (and the practitioner) to imply that you didn't communicate reports to the practitioner. If you're unable to get in touch with the physician after reasonable attempts, document the times and number of attempts. Follow facility policy for activating the chain of command. Notify the charge nurse and nursing supervisor for assistance with this procedure.

Essential documentation

Your note should include the date and time you notified the practitioner, the means you used to communicate (such as telephone or fax), the practitioner's name, and what you reported. If you left a message for the practitioner or gave a result to someone else, such as an office nurse, record that person's name as well. Record the practitioner's response and any orders given. If no orders are given, document that as well. If multiple attempts to notify the practitioner were unsuccessful, document the times the attempts were made, if the chain of command was initiated, and the outcome of these actions. Complete an incident report per facility policy.

1/13/08	2215	Called Dr. Derrick Spencer at 2200 to report increased serous drainage from pt.'s ⓇL chest tube. Dr. Spencer's order was to observe the drainage for 1 more hr and then call him back. ——————————— Danielle Bergeron, RN

Police custody of patient

A prisoner in police custody may be admitted for medical or surgical treatment or involuntarily for psychiatric assessment and care. Follow your facility's policy for caring for a patient in police custody. Safety considerations include removal of objects that the patient could use to harm himself or others.

The accompanying police officer isn't permitted to make decisions regarding the patient's medical care and treatment. The patient is afforded the rights of confidentiality, informed consent, refusal of treatment, and review of documents that describe his condition and care. All care must be delivered without discrimination against the patient. The nurse serves as the patient's advocate, protecting his rights to health care as she would the rights of any other patient. As the patient advocate, the nurse must protect him from physical, spiritual, or mental harm. The patient in police custody, if determined competent, also has the right to make his treatment decisions and such decisions must be respected. (See *When a prisoner refuses treatment.*)

LEGAL LOOKOUT

When a prisoner refuses treatment

Several courts have stated that individuals have a constitutional right to privacy based on a high regard for human dignity and self-determination. That means any competent adult may refuse medical care, even lifesaving treatments. A suspected criminal may refuse unwarranted bodily invasions. However, an arrested suspect or convicted criminal doesn't have the same right to refuse lifesaving measures. In *Commissioner of Correction v. Myers (1979)*, a prisoner with renal failure refused hemodialysis unless he was moved to a minimum security prison. The court disagreed, saying that although the defendant's imprisonment didn't divest him of his right to privacy or his interest in maintaining his bodily integrity, it did impose limitations on those constitutional rights.

As a practical matter, any time a patient refuses lifesaving treatments, inform your facility's administration. In the case of a suspect or prisoner, notify law enforcement authorities as well.

If blood, urine, or other specimens are collected, make sure they aren't left unattended. Follow your facility's guidelines for using a chain of custody form. The form should serve as an uninterrupted log of the whereabouts of the evidence.

Essential documentation

Documentation of care should be equivalent to that provided for any patient. Special attention is required for documentation related to the presence of the police officer and visitors.

Be especially careful and precise in documenting medical and nursing procedures when you care for a suspected criminal. Document that the patient's rights were protected. Note any blood work that was done, and list all treatments and the patient's responses to them.

If you turn over anything to police or administration, record what it is and the name of the person receiving it. Record a suspect's statements that are directly related to his care, such as "I think I was shot in the leg by a cop."

When the patient is discharged, document all specific instructions given for follow-up care. Such documentation may be critical, especially if the patient claims he was mistreated. Give a copy of the discharge instructions to the police officer.

4/2/08	0800	Pt. admitted to ED at 0730 with head laceration from
		MVA accompanied by San Antonio police officer B. Starr,
		badge #4532. Pt. placed in private exam room with officer
		in attendance at all times. Pt. A & O X 3. Speech clear and
		coherent. PERRLA. Lungs clear on auscultation, normal heart
		sounds, all peripheral pulses palpable. HR 82, BP 138/74,
		RR 18 and unlabored, oral T 97.7° F. MAE X 4, no deformities
		noted. No c/o nausea, vomiting, dizziness, diplopia, pain,
		except for sore forehead. Dr. Peter Lawson in to see pt
		at 0740. Cleaned head wound and applied sterile 4" X 4"
		dressing to 2-cm cut on Ⓡ side of forehead. Orders
		written for pt. discharge. Explained wound care to pt. and
		police officer, s/s to report to doctor. Written instructions
		for wound care and head injury given to pt. and police
		officer. Both pt. and police officer verbalized understanding
		of instructions. ——————————————— Joshua Jones, RN

Postoperative care

After surgery, when your patient recovers sufficiently from the effects of anesthesia, he can be transferred from the postanesthesia care unit (PACU) to his assigned unit for ongoing recovery and care. Your documentation should reflect your frequent assessments and interventions.

Essential documentation

Record the date and time of each entry. Avoid block charting. The frequency of your assessments depends on your facility's policy, practitioner's orders, and your patient's condition. Compare your assessments to preoperative and PACU assessments. Your documentation should include:

■ time the patient returned to your nursing unit and in what manner (stretcher, wheelchair)
■ assessment of airway and breathing, including breath sounds, positioning to maintain a patent airway, use of oxygen, and respiratory rate, rhythm, and depth
■ vital signs and pulse oximetry
■ neurologic assessment, including level of consciousness
■ pain assessment, including the use of 0 to 10 rating scale, need for analgesics and patient's response, and use of other comfort measures
■ wound assessment, including the appearance of dressing, drainage, bleeding, and skin around site, if possible (Note the presence of drainage tubes and amount, type, color, and consistency of drainage; chart the type and amount of suction, if applicable.)

- cardiovascular assessment, including heart rate and rhythm, peripheral pulses, skin color, and temperature
- renal assessment, including urine output, patency of catheter, and bladder distention
- GI assessment, including bowel sounds, presence and condition of nasogastric tube, abdominal distention, and nausea or vomiting
- safety measures, such as placement of call bell within reach, bed in low position, proper positioning, and use of side rails
- fluid management, including intake and output, type and size of I.V. catheter, location of I.V. line, I.V. solution, flow rate, and condition of I.V. site
- use of antiembolism stockings, sequential compression device, early ambulation, and prophylactic anticoagulants
- patient education and understanding, such as turning and positioning, coughing and deep breathing, incentive spirometry, splinting the incision, pain control, and the importance of early ambulation
- emotional support provided.

Document drugs given—the dosage, frequency, and route—and the patient's response. Record the name of the practitioner whom you notified of changes in the patient's condition, the time of notification, orders given, your actions, and the patient's responses. Use flow sheets to record your frequent assessments of vital signs, intake and output, I.V. therapy, and laboratory values.

| 1/8/08 | 1100 | Pt. returned from PACU at 1030 S/P laparoscopic laser cholecystectomy. HR 88 and regular, BP 112/82, RR 18, tympanic T 98.2° F. Breath sounds clear on auscultation, skin pink and warm, capillary refill less than 3 sec. Sleeping but easily arousable and oriented to time, place, and person. Speech clear and coherent. PERRLA. S₁S₂ heart sounds, strong radial and dorsalis pedis pulses bilaterally. Bladder nondistended, denies urge to void, normal bowel sounds in all 4 quadrants. Abdomen slightly distended, no c/o nausea. Has 4 abdominal puncture wounds covered with 4" X 4" gauze. Dressings without blood or drainage. Pt. c/o of abdominal discomfort 3/10, refusing analgesics at this time. Pt. placed in semi-Fowler's position, bed in low position, call bell within reach and pt. verbalized understanding of its use. I.V. of 1000 ml D₅/0.45 NS infusing at 75 ml/hr in Ⓡ forearm via infusion pump. See flow sheets for frequent VS, I.V. therapy, and I/O. Explained coughing and deep-breathing exercises to pt. and showed how to splint abdomen with pillow when coughing. Pt. able to give return demo. Told her to call if she feels she needs pain medication. ———————— *Christina Gault, RN* |

Preoperative care

Effective nursing documentation during the preoperative period focuses on two primary elements—the baseline preoperative assessment and patient teaching. Documenting these elements enhances communication among caregivers. Most facilities use a preoperative checklist to verify that a consent form has been signed, the required data have been collected and are available on the chart, and prescribed procedures and safety precautions have been executed. Preoperative teaching and patient understanding may need to be charted on a teaching plan form or in your nurse's notes.

Essential documentation

To use the preoperative checklist, place a check mark and initials in the appropriate column to indicate that a procedure has been performed (for example, checking that the patient is wearing an identification band or that the informed consent form has been signed). If an item doesn't apply to your patient, write "N/A," indicating that the item isn't applicable (such as the use of antiembolism stockings in a patient undergoing a minor surgical procedure). Make sure your full name, credentials, and initials appear on the form. Chart the patient's baseline vital signs on the form. Before the patient leaves for surgery, check the appropriate boxes to indicate that the patient has been properly and positively identified.

Be sure to document the time, date, and name of the person you notified of abnormalities that could affect the patient's response to the surgical procedure or deviations from facility standards.

See *Preoperative checklist and surgical identification form* for an example of preoperative documentation.

11/07/08	0730	Pt. for OR @ 0800. Preoperative checklist complete. Signed
		consent on chart. Pt. anxious; reassurance provided. Preoperative
		teaching on coughing, deep breathing, and use of incentive
		spirometry reinforced. Pt. states understanding. All questions
		answered. Pt. to be transported in bed by OR tech. ————
		———————————————————— F. May, RN

Preoperative checklist and surgical identification form

To document preoperative procedures, data collection, and teaching, most facilities use a checklist such as the one below.

Woodview
Hospital

**Pre-Operative Checklist
and Surgical Identification Form**

Instructions: All items checked "No" requires follow up. Follow up is to be documented. In "Additional Information / Comment" section until resolved.

Date: 3/28/08

Patient name: Zachary, Timothy

Medical record number: 987654

Pre-Op Checklist	Yes	No	Resolved	Initials
ID Band On	✓			NRC
Allergies Noted / Bracelet	✓			NRC
History & Physical (Present & Reviewed)	✓			NRC
Surgical Informed Consent Signed	✓			NRC
Anesthesia Informed Consent	✓			NRC
Pre-Op Teaching	✓			NRC
Prep. as Ordered	N/A			
NPO After Midnight	✓			NRC
Dentures, Capped Teeth, Cosmetics, Glasses, Contact Lenses, Wig Removed	N/A	✓		
Voided/Catheter Inserted	✓			NRC
Medical Clearance/Physician's Name	✓			NRC
TEDS, as Ordered	N/A			
SCD, as Ordered	N/A			
PCA Teaching, as Ordered	✓			NRC
Type & Cross/Screen Drawn (If Ordered)	N/A			
Must Have Blood Informed Consent Signed)				
**Blood Informed Consent Signed				
*Lab Results on Chart	✓			NRC
*ECG on Chart	✓			NRC
*Chest X-ray on Chart	✓			NRC

*Abnormal Results Reported To H&H Dr. Schoblitz
Time & Date 3/28/08 0800
Reported By NRC

Temp. 98.6° Pulse 84 Resp. 18 B/P 132/82

Valuables

Destination: ☐ To Safe ☐ To Family, Name _____

✗ Norma R. Clay, RN   NRC
Signature of Nurse   Initials

✗ _____
Signature of Transferring RN   Date   Time

Additional Information /Comments

Surgical Patient Identification Form

Nursing Floor RN Patient Identification

☑ Patient I.D. Bracelet Personally Observed
☑ Patient Questioned Verbally Regarding I.D., Procedure & Site
☑ Patient's Chart Reviewed to Verify I.D., Procedure & Site

✗ Norma R. Clay, RN   3/28/08   0800
R.N.'s Signature   Date   Time

Pre-Op Anesthesia Patient Identification

☐ Patient's I.D. Bracelet Personally Observed
☐ Patient Questioned Verbally Regarding I.D., Procedure & Site
☐ Patient's Chart Reviewed to Verify I.D., Procedure & Site

✗ _____
Anesthesiologist/Anesthetist's Signature   Date   Time

Operating Room and Anesthesia Personnel Patient Identification

Operative Procedure & Site: _____

ANES	CIRC Nurse	
☐	☐	Patient I.D. Bracelet Personally Observed
☐	☐	Patient Questioned Verbally Regarding I.D., Procedure & Site
☐	☐	Patient's Chart Reviewed to Verify I.D., Procedure & Site
☐	☐	Surgical Site Confirmed

✗ _____
Anesthesiologist/Anesthetist's Signature   Time

✗ _____
CIRC Nurse's Signature   Time

Surgeon's Patient Identification Statement

☐ Patient I.D. Bracelet Personally Observed
☐ Patient Questioned Verbally Regarding I.D., Procedure & Site
☐ Surgical Site Marked

✗ _____
Surgeon's Signature   Time

Pressure ulcer assessment

Pressure ulcers develop when pressure impairs circulation, depriving tissues of oxygen and life-sustaining nutrients. This process damages skin and underlying structures. The pressure may be of short duration with great force, or it may have been present for a longer period of time with lesser force.

Most pressure ulcers develop over bony prominences where friction and shearing force combine with pressure to break down skin and underlying tissue. Common sites include the sacrum, coccyx, ischial tuberosities, and greater trochanters. In bedridden and relatively immobile patients, pressure ulcers develop over the vertebrae, scapulae, elbows, knees, and heels. Untreated pressure ulcers may lead to serious systemic infection.

To select the most effective treatment plan for pressure ulcers, the nurse first assesses the pressure ulcer and stages it based on the guidelines of the National Pressure Ulcer Advisory Panel and the Agency for Healthcare Research and Quality.

In addition to assessing the pressure ulcer, perform an assessment to determine the patient's risk of developing pressure ulcers. The Braden scale is one of the most reliable instruments. The Braden scale assesses sensory perception, moisture, activity, mobility, nutrition, and friction and shear. The lower the score, the greater the risk. (See *Braden Scale for predicting pressure sore risk,* pages 334 and 335.)

Documentation of pressure ulcer assessments assists the nurse in detecting changes in a patient's skin condition, determining the response to treatment, identifying at-risk patients, and reducing the incidence of pressure ulcers through early independent interventions and treatment.

Essential documentation

Documentation of your pressure ulcer assessment should include the patient's history and risk factors leading to the formation of a pressure ulcer, using a tool such as the Braden scale. If the patient has or develops a pressure ulcer, in your note, describe the pressure ulcer, including its location, size and depth (in centimeters), stage, color, and appearance; presence of necrotic or granulation tissue, drainage, and odor; length of any undermining; and condition of the surrounding tissue. A photo of the wound should be obtained as soon as the pressure ulcer is discovered. Assess the pressure ulcer with each dressing change or at least weekly for the patient at home. Obtain another photo of the pressure ulcer when the patient is discharged.

1/18/08	1100	Pt. admitted to 6 South from Green Brier Nursing Home. Pt. has stage 2 pressure ulcer on coccyx, approx. 2 cm X 1 cm X 0.5 cm. No drainage noted. Base has deep pink granulation tissue. Skin surrounding ulcer pink, intact, well-defined edges. Irrigated ulcer with NSS. Skin around ulcer dried and ulcer covered with transparent dressing. Braden score 14 (see Braden Pressure Ulcer Risk Assessment Scale). Photo placed on chart ———————————————————————— Joan Norris, RN

Pulse oximetry

Pulse oximetry is a noninvasive procedure used to monitor a patient's arterial blood oxygen saturation (SpO_2). It's a significant tool in identifying respiratory failure and initiating measures to improve oxygenation.

A sensor containing two light-emitting diodes (LEDs)—one red and one infrared—and a photodetector placed opposite these LEDs across a vascular bed are attached to the skin with adhesive or clips. The sensor is placed across a pulsating arteriolar bed, such as a finger, toe, nose, or earlobe. Selected wavelengths of light are absorbed by hemoglobin and transmitted through tissue to the photodetector. The pulse oximeter computes SpO_2 based on the relative amounts of light that reach the photodetector. The normal value is between 95% and 100%. Pulse oximetry may be performed intermittently or continuously.

Essential documentation

Record the date and time of pulse oximetry readings. Frequent SpO_2 readings may be documented on a flow sheet. Document the reason for use of pulse oximetry and whether readings are continuous or intermittent. If SpO_2 readings are continuous, record the alarm setting and readings with each vital sign check and when significant changes occur. If the patient is receiving oxygen, record the concentration and mode of delivery. Describe events precipitating acute oxygen desaturation, your actions, and the patient's response. Record activities or

(Text continues on page 336.)

Braden Scale for predicting pressure sore risk

The Braden scale, shown below, is the most reliable of several instruments for assessing the older patient's risk of developing pressure ulcers. The lower the score, the greater the risk.

Patient's name ___Kevin Lawson___   Medical record # ___654321___

SENSORY PERCEPTION Ability to respond meaningfully to pressure-related discomfort	I. Completely limited: Is unresponsive (doesn't moan, flinch, or grasp in response) to painful stimuli because of diminished level of consciousness or sedation OR Has a limited ability to feel pain over most of body surface	2. Very limited: Responds only to painful stimuli; can't communicate discomfort except through moaning or restlessness OR Has a sensory impairment that limits ability to feel pain or discomfort over half of body
MOISTURE Degree to which skin is exposed to moisture	I. Constantly moist: Skin kept moist almost constantly by perspiration, urine, or other fluids; dampness detected every time patient is moved or turned	2. Very moist: Skin often but not always moist; linen must be changed at least once per shift
ACTIVITY Degree of physical activity	I. Bedridden: Confined to bed	2. Chairfast: Ability to walk severely limited or nonexistent; can't bear own weight and must be assisted into chair or wheelchair
MOBILITY Ability to change and control body position	I. Completely immobile: Doesn't make even slight changes in body or extremity position without assistance	2. Very limited: Makes occasional slight changes in body or extremity position but is unable to make frequent or significant changes independently
NUTRITION Is NPO or maintained on clear liquids or I.V. fluids for more than 5 days	I. Very poor: Never eats a complete meal; rarely eats more than one-third of any food offered; eats two servings or less of protein (meat or dairy products) per day; takes fluids poorly; doesn't take a liquid dietary supplement OR Is NPO or maintained on clear liquids or I.V. fluids for more than 5 days	2. Probably inadequate: Rarely eats a complete meal and generally eats only about half of any food offered; protein intake includes only three servings of meat or dairy products per day; occasionally will take a dietary supplement OR Receives less than optimum amount of liquid diet or tube feeding
FRICTION AND SHEAR Ability to assist with movement or to be moved in a way that prevents skin contact with bedding or other surface	I. Problem: Requires moderate to maximum assistance in moving; complete lifting without sliding against sheets is impossible; frequently slides down in bed or chair, requiring frequent repositioning with maximum assistance; spasticity, contractures, or agitation leads to almost constant friction	2. Potential problem: Moves feebly or requires minimum assistance during a move; skin probably slides to some extent against sheets, chair restraints, or other devices; maintains relatively good position in chair or bed most of the time but occasionally slides down

Evaluator's name   _Joan Norris, RN_

		DATE OF ASSESSMENT	3/21/08		
3. Slightly limited: Responds to verbal commands but can't always communicate discomfort or need to be turned	4. No impairment: Responds to verbal commands; has no sensory deficit that would limit ability to feel or voice pain or discomfort		3		
3. Occasionally moist: Skin occasionally moist, requiring an extra linen change approximately once per day	4. Rarely moist: Skin usually dry; linen only requires changing at routine intervals		3		
3. Walks occasionally: Walks occasionally during day, but for very short distances, with or without assistance; spends majority of each shift in bed or chair	4. Walks frequently: Walks outside room at least twice per day and inside room at least once every 2 hours during waking hours		2		
3. Slightly limited: Makes frequent though slight changes in body or extremity position independently	4. No limitations: Makes major and frequent changes in body or extremity position without assistance		2		
3. Adequate: Eats more than half of most meals; eats four servings of protein (meat and dairy products) per day; occasionally refuses a meal but will usually take a supplement if offered OR Is on a tube feeding or total parenteral nutrition regimen that probably meets most nutritional needs	4. Excellent: Eats most of every meal and never refuses a meal; usually eats four or more servings of meat and dairy products per day; occasionally eats between meals; doesn't require supplementation		2		
3. No apparent problem: Moves in bed and in chair independently and has sufficient muscle strength to lift up completely during move; maintains good position in bed or chair at all times			2		
		Total	14		

interventions affecting SpO_2 values. Document patient teaching and understanding related to pulse oximetry.

3/13/08	1100	At 1040 pt. gasping and SOB. HR 128, BP 140/96, RR 34, tympanic T 97.3° F. Having difficulty speaking. O_2 NC resting on bedside table. Wife states, "He took it off because it hurts his ears." Pulse oximetry 86%. NC reapplied at 6 L/min. Pt. less dyspneic, able to speak in sentences. HR 100, BP 136/90, RR 26. Pulse oximetry 93%. Pt. and wife instructed to leave NC in place in nostrils. Tubing padded around earpieces for comfort. Pt. instructed to call the nurse if tubing becomes uncomfortable rather than removing it. Pt. and wife verbalized understanding of the need for O_2 and oximetry monitoring. —————— *Terry Delmonico, RN*

Q

Quality of care, family questions about

At times, the family of a patient may have questions about the quality of care that a family member is receiving. These concerns should be taken seriously—don't argue with the family, and avoid defending yourself, a coworker, the practitioner, or the facility.

When family members question the quality of care, show that you're concerned and ask them to clarify what they believe to be the problem. Provide education about nursing routines, policies, procedures, and within the limits of confidentiality, the patient's care plan. The Joint Commission standards state that the patient must be informed of the conflict resolution process of the facility. Report conflicts or unresolved issues to the practitioner, charge nurse, nurse manager, nursing supervisor, risk manager, or another appropriate person who may assist with resolving the problem. Have the appropriate person speak with the family to help obtain resolution of any concerns or problems.

Essential documentation

Record the date and time of your initial conversation. Include the names of the family members present. Document the concerns using their own words, in quotes, if possible. Describe your answers and the family members' responses. Record the names of the people you notified of the family's concerns, including the practitioner, charge nurse,

nurse manager, nursing supervisor, and risk manager, and the time of notification. Document your conversation and their responses, in quotes. Document any resolution that occurs or follow-up that remains.

3/22/08	1600	Pt.'s daughter, Emily Jones, verbalized concerns regarding
		mother's hygiene. She stated,"I don't think my mother is
		receiving her showers. Her hair and fingernails are dirty."
		After reviewing the shower schedule, explained to Mrs. Jones
		that her mother has been refusing 1 of her 2 scheduled
		showers each week since admission 2 weeks ago and has been
		receiving sponge baths instead. Nurses' notes indicate that
		resident stated,"I've never taken more than 1 shower per
		week in my entire life and I don't intend to start now."
		Records also show that for the last 2 days resident has been
		participating in planting flower boxes around the facility.
		Mrs. Jones spoke with her mother and reported that her
		mother will continue to shower once per week, sponge bathe
		on a daily basis, and have an appointment at the facility
		beauty salon once per week. Care plan amended to reflect
		this. —————————————————————— Liz Mazerka, RN

R

Request for patient information from media

You have a professional and ethical responsibility to protect your patient's privacy. The American Nurses Association's Code for Nurses states that you must safeguard the patient's right to privacy "by judiciously protecting information of a confidential nature." Moreover, the American Hospital Association's Patient's Bill of Rights upholds a patient's right to privacy. This means that you may not disclose any medical or personal information about the patient to anyone, including the media. Also, the Health Insurance Portability and Accountability Act provides safeguards against the inappropriate use and release of personal medical information. Violations of protecting privacy can result in fines. If medical information is released, it's done with the approval of the patient. In certain instances, the public feels it has the right to this information. (See *The public's right to know,* page 340.) If you become involved in a media situation, notify the nurse manager, nursing supervisor, risk manager, or public relations liaison for assistance. If the media become a problem on your unit, notify security for assistance in escorting them from the building.

Essential documentation

If the media arrive on your unit requesting information on a patient, record the date and time, the name of the individuals and their organizations, and the information requested. Document the outcome of the

LEGAL LOOKOUT

The public's right to know

The newsworthiness of an event or person can make some disclosure acceptable. For example, newspapers routinely publish the findings of the president's annual physical examination in response to the public's demand for information.

Other events for which the public's right to know may outweigh the patient's right to privacy include breakthroughs in medical technology (the first successful hand transplant) and product tampering cases, for example. In 1999, the national media gave wide exposure to an incident in New York state in which nine people died from St. Louis encephalitis transmitted by mosquito bites.

situation. Document who was notified about the situation, being sure to include names and titles. If the media call your unit about a patient, document the date and time of the call, their names and organizations, and the outcome of the call. Complete an incident report per facility policy.

| 1/13/08 | 1745 | *Post Tribune reporter James Smith, appeared at the nurse's station at 1730 requesting information about pt. Told Mr. Smith that no information could be given out about any pt., to contact the hospital's public affairs office in the morning, and to please leave the hospital immediately. Mr. Smith refused to leave. Security called at 1735. Security officer, Steven Tully, arrived on unit at 1737 and escorted Mr. Smith off the unit. Nursing supervisor, Betty Blakemore, RN, notified of incident at 1740. ———————— Catherine Watts, R.N* |
| | | |

Respiratory arrest

Respiratory arrest is defined as the absence of adequate respirations. If a patient is found without adequate respirations, rapid intervention is critical because brain death occurs within 4 minutes after respirations cease. Immediately call for a coworker to call the code team, or use the telephone in the patient's room to call for help. After assessing the patient's airway and breathing, check for a pulse. If you detect a pulse, begin rescue breathing (using a pocket facemask) and continue until respirations return spontaneously or ventilatory support via endotracheal intubation and mechanical ventilation can be instituted.

Essential documentation

Most facilities use a special form to facilitate documentation of a code event. (For more on code sheets, see "Cardiopulmonary arrest and resuscitation," page 206.) Your charting should include the date and time that the patient was found unresponsive and without respirations, and the name of the person who found the patient. Include whether the event was witnessed. Record the name of the person who initiated cardiopulmonary resuscitation (CPR) and the time CPR was initiated, as well as the names of the other members of the code team. Make a notation in your note to "see the code sheet" for detailed information. Describe the outcome of the code. For example, did the patient resume spontaneous respirations, is he receiving mechanical ventilation, or did he die? If the patient was transferred to a specialty unit, note the time and method of transfer and who accompanied the patient. Document notification of the primary practitioner. Note whether the family was present or the time that the family was notified of the event.

1/3/08	1440	Found pt. unresponsive on floor next to his bed at 1428.
		Airway opened, no respirations noted. Code called. Ventilation
		attempt via pocket facemask unsuccessful. Head repositioned
		but still unable to deliver breath. No foreign bodies noted in
		mouth. After delivery of 3rd abdominal thrust, piece of meat
		was expelled. Pt. still without respirations; carotid pulse
		palpable. Rescue breathing initiated via facemask. Code team
		arrived at 1433 and continued resuscitative efforts. See code
		record. ———————————————— Fran Vitello, RN
	1450	Pt. resumed spontaneous respirations and opened eyes. HR
		68, BP 102/52, RR 32 unlabored. Placed on O₂ 2 L/min via
		NC. Pt. being transferred to ICU for observation. Report
		called to Peggy Wallace, RN, at 1445. Family notified of pt.'s
		condition and transfer to ICU. Dr. Martin Jones notified of
		pt. condition and transfer. ———————— Fran Vitello, RN

Restraints

Restraints are defined as any method of physically restricting a person's freedom of movement, physical activity, or normal access to his body. Restraints can cause numerous problems, including limited mobility, skin breakdown, impaired circulation, incontinence, psychological distress, and death.

There are two reasons for restraints, behavioral and medical. Behavioral restraints are initiated when the patient demonstrates harmful behavior to himself or others. Medical restraints are needed when the patient may cause harm to himself by interrupting treatment or removing devices, such as an endotracheal tube. Most facilities are striving to become restraint-free. Some policies require restraint initiation to be reviewed by more than one registered nurse in order to verify its need. It's important to know and follow your facility's policy on the use of restraints.

Time limitations have also been set on the use of restraints. Within 4 hours of placing a patient in restraints, a practitioner must give an order for restraints; however, if the need for restraints is due to a significant change in the patient's condition, the practitioner must examine the patient immediately. This order must be renewed every 24 hours.

The Joint Commission standards require continuous monitoring of the restrained patient to ensure patient safety, including monitoring the patient's vital signs, nutrition and hydration needs, circulation, and hygiene and toileting needs. The patient's family members must also be notified of the use of restraints if the patient consented to have them informed of his care. Moreover, the patient must be informed of the conditions necessary for his release from restraints.

Essential documentation

Document each episode of the use of restraints, including the date and time they were initiated. Your facility may have a special form or flow sheet for this purpose. Record the circumstances resulting in the use of restraints and alternative interventions attempted first. Describe the rationale for the specific type of restraints used. Chart the name of the practitioner who ordered the restraints. If a verbal order was given for the restraints, it must be signed within 12 hours by the ordering practitioner. Document restraint use according to facility policy. Record 15-minute assessments of the patient, including signs of injury, nutrition, hydration, circulation, range of motion, vital signs, hygiene, elimination, comfort, physical and psychological status, and readiness for removing the restraints. Record your interventions to help the patient meet the conditions for removing the restraints. Note that the patient was continuously monitored. Document any injuries or complications that occurred, the time they occurred, the name of the practitioner notified, and the results of your interventions or actions. Document patient and family teaching about restraint use.

1/13/08	0800	Pt. became agitated and extubated self @ 0630. Pulse oximetry decreased to 85%. Pt. reintubated by Dr. Matthew McHardy and placed back on ventilator on previous vent settings. Soft bilateral wrist restraints applied per order of Dr. McHardy. Pt. sedated with Ativan 1 mg I.V. ———————— K. Goodman, RN

S

Seizure management

Seizures are paroxysmal events associated with abnormal electrical discharges of neurons in the brain. Partial seizures are usually unilateral, involving a localized or focal area of the brain. Generalized seizures involve the entire brain.

When your patient has a generalized seizure, observe the seizure characteristics to help determine the area of the brain involved; administer anticonvulsants as ordered; protect him from injury; and prevent serious complications, such as aspiration and airway obstruction. When caring for a patient at risk for seizures, take precautions to prevent injury and complications in the event of a seizure.

Essential documentation

If a patient is at risk for seizures, document all precautions taken, such as padding the side rails, headboard, and footboard of the bed; keeping the bed in low position; raising side rails while the patient is in bed; placing an airway at the bedside; and having suction equipment nearby. Record that seizure precautions have been explained to the patient.

If your patient has a seizure, record the date and time it began as well as its duration and any precipitating factors. Identify any sensation that may be considered an aura. Describe involuntary behavior occurring at the onset, such as lip smacking, chewing movements, or hand and eye movements. Record any incontinence, vomiting, or salivation during the seizure. Describe where the movement began and the parts of the body involved. Note any progression or pattern to the activity. Document whether the patient's eyes deviated to one side and whether the pupils changed in size, shape, equality, or reaction to light. Note whether the patient's teeth were clenched or open.

Document the patient's response to the seizure, drugs given, complications, and interventions. Record the name of the practitioner you notified, the time of notification, and any orders given. Finally, record your assessment of the patient's postictal mental and physical status every 15 minutes for 1 hour, every 30 minutes for 1 hour, and then hourly as long as there are no further complications, or according to your facility's policy.

Document patient teaching that you provide for the patient or his family, including patient and family understanding of the teaching.

1/19/08	1730	At 1712, pt. had generalized seizure that lasted 2½ min.
		Breathing was labored during seizure, no cyanosis noted. Pt.
		sleeping at time of onset. Pt. incontinent during seizure, but
		no vomiting or salivation noted. Padded side rails, head-
		board, and footboard in place prior to seizure; bed in low
		position. Pt. placed on Ⓛ side, airway patent, breath sounds
		clear bilaterally. Dr. Peter Gordon notified of seizure at 1716
		and came to see pt. at 1720. Pt. currently sleeping, confused
		when aroused, not oriented to time or place. HR 94, BP 142/88,
		RR 18 and regular, tympanic T 97.7° F. See flow sheets for
		frequent VS and neurologic assessments, per policy. ————
		—————————————————— Gale Hartman, RN

Sexual advance by a colleague

The Equal Employment Opportunity Commission defines sexual harassment as an unwelcome sexual advance, a request for sexual favors, and other verbal, nonverbal, or physical conduct of a sexual nature. Sexual harassment is a subtle but real form of sexual abuse. (See *Myths about sexual harassment,* page 346.)

An unwanted sexual advance by a colleague should be addressed immediately. Decline the advance in a direct and honest manner. Inform the harassing individual that the attention is unwanted and unwelcome. If your colleague's behavior persists, or if the initial advance consists of sexually charged, degrading, or vulgar words or makes you a target of sexual jokes, touching, or pinching, further action should be taken.

Employers are required to act on complaints of sexual harassment. Most facilities have a policy for filing a complaint. If your facility doesn't have a policy, inform your immediate supervisor or the human

Myths about sexual harassment

Common myths about sexual harassment include:
- If women would just say "No," it would stop.
- Harassment will stop if a person just ignores it.
- If women watched the way they dress, there wouldn't be a problem with sexual harassment.
- Only women can be sexually harassed.
- Sexual harassment is no big deal — it's the natural way men and women express affection and friendship.
- Most people enjoy sexual attention at work. Teasing and flirting make work fun.
- Sexual harassment is harmless. Persons who object have no sense of humor or don't know how to accept a compliment.
- Sexual harassment policies will negatively affect friendly relationships.
- Nice people couldn't possibly be harassers.

resources department that the behavior you experienced constitutes sexual harassment, and ask how to proceed with a complaint.

The human resources department will contact the accused employee and inform him that a complaint has been filed against him. It's the responsibility of your employer to follow through according to local and federal guidelines. Confidentiality is important, and the privacy of individuals reporting or accused of sexual harassment must be protected as much as possible. A complaint may also be filed with the state Human Rights Commission or with the federal Equal Employment Opportunity Commission.

Essential documentation

States vary in the way that sexual harassment issues are addressed and resolved. The human resources department in your facility can help you with documentation that complies with local and federal law and facility policy. In general, documentation should include:
- description of the incident, including the date, time, and location
- statements made by both parties (in quotes)
- names of individuals that you informed about the incident, such as the nursing supervisor and human resources manager, and their responses

■ date, time, and location where the information was shared as well as any counseling or referral offered to you

■ names of witnesses, if any

■ names of anyone who supports your charge (other victims or witnesses).

Document each instance of harassment. Keep a copy of all the documentation at home. This will be useful if legal action is taken. Also complete an incident report per facility policy.

To: Tom Cooke, RN, Nursing Supervisor
    Martin Hillman, Director of Human Resources
From: Martha Clark, RN
      MICU
Date: 3/22/08
Time: 1320
At 1240, Dr. James Parker asked me to go with him to a movie. I refused, saying I was busy. He said, "You don't have to be such a snob." I responded by repeating that I had other plans. He then began to follow me down the hall saying loudly, "Why won't you go out with me? Come on answer me. What's the matter? Are you frigid?" I requested that he stop speaking to me in this manner and, when he persisted, I called Tom Cooke, RN, nursing supervisor, at 1245 and asked him to address the situation. J. Smith, K. Brown, P. Green, and M. Carter were in the hallway and heard this exchange. The nursing supervisor arrived on the unit at 1310 and after speaking with me, instructed Dr. Parker to stop speaking loudly to me and advised me that I should report the incident to the human resources dept. He also asked that I put the event in writing. Dr. Parker did stop his behavior and apologized to me. He said, "I'm sorry I bothered you. I won't bother you again."

Sexual advance by a patient

Several studies show that more than 50% of nurses have experienced sexual harassment on the job and more than 25% admit being victimized while on the job. Patients were the most frequent sources of sexual harassment and physical assault. Nursing, by its very nature of having to care for a patient's bodily needs, transgresses normal social rules regarding physical contact. A patient who relies on a nurse's caring attitude may exploit this. In addition, the intimacy of the nurse-patient relationship can mislead a patient into believing that a nurse might be receptive to such an advance.

The patient's motivation for making a sexual advance may be a need for friendliness or attention, a demonstration of anger, or a plea for reassurance about sexual attractiveness. In many cases, when a sexual advance by a patient occurs, the nurse will typically ignore it, pretend she hasn't heard it, or withdraw from contact with the patient. However, a better way to handle this type of behavior is to address it immediately and to be honest and direct with the patient, making a comment such as "I'm uncomfortable when you speak to me like that. Let's talk about something else." Or "I don't want you to touch me that way."

If a verbal warning isn't effective in changing the patient's behavior, inform your charge nurse, nursing supervisor, or nurse manager and have a colleague present when care is delivered. In addition, speak with the patient's practitioner about the patient's behavior. Be sure to maintain the patient's privacy and confidentiality, discussing his behavior only with caregivers who need to know.

Essential documentation

Follow your facility's policy for documenting a sexual advance by a patient. In addition to documenting the incident in the medical record, you may be required to fill out an incident report.

Record the date and time that the sexual behavior took place. Carefully document the care that the patient received as well as the inappropriate behavior. Record what the patient said, using his words in quotation marks. List staff members who witnessed the behavior. Document your response to the patient's behavior, putting your exact statements in quotes. Record the time that you notified the charge nurse, nursing supervisor, nurse manager, or practitioner, their names, and their response.

1/14/08	0900	While taking the pt.'s VS at 0830, he touched my breast and asked me to "get in here and cuddle." I stepped back from the bed and told the pt., "I'm not comfortable when you touch me like that or speak in that way. I prefer that you not do it." Pt. persisted in his remarks, and I left the room and returned at 0835 with Jan Smith, RN. Pt. made no further comments or sexual approaches. VS completed at 0840. Dr. Robert Hope and K. Smith, RN, nursing supervisor, informed at 0845 of incident. ———————— Monica Smith, RN

Skin assessment

Skin assessment begins with the admission of a patient to a facility. Because of the number of complications that can occur due to a break in skin integrity, skin assessment should be done with all direct patient care and should occur on a continuous basis throughout the patient's stay. The Braden scale is a reliable tool used to assess risk of pressure ulcer development used by many institutions to initiate additional skin care measures. (See *Braden Scale for predicting pressure sore risk,* pages 334 and 335.)

Essential documentation

Document the patient's skin condition on admission to the facility. Describe its condition, noting color, temperature, texture, tone, turgor, thickness, moisture, and integrity. If the patient is admitted with a pressure ulcer, document all information regarding the pressure ulcer and obtain a photograph and place it on the chart. (See "Pressure ulcer assessment," page 332.) If an area of the skin has changed since the last assessment, document if the practitioner was notified and any skin care performed.

| 04/04/08 | 2100 | PM care completed. ℚ heel slightly red. Lotion applied and |
| | | heels elevated with pillow. ———————————— M. Jones, RN |

Skin care

In addition to helping shape a patient's self-image, the skin performs many physiologic functions. It protects internal body structures from the environment and potential pathogens, regulates body temperature and homeostasis, and serves as an organ of sensation and excretion. As a result, meticulous skin care helps maintain skin integrity and is essential to overall health. Keeping the skin clean and dry, performing massage, and repositioning, all constitute forms of skin care and help maintain skin integrity.

Essential documentation

Record the date and time of your entry. Document your assessment of your patient's skin condition. Describe your interventions related to skin care and the patient's response. Note the time that you notified the practitioner of any changes, his name, the orders given, your actions, and the patient's response. Document repositioning of the

patient, because this is a component of skin care. Describe patient
teaching given regarding skin care and patient understanding.

2/22/08	1000	Pt. c/o itchy skin. Pt.'s skin dry and flaking, warm to touch. Skin
		tents when pinched. Lotion applied. Explained the importance
		of drinking more fluids and using lotion. Encouraged pt.
		not to scratch skin and to report intense itching to nurse.
		Dr. Harry Johnson notified at 0945 and order given for
		Benadryl 0.25 mg P.O. q 6hr prn for intense itching. ————
		———————————————————————— Jason Dickson, RN

Skin graft care

A skin graft consists of healthy tissue taken from one area on the
patient (autograft) or a donor (allograft) that's then applied to the damaged area on the patient's body. A graft resurfaces an area damaged by
burns, traumatic injury, or surgery. Care procedures for an autograft or
allograft are essentially the same. However, an autograft requires care
for two sites: the graft site and the donor site.

Successful grafting depends on various factors, including clean
wound granulation with adequate vascularization, complete contact of
the graft with the wound bed, sterile technique to prevent infection,
adequate graft immobilization, and skilled care. Depending on your
facility's policy, a practitioner or specially trained nurse may change
graft dressings.

Essential documentation

Record the date and time of each dressing change. Note the location,
size, and appearance of the graft site. Describe the condition of the
graft, and note any signs of infection or rejection. Chart the name of
the practitioner you notified, the time of notification, and any concerns or complications discussed. Record the specific care given to the
graft site, including how it was covered. Document any patient and
family teaching that you provide and evidence of their understanding.
Note the patient's reaction to the graft and emotional support that you
provided.

3/17/08	1300	Dressings removed from ® anterior thigh skin graft site.
		Site is 4 cm X 4 cm, pink, moist, and without edema or
		drainage. Area irrigated with NSS. Xeroflo placed over site
		and covered with burn gauze and a roller bandage. Pt.
		instructed not to touch dressing, to report if dressing
		becomes loose, and to avoid placing any weight on the site.
		Pt. verbalized understanding of the instructions. ————
		———————————————————————— Brian Wilcox, RN

Smoking

It's an established fact that smoking has adverse effects on health. Yet people continue to smoke—even while hospitalized. Explain your facility's smoking policy to the patient on admission, and provide him with a written set of facility rules, if available. If you find your patient smoking in a nonsmoking area, remind him of the facility's smoking policy. Ask him to extinguish his smoking materials and to move to a designated smoking area, if possible. Alert the practitioner if your patient is smoking against medical advice.

Talk to your patient about smoking cessation. If the patient is interested in quitting, discuss strategies for smoking cessation, including smoking cessation programs and nicotine replacement therapy. Alert the practitioner about your patient's smoking habits.

Essential documentation

Smoking information is commonly obtained while completing the nursing admission assessment form. Document that the patient received information upon his admission regarding facility policies on smoking. Record the number of years he has smoked and the number of cigarettes he smokes per day. Describe his feelings about quitting and his experience with smoking cessation programs. Record patient teaching, such as discussing the hazards of smoking, the use of nicotine replacement therapy, and available information on smoking cessation programs and support groups. Describe the patient's response to teaching and any smoking cessation plans. Include any written materials given to the patient.

If your patient is smoking against facility policy, chart the date and time of the incident and where he was found smoking. Record what you told the patient and his response. Document any education that took place regarding smoking cessation and the patient's response. If the practitioner was notified, record that you notified him, the time, his name, and any orders given. Describe any arrangements made for the patient to smoke. Some facilities may require you to complete an incident report.

3/18/08	1400	Pt. found smoking in bathroom. Reinforced the facility's no smoking policy. Explained that if pt. wished to smoke, he would need his dr.'s order to be escorted outdoors to a designated area. Pt. asked about the use of a nicotine patch. Dr. George Pasad notified. Order given for nicotine patch. Use of nicotine patch, frequency, dosage, adverse effects, dangers of smoking while wearing patch, and s/s to report to dr. explained to pt. Pt. states understanding. Pt. information dispensed with patch given to pt. to read. ——————————————— Bruce Mailor, RN

Substance abuse by a colleague, suspicion of

An estimated 10% of nurses are addicted to alcohol or drugs and approximately 6% to 8% of nurses engaged in substance abuse have impaired judgment while working. This addiction may be a result of a family history of emotional impairment, stress, alcoholism, emotional abuse, or overwork. Availability of abusive substances in the workplace is also a factor. The suspicion of substance abuse may not be limited to nursing colleagues but may include other members of the health care team, such as practitioners, assistive personnel, or multidisciplinary team members. (See *Reporting a colleague's substance abuse: Your obligations.*)

If you detect signs of substance abuse, make sure that your suspicions are as accurate as possible. (See *Signs of drug or alcohol abuse in*

 LEGAL LOOKOUT
Reporting a colleague's substance abuse: Your obligations

Although the decision to report a coworker is never easy, you have an ethical obligation to intervene if you suspect that a colleague is abusing drugs or alcohol. Intervening enables you to fulfill your moral obligation to your colleague: By reporting abuse, you compel her to take the first step toward regaining control over her life and undergoing rehabilitation. You also fulfill your obligation to patients by protecting them from a nurse whose judgment and care don't meet professional standards.

LEGAL LOOKOUT
Signs of drug or alcohol abuse in a colleague

Signs of drug or alcohol abuse may include:
- rapid mood swings, usually from irritability or depression
- frequent absences, lateness, and use of private quarters such as bathrooms
- frequent volunteering to administer drugs
- excessive errors or problems with controlled substances, such as reports of broken vials or spilled drugs
- illogical or sloppy charting
- inability to meet deadlines or minimum job requirements
- increased errors in treatment
- poor personal hygiene
- inability to concentrate or remember details
- odor of alcohol on the breath
- discrepancies in opioid supplies
- slurred speech, unsteady gait, flushed face, or red eyes
- patient complaints of no relief from opioids supposedly administered when the nurse is on duty
- social withdrawal.

a colleague.) Be aware that allegations of substance abuse are serious and potentially damaging. Follow your facility's policy for reporting suspicions of substance abuse. Use the appropriate channels for your facility and report your suspicions to your nurse manager or nursing supervisor. You'll be asked to document your suspicion on the appropriate form for your facility, possibly an incident or variance report. Most states require reporting to the nursing board, which is usually done by the nurse manager.

Essential documentation

Record the date, time, and location of the incident. Include a description of what you observed and what was said, using direct quotes. Write down the names of any witnesses. Record only objective facts, and be sure to leave out opinions and judgments. Document the name of the nurse manager or nursing supervisor you notified of the incident, and record any instructions given.

To: *Theresa Stiller, RN*
  Nursing supervisor
  Jane McFadden, Nurse Manager, ICU
From: *Pamela Stevens, RN*
Date: *12/3/07*
Time: *2245*
At about *2100* on *12/1/07*, *Janet Fox* in room *501* told me "Your injections of morphine are much better than those the other nurse gives." I asked her what she meant. She told me, "Nurse Barrett's injections never do much for me, but yours always do." Two nights later, at *2215*, I went to the restroom. When I opened the door, I saw Ms. Barrett injecting some solution into her thigh using a syringe. I immediately notified Theresa Stiller, RN, nursing supervisor.

Suicide precautions

Patients who have been identified as at risk for self-harm or suicide are placed on some form of suicide precautions. If your patient has suicidal ideations or makes a suicidal threat, gesture, or attempt, contact the practitioner and charge nurse or nursing supervisor immediately and institute suicide precautions. The Joint Commission National Patient Safety Goal 15 requires that organizations identify patients at risk for suicide. Follow any established risk assessment for suicide in your facility and initiate precautions according to policy. Also follow your facility's policy when caring for a potentially suicidal patient.

Essential documentation

Record the date and time that suicide precautions were initiated and the reasons for the precautions. Chart the time that you notified the practitioner, the practitioner's name, and orders given. Also include the names of other people involved in making this decision. Document the measures taken to reduce the patient's risk of self-harm; for example, removing potentially dangerous items from the patient's environment, accompanying the patient to the bathroom, and placing him in a room by the nurses' station with sealed windows. Record the level of observation, such as close or constant observation, and who's performing the observation. Chart that the patient was instructed about the suicide precautions and his response. Throughout the period of suicide precautions, maintain a suicide precautions flow sheet that includes observations of the patient at designated intervals, usually every 15 minutes.

1/17/08	1600	Pt. stated, "Every year about this time, I think about offing
		myself." History of self-harm 1 year ago. States that he has
		been thinking about cutting his wrists again. Dr. Michael
		Gordon notified and pt. placed on suicide precautions. Leah
		Halloran, RN, nursing supervisor, and Michael Stone, charge
		nurse, notified. Pt. placed in room closest to nurses' station,
		verified that the sealed window can't be opened. With pt.
		present, personal items inventoried and those potentially
		injurious were placed in the locked patient belongings
		cabinet. Instructed pt. that he must remain in sight of
		the assigned staff member at all times, including being
		accompanied to the bathroom and on walks on the unit. CNA
		to sit with pt. See precaution sheet for pt. observation.
		———————————————————— Sandy Peres, RN

Surgical incision care

In addition to documenting vital signs, level of consciousness, and pain level when the patient returns from surgery, pay particular attention to maintaining records pertaining to the surgical incision and drains and the care that you provide. Also, read the records from the postanesthesia care unit. Look for a practitioner's order indicating who will perform the first dressing change.

Essential documentation

Chart the date, time, and type of wound care performed. Describe the wound's appearance (size, condition of margins, and necrotic tissue, if any), odor (if any), location of any drains, drainage characteristics (type, color, consistency, and amount), and the condition of the skin around the incision. Record the type of dressing and tape applied. Document additional wound care procedures provided, such as drain management, irrigation, packing, or application of a topical medication. Record the patient's tolerance of the procedure. Chart the time that you notified the practitioner of any abnormalities or concerns. Record the practitioner's name and orders given. Note explanations or instructions given to the patient.

Record special or detailed wound care instructions and pain management measures on the nursing care plan. Document the color and amount of measurable drainage on an intake and output form. If the patient will need wound care after discharge, provide and document appropriate instructions. Record that you explained sterile technique, described how to examine the wound for signs of infection and other complications, demonstrated how to change the dressing, and provided written instructions for home care. Include the patient's understanding of your instructions.

2/10/08	0830	Dressing removed from 8-cm midline abdominal incision; no
		drainage noted on dressing. Incision well-approximated and intact
		with staples. Margin ecchymotic. Skin around incision without
		redness, warmth, or irritation. Small amt. of serosanguineous
		drainage cleaned from lower end of incision with NSS. Sterile
		4" X 4" gauze pads applied. Jackson Pratt drain intact in LLQ
		draining serosanguineous fluid, emptied 40 ml. Jackson Pratt
		insertion site without redness or drainage. 4" X 4" gauze applied
		around Jackson Pratt drain. Pt. stated he had only minor dis-
		comfort and that he didn't need any pain meds. Pt. instructed to
		call nurse if dressing becomes loose or soiled and for incision
		pain. Pt. demonstrated how to splint incision with pillow during
		C&DB exercises. ———————————— Grace Feder, R.N.

Surgical site identification

To prevent wrong-site surgery and improve the overall safety of patients undergoing surgery, The Joint Commission launched Universal Protocol for Preventing Wrong Site, Wrong Procedure, Wrong Person Surgery in 2004. This protocol encompasses three important steps:

■ A preoperative verification process ascertains that all important documents and tests are on hand before surgery and that these material are evaluated and consistent with one another as well as with the patient's expectations and the surgical team's understanding of the patient, surgical procedure, surgical site, and any implants that may be used. All missing information and inconsistencies must be resolved before starting surgery.

■ Mark the operative site—by the surgeon performing the surgery and with the involvement of the awake and aware patient, if possible. The mark should be the surgeon's initials or "yes."

■ Take a "time out" immediately before surgery is started, in the location where the surgery is to be performed, so that the entire surgical team can confirm the correct patient, surgical procedure, surgical site, patient position, and any implants or special equipment requirements.

Preoperative surgical identification checklist

A preoperative surgical identification checklist such as the one below is commonly used to ensure the safety of patients undergoing surgery.

PREOPERATIVE SURGICAL IDENTIFICATION CHECKLIST

Patient's name _Thomas Smith_   Date _1/6/08_   Time _1032_
Medical record number _123456_   Initials _MC_

	HEALTH TEAM MEMBER INITIALS	DATE	TIME
Preoperative verification			
Patient identified using two identifiers	MC	1/6/08	1032
Informed consent with surgical procedure and site (side/level) signed and in chart	MC	1/6/08	1045
History and physical complete and in chart	MC	1/6/08	1045
Laboratory studies reviewed and in chart	MC	1/6/08	1045
Radiology and ECG reports reviewed and in chart	MC	1/6/08	1045
Medications listed in chart	MC	1/6/08	1045
Patient/family member/guardian verbalizes surgical procedure and points to surgical site	MC	1/6/08	1055
Surgical site marked	HD	1/6/08	1100
Patient, surgery, and marked site verified by patient/family/guardian	MC	1/6/08	1100
Surgical procedure and site, medical record, and tests are consistent	MC	1/6/08	1100
Proper equipment and implants available	MC	1/6/08	1100
Describe any discrepancies and actions taken:	N/A		
"Time out" verification			
Patient verification with two identifiers	BT	1/6/08	1135
Surgical site verified	BT	1/6/08	1135
Surgical procedure verified	BT	1/6/08	1135
Implants and equipment available	N/A		
Verbal verification of team obtained	BT	1/6/08	1135
Describe any discrepancies and actions taken:	N/A		

Signature _Mary Cooke, RN_   Initials _MC_   Signature _Beverly Thomas, RN_   Initials _BT_
Signature _Howard Dunn, MD_   Initials _HD_   Signature _____   Initials _____

Essential documentation

Most facilities use a detailed checklist to ensure that all steps of the verification process have been completed. Each member of the intra-operative team should document the checks that they performed to ensure proper surgical site verification. All documents on the checklist should include the date, time, and initials of the team member providing the check. When using initials on a checklist, make sure that you sign your full name and initials in the signature space provided. Any discrepancies in the verification process should be noted on the checklist with a description of actions taken to rectify the discrepancy. Include the names of any people notified and their actions. (See *Preoperative surgical identification checklist,* page 357.)

T

Termination of life support

According to the right-to-die laws of most states, a patient has the right to refuse extraordinary life-supporting measures if he has no hope of recovery. If the patient can't make this decision, the patient's next of kin is usually permitted to decide if life support should continue. A written statement of the patient's wishes is always preferable. Because of the Patient Self-Determination Act, each health care facility is required to ask the patient upon admission whether he has an advance directive. (See "Advance directive," page 182.) An advance directive is a statement of the patient's wishes that becomes valid if he's unable to make decisions for himself. An advance directive may include a living will, which goes into effect when the patient can't make decisions for himself, as well as a durable power of attorney for health care, which names a designated person to make health care decisions when the patient can't. The Patient Self-Determination Act also states that the patient must receive written information concerning his right to make decisions about his medical care.

If life support is to be terminated, read the patient's advance directive to ensure that the present situation matches the patient's wishes, and verify that the risk manager has reviewed the document. Check that the appropriate consent forms have been signed. Ask the patient's family whether they would like to see the chaplain and whether they would like to be with the patient before, during, and after life support termination.

Essential documentation

Document whether an advance directive is present and whether it matches your patient's present situation and life support wishes. Note that your facility's risk manager has reviewed the advance directive. Document that a consent form has been signed to terminate life support, according to facility policy. Document the names of persons who were notified of the decision to terminate life support and their responses. Describe physical care for the patient before and after life-support termination. Note whether the family was with the patient before, during, and after termination of life support. Record whether a chaplain was present. Document the time of termination, name of the practitioner who turned off the equipment, and names of people present. Record vital signs after extubation as well as the time the patient stopped breathing, the time he was pronounced dead, and who made the pronouncement. Document the family's response, your interventions for them, and postmortem care for the patient.

1/02/08	1800	Advance directive on chart. Wife signed consent form to terminate
		life support. Wife with pt. when life support terminated at 1730
		by Dr. Emmet Brown. VS after extubation: HR 50, BP 50/20, no
		respiratory effort noted. Pronounced dead at 1737. Chaplain
		Greene and wife present. Post-mortem care done. — Lucy Danios, RN

Thoracentesis

Thoracentesis involves the aspiration of fluid or air from the pleural space. It relieves pulmonary compression and respiratory distress by removing accumulated air or fluid that results from injury or such conditions as tuberculosis and cancer. It also provides a specimen of pleural fluid or tissue for analysis and allows the instillation of chemotherapeutic agents or other drugs into the pleural space.

Essential documentation

Note that the procedure, its risks and advantages, alternative treatments, and the consequences of no treatment have been explained to the patient and that a consent form has been signed. Record the date and time of the thoracentesis and the name of the person performing the procedure. Document the location of the puncture site, the volume and description (color, viscosity, and odor) of the fluid withdrawn, and specimens sent to the laboratory. Chart your patient's vital signs and respiratory assessment before, during, and after the procedure. Record any postprocedural tests such as a chest X-ray study. Note any complications (such as pneumothorax, hemothorax, or subcutaneous hematoma), the name of the practitioner notified and the time of notification, orders given, your interventions, and the patient's response. Also record the patient's reaction to the procedure.

After the procedure, record the patient's vital signs every 15 minutes for 1 hour. Then continue to record the patient's vital signs and respiratory status as indicated by his condition. These frequent assessments may be charted on a frequent vital signs flow sheet.

1/10/08	1100	Procedure risks and benefits, alternatives, and consequences
		of no treatment explained to pt. and written consent obtained
		by Dr. Brent McCall. Breath sounds decreased in RLL and pt.
		SOB. Pulse oximetry 88% on 4 L O₂ by NC. P 102, BP 148/84.
		RR 32 and labored. Pt. positioned over secured bedside table.
		RLL thoracentesis performed without incident. Sterile 4" X 4"
		dressing applied to site. Site clean and dry, no redness or
		drainage present. 900 ml of blood-tinged serosanguineous
		fluid aspirated. Specimen sent to lab as ordered. During
		procedure HR 108, BP 144/82, RR 30, pt. SOB, pulse oximetry
		90%. Postprocedure P 98, BP 138/80, RR 24, breath sounds
		clear bilaterally, no dyspnea noted. Pt. denies SOB. Pulse
		oximetry 96% on 4 L O₂ by NC. No c/o pain or discomfort
		at puncture site. CXR done at 1045, results pending. See
		frequent VS sheet for q15min VS and respiratory assessments.
		———————————————— Ellen Pritchett, RN

Tracheostomy care

Tracheostomy care is performed to ensure airway patency of the tracheostomy tube by keeping it free from mucus buildup, maintain mucous membrane and skin integrity, prevent infection, and provide psychological support. The patient may have one of three types of tracheostomy tubes: uncuffed, cuffed, or fenestrated. An uncuffed tracheostomy tube, which may be plastic or metal, allows air to flow freely around the tube and through the larynx, reducing the risk of tracheal damage. A cuffed tube, made of plastic, is disposable. The cuff and the tube won't separate accidentally because they're bonded. A cuffed tube also doesn't require periodic deflating to lower pressures, and it reduces the risk of tracheal damage. A fenestrated tube, also made of plastic, permits speech through the upper airway when the external opening is capped and the cuff is deflated. It also allows easy removal of the inner cannula for cleaning. However, a fenestrated tracheostomy tube may become occluded. When using any one of these tubes, use sterile technique to prevent infection until the stoma has healed. When caring for a recently performed tracheotomy, use sterile gloves at all times. After the stoma has healed, clean gloves may be used.

Essential documentation

Record the date and time of tracheostomy care. Document the type of care performed. Describe the amount, color, consistency, and odor of secretions. Chart the condition of the stoma and the surrounding skin. Note the patient's respiratory status. Record the duration of any cuff deflation, amount of any cuff inflation, and cuff pressure readings and specific body position. Note any complications, the time that you notified the practitioner, the practitioner's name, and orders given. Record your interventions and the patient's response. Document the patient's tolerance of the procedure. Be sure to report any patient or family teaching and their level of comprehension. Depending on your facility's policy, patient teaching may be recorded on a patient-teaching record.

1/19/08	2200	Trach. care performed using sterile technique and applied sterile trach. dressing. Skin around stoma intact, no redness. Small amount creamy-white, thick, odorless secretions noted. Trach. ties clean and secure. Pt. verbalized no discomfort or respiratory distress. Pt.'s wife verbalized desire to assist with procedure when next scheduled to be performed. ——— Laurie Willes, RN

Tracheostomy suctioning

Tracheostomy suctioning involves the removal of secretions from the trachea or bronchi by means of a catheter inserted through the tracheostomy tube. In addition to removing secretions, tracheostomy suctioning also stimulates the cough reflex. This procedure helps maintain a patent airway to promote the optimal exchange of oxygen and carbon dioxide and to prevent pneumonia that results from pooling of secretions. Requiring strict sterile technique, tracheostomy suctioning should be performed as frequently as the patient's condition warrants.

Essential documentation

Record the date and time that you performed tracheostomy suctioning as well as the reason for suctioning. Document the amount, color, consistency, and odor of the secretions. Note any complications as well as nursing actions taken and the patient's response to them. Record any pertinent data regarding the patient's response to the procedure.

1/19/08	2145	Pt. coughing but unable to expel secretions. Skin dusky
		HR 98, BP 110/78, RR 30 noisy and labored. Explained
		suction procedure to pt. Using sterile technique, suctioned
		moderate amount of creamy, thick, odorless secretions
		from tracheostomy tube. After suctioning, skin pink,
		respirations quiet. P 88, BP 112/74, RR 24. Breath sounds
		clear. Pt. resting comfortably in bed. —— Ken Wallings, RN

Transcutaneous electrical nerve stimulation

Transcutaneous electrical nerve stimulation (TENS) involves a portable, battery-powered device that transmits a painless electric current to peripheral nerves or directly to a painful area over large nerve fibers. By blocking painful stimuli traveling over smaller fibers, the patient's perception of pain is altered. TENS reduces the need for analgesic drugs when used after surgery or for chronic pain. A typical course of treatment is 3 to 5 days. (See *Current uses of TENS,* page 364.)

Essential documentation

In the medical record and nursing care plan, record the electrode sites and control settings. Document the patient's tolerance to treatment. Also, during each shift, document your evaluation of pain control.

3/21/08	1730	TENS electrodes placed over ® and Ⓛ posterior superior iliac
		spines and ® and Ⓛ gluteal folds for lower back pain.
		Stimulation frequency set at 80 Hz. Pt. verbalizes discomfort
		as 3/10. Pt. verbalizes satisfaction with level of pain control at
		this time. ———————————————— Lydia Vrubel, RN

Current uses of TENS

Transcutaneous electrical nerve stimulation (TENS) must be prescribed by a physician and is most successful if it's administered and taught to the patient by a therapist skilled in its use. TENS has been used for temporary relief of acute pain, such as postoperative pain, and for ongoing relief of chronic pain, such as sciatica. Among the types of pain that respond to TENS are:

- arthritis
- bone fracture pain
- bursitis
- cancer-related pain
- lower back pain
- musculoskeletal pain
- myofascial pain
- neuralgia and neuropathy
- phantom limb pain
- postoperative incision pain
- sciatica
- whiplash.

Tube feeding

Tube feeding involves the delivery of a liquid feeding formula directly to the stomach (known as *gastric gavage*), duodenum, or jejunum. Gastric gavage is typically indicated for a patient who can't eat normally because of dysphagia or oral or esophageal obstruction or injury. Gastric feedings may also be given to an unconscious or intubated patient or to a patient recovering from GI tract surgery who can't ingest food orally.

Duodenal or jejunal feedings decrease the risk of aspiration because the formula bypasses the pylorus. Jejunal feedings reduce pancreatic stimulation; thus the patient may require an elemental diet. Patients usually receive gastric feedings on an intermittent schedule. However, for duodenal or jejunal feedings, most patients tolerate a continuous slow drip.

Liquid nutrient solutions come in various formulas for administration through a nasogastric tube, small-bore feeding tube, gastrostomy or jejunostomy tube, percutaneous endoscopic gastrostomy or jejunostomy tube, or gastrostomy feeding button. Tube feedings are contraindicated in patients who have no bowel sounds or a suspected intestinal obstruction.

Essential documentation

On the intake and output sheet, record the date, volume of formula, and volume of water. (See "Intake and output," page 268.) In your note, document abdominal assessment findings (including tube exit site, if appropriate); amount of residual gastric contents; verification of tube placement; amount, type, strength, and time of feeding; and tube patency. Discuss the patient's tolerance of the feeding, including complications, such as nausea, vomiting, cramping, diarrhea, or distention.

Note the result of any laboratory tests, such as urine and serum glucose, serum electrolyte, and blood urea nitrogen levels as well as serum osmolality. Document the time that you notified the practitioner of complications, such as hyperglycemia, glycosuria, and diarrhea as well as the practitioner's name. Be sure to include any orders given, your actions, and the patient's response. Record the patient's hydration status and any drugs given through the tube. Note any drugs or treatments to relieve constipation or diarrhea. Include the date and time of administration set changes and the results of specimen collections. Describe any oral and nasal hygiene and dressing changes provided.

1/25/08	0700	Full-strength Pulmocare infusing via Flexiflow pump through
		Dobhoff tube in Ⓡ nostril at 50 ml/hr. Tube placement
		confirmed by air bolus. 5 ml residual noted. HOB maintained
		at 45-degree angle. Pt. denies N/V, abdominal cramping.
		Normal bowel sounds auscultated in all 4 quadrants, no
		abdominal distention noted. Nares cleaned with NSS. Water-
		soluble lubricant applied to nares and lips. Skin around nares
		intact, no redness around tape noted. Helped pt. to brush
		teeth. Tube flushed with 30 ml H_2O, as ordered. Instructed
		pt. to tell nurse of any abdominal discomfort or nausea. Pt.
		verbalized understanding. ———————— *Sandra Mann, RN*

U

Urinary catheter insertion, indwelling

Also known as a *Foley* or *retention catheter,* an indwelling urinary catheter remains in the bladder to provide continuous urine drainage. A balloon inflated at the catheter's distal end prevents it from slipping out of the bladder after insertion.

An indwelling catheter is inserted using sterile technique and only when absolutely necessary. Insertion should be performed with extreme care to prevent injury to the patient and possible infection.

An indwelling catheter is most commonly used to relieve bladder distention caused by urine retention and allow continuous urine drainage when the urinary meatus is swollen from childbirth, surgery, or local trauma. Other indications for an indwelling catheter include urinary tract obstruction caused by a tumor or enlarged prostate, urine retention or infection from neurogenic bladder paralysis caused by spinal cord injury or disease, and any illness in which the patient's urine output must be closely monitored.

Essential documentation

Record the date and time that the indwelling urinary catheter was inserted. Note the size and type of catheter used. Also, describe the amount, color, and other characteristics of the urine emptied from the bladder. Intake and output should be recorded on the patient's intake and output record. (See "Intake and output," page 268.) If large volumes of urine have been emptied, describe the patient's tolerance for the procedure. Note whether a urine specimen was sent for laboratory analysis. Document any patient teaching performed.

2/12/08	1115	Explained reason for insertion of indwelling urinary catheter to
		pt. prior to hysterectomy. Pt. stated she understood. Demonstrated
		how to do breathing exercises during insertion. #16 Fr. Foley
		catheter inserted using sterile technique at 1045. Emptied 450 ml
		from bladder. Urine dark amber, no odor, or sediment. Specimen
		sent to lab for U/A. Pt. states she has no discomfort. See I/O
		flow sheet. ———————————————— Molly Malone, RN

V

Vascular access device, accessing

Surgically implanted under local anesthesia by a physician, a vascular access device consists of a silicone catheter attached to a reservoir, which is covered with a self-sealing silicone rubber septum. It's used most commonly when an external central venous catheter isn't desirable for long-term I.V. therapy. The most common type of vascular access device is a vascular access port (VAP). Typically, VAPs deliver intermittent infusions. They're used to deliver chemotherapy and other drugs, I.V. fluids, and blood. They can also be used to obtain blood.

To access a VAP, a noncoring or Huber needle is inserted into the reservoir. An extension set is flushed with normal saline solution and then attached to the needle. After checking for blood return, the port is flushed with normal saline solution, according to your facility's policy.

While the patient is hospitalized, a luer-lock injection cap may be attached to the end of an extension set to provide ready access for intermittent infusions. In addition to saving time, a luer-lock cap reduces the discomfort of accessing the port and prolongs the life of the port septum by decreasing the number of needle punctures.

Essential documentation

Record the date and time that the port was accessed. Note whether signs or symptoms of infection or skin breakdown are present. Describe any pain or discomfort that the patient experienced when the port was accessed. If you used ice or local anesthetic, be sure to chart it. Describe how the area was cleaned before accessing the port. Note whether resistance was met when inserting the needle and whether you obtained a blood return. Include the number of attempts made to access the port. Record any problems with the normal saline flush, such as swelling or pain. Chart the time that the practitioner was notified of any problems, the practitioner's name, any orders given, your interventions, and the patient's response. Also document any patient education performed.

1/20/08	1200	No breakdown, redness, warmth, or drainage noted at VAP
		access site in Ⓡ chest. Pt. states he doesn't use a local anesthetic
		to access the site. Site cleaned with chlorhexidine, per protocol,
		and anchored by hand while noncoring needle was inserted
		perpendicular to port septum on first attempt. No resistance
		noted. Blood return observed and device flushed with NSS, per
		protocol. Antibiotic infusing without problem. Pt. has been using
		VAP at home for 3 months and verbalized understanding of its
		use. Pt. will access device with next drug infusion, with nurse
		watching to evaluate his technique. ——— *Chelsea Burton, R.N.*

Vital signs, frequent monitoring of

A patient may require frequent monitoring of vital signs after surgery or certain procedures and diagnostic tests or during a critical illness. A frequent vital signs flow sheet allows you to quickly document vital signs the moment you take them without having to take the time to write a progress note. A flow sheet also allows you to readily detect changes in the patient's condition.

Sometimes, recording only vital signs isn't sufficient to give a complete picture of the patient's status. In such a case, you'll also need to write a progress note. Make sure the data on the vital signs flow sheet are consistent with the data in your progress note.

Essential documentation

Record the date on the flow sheet. Chart the specific time each set of vital signs is taken. If there's a significant change in vital signs, write a progress note documenting the change, the time the practitioner was notified, the practitioner's name, any orders given, your actions, and the patient's response. (See *Frequent vital signs flow sheet,* page 370.)

Frequent vital signs flow sheet

When the patient requires frequent vital sign assessments, a flow sheet such as this may help facilitate documentation by eliminating the need to continually make entries in the notation section of the chart. In the example below, blood pressure is monitored every 15 minutes.

FREQUENT VITAL SIGNS FLOW SHEET

DATE	TIME	KEY	BP	P	RR	T	CVP	PAP S/D	M	W	COMMENTS	TITRATED I.V.'S	MEDS STAT AND PRN	INITIALS
11/13/08	0900	S	122/84	98	18	986								MC
	0915	S	124/82	94	18									MC
	0930	S	122/78	92	20									MC
	0945	S	120/80	94	18									MC
	1000	S	128/78	94	20									MC

Key: S = Stethoscope D = Doppler P = Palpation T = Transducer

Signature: *M. Clark, RN*

WXYZ

Wound assessment

When caring for a patient with a wound, complete a thorough assessment so that you'll have a clear baseline from which to evaluate healing and the appropriateness of therapy. Care may need to be altered if the wound doesn't respond to therapy. Many facilities have a specific wound care protocol that specifies different treatment plans based on wound assessment. A wound should be assessed with each dressing change.

Essential documentation

Record the date and time of your entry. Be sure to include the following points when documenting wound assessment:
- wound size, including length, width, and depth in centimeters
- wound shape
- wound site, drawn on a body plan to document exact location
- wound stage
- characteristics of drainage, if any, including amount, color, and presence of odor
- characteristics of the wound bed, including description of tissue type, such as granulation tissue, slough, or epithelial tissue, and percentage of each tissue type
- character of the surrounding tissue
- presence or absence of eschar

Wound and skin assessment tool

When performing a thorough wound and skin assessment, a pictorial demonstration is usually helpful to identify the wound site or sites. Using the wound and skin assessment tool below, the nurse identified the left second toe as a partial-thickness wound, vascular ulcer, that's red in color using the classification of terms that follow.

PATIENT'S NAME (LAST, FIRST)	ATTENDING PHYSICIAN	ROOM NUMBER	ID NUMBER
Brown, Ann	Dr. A. Dennis	123-2	01726

WOUND ASSESSMENT:

NUMBER	1	2	3	4	5	6
DATE	1/03/08					
TIME	1215					
LOCATION	Ⓛ second toe					
STAGE	II					
APPEARANCE	G					
SIZE-LENGTH	0.5 cm					
SIZE-WIDTH	1 cm					
COLOR/FLR.	RD					
DRAINAGE	0					
ODOR	0					
VOLUME	0					
INFLAMMATION	0					
SIZE INFLAM.	0					

KEY

Stage:
- I. Red or discolored
- II. Skin break/blister
- III. Subcutaneous tissue
- IV. Muscle and/or bone

Appearance:
- D = Depth
- E = Eschar
- G = Granulation
- IN = Inflammation
- NEC = Necrotic
- PK = Pink
- SL = Slough
- TN = Tunneling
- UND = Undermining
- MX = Mixed (specify)

Color of Wound
Floor:
- RD = Red
- Y = Yellow
- BLK = Black
- MX = Mixed (specify)

Drainage:
- 0 = None
- SR = Serous
- SS = Serosanguineous
- BL = Blood
- PR = Purulent

Odor:
- 0 = None
- MLD = Mild
- FL = Foul

Volume:
- 0 = None
- SC = Scant
- MOD = Moderate
- LG = Large

Inflammation:
- 0 = None
- PK = Pink
- RD = Red

Wound and skin assessment tool *(continued)*

WOUND ANATOMIC LOCATION:

(circle affected area)

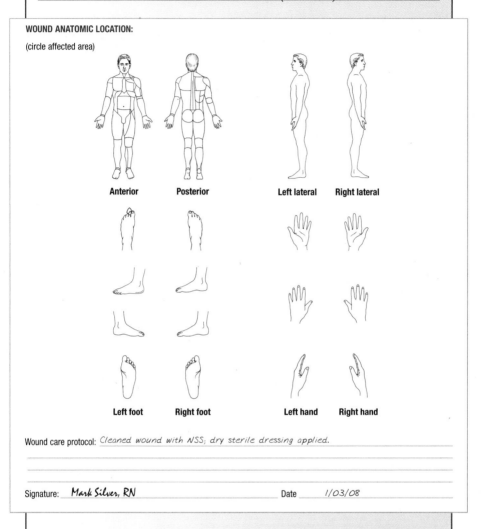

Anterior   Posterior   Left lateral   Right lateral

Left foot   Right foot   Left hand   Right hand

Wound care protocol: *Cleaned wound with NSS; dry sterile dressing applied.*

Signature: *Mark Silver, RN*   Date *1/03/08*

- presence or absence of pain
- presence or absence of undermining or tunneling (in centimeters).

Many facilities also have a special form or flow sheet on which to document wounds. (See *Wound and skin assessment tool.*)

2/14/08	1330	Pt. admitted to unit for fem-pop bypass in A.M. Pt. has open
		wound at tip of 2nd ℚ toe, approx. 0.5 cm X 1 cm X 0.5 cm
		deep. Wound is round with even edges. Wound bed is pale
		with little granulation tissue. No drainage, odor, eschar, or
		tunneling noted. Pt. reports pain at wound site, rates pain as
		4/10. Surrounding skin cool to touch, pale, and intact. Pt.
		understands not to cross legs or wear tight garments. ———
		——————————————————————————— Mark Silver, RN

Wound care

When caring for a surgical wound, your intent is to help prevent infection by stopping pathogens from entering the wound. In addition to promoting patient comfort, such procedures protect the skin surface from maceration and excoriation caused by contact with irritating drainage. They also allow you to measure wound drainage to monitor fluid and electrolyte balance.

The two principal methods for managing a draining wound are dressing and pouching. Dressing is the best choice when skin integrity isn't compromised by caustic or excessive drainage. Lightly seeping wounds with drains as well as wounds with minimal purulent drainage can usually be managed with packing and gauze dressings. Copious, excoriating drainage calls for pouching to protect the skin.

Essential documentation

Document the date and time of the procedure as well as the type of wound management. Record the amount of soiled dressing and packing removed. Describe wound appearance (size, condition of margins, and presence of necrotic tissue) and odor (if present). Chart the type, color, consistency, and amount of drainage for each wound. Indicate the presence and location of drains. Note any additional procedures, such as irrigation, packing, or application of a topical medication. Record the type and amount of new dressing or pouch applied. Note the patient's tolerance of the procedure and any instructions given.

Document special or detailed wound care instructions and pain management steps on the care plan. Record the color and amount of drainage on the intake and output sheet.

1/17/08	1030	Dressing removed from ℞ mastectomy incision. 1.5 cm round
		area of serosanguineous drainage noted on dressing. No odor
		noted. 11-cm incision well-approximated, staples intact. Skin
		around incision intact, no redness. Site cleaned with sterile
		NSS. Sterile 4" X 4" gauze pads applied. Jackson Pratt drain at
		lateral edge of incision emptied for 10 ml serosanguineous
		fluid, no odor noted. Explained dressing change and signs and
		symptoms of infection to report. Pt. verbalized understanding.
		Pt. states incision is tender but doesn't require pain medication.
		———————————————————————— Deborah Liu, RN

Appendix
Selected references
Index

NANDA-I nursing diagnoses by domain

The following is a list of the 2007-2008 current nursing diagnosis classifications according to domain. The 2007 revised and new diagnoses are in *italics*.

1. Domain: Health promotion

- Effective therapeutic regimen management
- Health-seeking behaviors (specify)
- Impaired home maintenance
- Ineffective community therapeutic regimen management
- Ineffective family therapeutic regimen management
- Ineffective health maintenance
- Ineffective therapeutic regimen management
- *Readiness for enhanced immunization status*
- Readiness for enhanced nutrition
- Readiness for enhanced therapeutic regimen management

2. Domain: Nutrition

- Deficient fluid volume
- Excess fluid volume
- Imbalanced nutrition: Less than body requirements
- Imbalanced nutrition: More than body requirements
- Impaired swallowing
- Ineffective infant feeding pattern
- Readiness for enhanced fluid balance
- Risk for deficient fluid volume
- Risk for imbalanced fluid volume
- Risk for imbalanced nutrition: More than body requirements
- *Risk for impaired liver function*
- *Risk for unstable glucose level*

3. Domain: Elimination/exchange

- Bowel incontinence
- Constipation
- Diarrhea
- Functional urinary incontinence
- Impaired gas exchange
- Impaired urinary elimination
- *Overflow urinary incontinence*
- Perceived constipation
- Readiness for enhanced urinary elimination
- Reflex urinary incontinence
- Risk for constipation
- Risk for urge urinary incontinence

- Stress urinary incontinence
- Total urinary incontinence
- Urge urinary incontinence
- Urinary retention

4. Domain: Activity/rest

- Activity intolerance
- Bathing or hygiene self-care deficit
- Decreased cardiac output
- Deficient diversional activity
- Delayed surgical recovery
- Dressing or grooming self-care deficit
- Dysfunctional ventilatory weaning response
- Energy field disturbance
- Fatigue
- Feeding self-care deficit
- Impaired bed mobility
- Impaired physical mobility
- Impaired spontaneous ventilation
- Impaired transfer ability
- Impaired walking
- Impaired wheelchair mobility
- Ineffective breathing pattern
- Ineffective tissue perfusion (specify: renal, cerebral, cardiopulmonary, gastrointestinal, peripheral)
- *Insomnia* (formerly Disturbed sleep pattern)
- *Readiness for enhanced self-care*
- Readiness for enhanced sleep
- Risk for activity intolerance
- Risk for disuse syndrome
- Sedentary lifestyle
- Sleep deprivation

- Toileting self-care deficit

5. Domain: Perception/cognition

- Acute confusion
- Chronic confusion
- Deficient knowledge (specify)
- Disturbed sensory perception (specify: visual, auditory, kinesthetic, gustatory, tactile, olfactory)
- Disturbed thought processes
- Impaired environmental interpretation syndrome
- Impaired memory
- Impaired verbal communication
- Readiness for enhanced communication
- *Readiness for enhanced decision making*
- Readiness for enhanced knowledge (specify)
- *Risk for acute confusion*
- Unilateral neglect
- Wandering

6. Domain: Self-perception

- Chronic low self-esteem
- Disturbed body image
- Disturbed personal identity
- Hopelessness
- Powerlessness
- *Readiness for enhanced hope*
- *Readiness for enhanced power*
- Readiness for enhanced self-concept
- *Risk for compromised human dignity*
- Risk for loneliness
- Risk for powerlessness

- Risk for situational low self-esteem
- Situational low self-esteem

7. Domain: Role relationships

- Caregiver role strain
- Dysfunctional family processes: Alcoholism
- Effective breast-feeding
- Impaired parenting
- Impaired social interaction
- Ineffective breast-feeding
- Ineffective role performance
- Interrupted breast-feeding
- Interrupted family processes
- Parental role conflict
- Readiness for enhanced family processes
- Readiness for enhanced parenting
- Risk for caregiver role strain
- Risk for impaired parent/infant/child attachment
- Risk for impaired parenting

8. Domain: Sexuality

- Ineffective sexuality pattern
- Sexual dysfunction

9. Domain: Coping/stress tolerance

- Anxiety
- Autonomic dysreflexia
- Chronic sorrow
- *Complicated grieving* (formerly Dysfunctional grieving)
- Compromised family coping
- Death anxiety

- Decreased intracranial adaptive capacity
- Defensive coping
- Disabled family coping
- Disorganized infant behavior
- Fear
- *Grieving* (formerly Anticipatory grieving)
- Ineffective community coping
- Ineffective coping
- Ineffective denial
- Post-trauma syndrome
- Rape-trauma syndrome
- Rape-trauma syndrome: Compound reaction
- Rape-trauma syndrome: Silent reaction
- Readiness for enhanced community coping
- Readiness for enhanced coping (individual)
- Readiness for enhanced family coping
- Readiness for enhanced organized infant behavior
- Relocation stress syndrome
- Risk for autonomic dysreflexia
- Risk for disorganized infant behavior
- *Risk for complicated grieving* (formerly Risk for dysfunctional grieving)
- Risk for post-trauma syndrome
- Risk for relocation stress syndrome
- *Risk prone health behavior* (formerly Impaired adjustment)
- *Stress overload*

10. Domain: Life principles

- Decisional conflict (specify)
- Impaired religiosity
- *Moral distress*
- Noncompliance (specify)
- *Readiness for enhanced decision making*
- *Readiness for enhanced hope*
- Readiness for enhanced religiosity
- Readiness for enhanced spiritual well-being
- Risk for impaired religiosity
- Risk for spiritual distress
- Spiritual distress

11. Domain: Safety/protection

- *Contamination*
- Hyperthermia
- Hypothermia
- Impaired dentition
- Impaired oral mucous membrane
- Impaired skin integrity
- Impaired tissue integrity
- Ineffective airway clearance
- Ineffective protection
- Ineffective thermoregulation
- Latex allergy response
- *Readiness for enhanced immunization status*
- Risk for aspiration
- *Risk for contamination*
- Risk for falls
- Risk for imbalanced body temperature
- Risk for impaired skin integrity
- Risk for infection
- Risk for injury
- Risk for latex allergy response
- Risk for other-directed violence
- Risk for perioperative positioning injury
- Risk for peripheral neurovascular dysfunction
- Risk for poisoning
- Risk for self-directed violence
- Risk for self-mutilation
- Risk for sudden infant death syndrome
- Risk for suffocation
- Risk for suicide
- Risk for trauma
- Self-mutilation

12. Domain: Comfort

- Acute pain
- Chronic pain
- Nausea
- *Readiness for enhanced comfort*
- Social isolation

13. Domain: Growth/development

- Adult failure to thrive
- Delayed growth and development
- Risk for delayed development
- Risk for disproportionate growth

Selected references

Austin, S. "Ladies and Gentlemen of the Jury, I Present....the Nursing Documentation," *Nursing* 36(11):56-63, January 2006.

ChartSmart: An A-to-Z Guide to Better Nursing Documentation, 2nd ed. Philadelphia: Lippincott Williams & Wilkins, 2006.

Childers, K. "Paying a Price for Poor Documentation," *Nursing* 35(11):32hn4-32hn6, November 2005.

Documentation in Action. Philadelphia: Lippincott Williams & Wilkins, 2006.

Ferrell, K.G. "Documentation, Part 2: The Best Evidence of Care," *AJN* 107(7):61-64, July 2007.

Mascolo, L. "Skin Care Team Improves Assessment and Documentation," *Nursing* 36(10):66-67, October 2006.

Monarch, K. "Documentation, Part 1: Principles for Self-protection," *AJN* 107(7):58-60, July 2007.

Smith, K., et al. "Evaluating the Impact of Computerized Clinical Documentation," *Computers, Informatics, Nursing* 23(3):132-38, May-June 2005.

Index

A

Abbreviations
  to avoid, 5-7t
  on flow sheets, 148
  standard, 4
Abuse, suspected, 174-176
  documentation of, 174, 176, 176i
  reporting, 177
  signs of, 175-176
  substance, 352-354
Access to health information
  computerization and, 110-111
  patient requests for, 307-308, 308i
  patient right of, 261
Accuracy of documentation, 8
Activities of daily living, 176-182
  Barthel index for, 180-181i
  checklists for, 176-177
  documentation of, 177-179, 182
  instrumental, 179
  Katz index for, 178i
  Lawton scale for, 179i
Activity level, 303-304
Acute care, 120-172
  clinical pathways in, 149-152
  dictated documentation in, 166-167
  discharge summary–patient instruction forms in, 163-165
  flow sheets in, 141-148
  graphic forms in, 139-141

Acute care *(continued)*
  Kardex in, 132-139
  miscellaneous forms in, 170-172
  nursing admission assessment forms in, 120-129
  patient self-documentation in, 167-170i
  patient-teaching forms in, 156-162
  patient-teaching plans in, 152-155
  progress notes in, 129-132
  rapid response documentation in, 170, 171i
Admission, patient's belongings at, 319-320
Admission assessment form, nursing, 120-129
  advantages and disadvantages of, 123-124
  completing, 121-123i
  data in, 121, 123
  documentation styles for, 124-128
  guidelines for, 128-129
  writing narrative, 125-128i
Admission database form, integrated, 22-30i
Advance directives, 77, 84-86, 182-184
  checklist for, 183i
  documentation of, 182, 184
  failure to honor, 85

---

i refers to an illustration; t refers to a table.

---

i refers to an illustration; t refers to a table.

---

i refers to an illustration; t refers to a table.

i refers to an illustration; t refers to a table.

i refers to an illustration; t refers to a table.

---

i refers to an illustration; t refers to a table.

---

i refers to an illustration; t refers to a table.

---

i refers to an illustration; t refers to a table.

---

i refers to an illustration; t refers to a table.

---

i refers to an illustration; t refers to a table.

i refers to an illustration; t refers to a table.

---

i refers to an illustration; t refers to a table.

i refers to an illustration; t refers to a table.

---

i refers to an illustration; t refers to a table.

i refers to an illustration; t refers to a table.

---

i refers to an illustration; t refers to a table.

i refers to an illustration; t refers to a table.

---

i refers to an illustration; t refers to a table.